DIAGNOSIS OF THE

Temporomandibular Joint

DIAGNOSIS OF THE
Temporomandibular Joint

RICHARD W. KATZBERG, MD

Professor and Chair
Department of Radiology
University of California, Davis
School of Medicine
Sacramento, California

PER-LENNART WESTESSON, DDS, PhD

Professor of Radiology and Associate Professor of
Clinical Dentistry
Head of Section for Maxillofacial and Oral Imaging
University of Rochester School of Medicine and Dentistry
Rochester, New York
Associate Professor of Orthodontics
Eastman Dental Center
Rochester, New York
Research Associate Professor of Oral Medicine
State University of New York at Buffalo
Buffalo, New York
Associate Professor (Docent) of Oral Radiology
University of Lund
Malmö, Sweden
Attending Radiologist and Dentist
Strong Memorial Hospital
Rochester, New York

W.B. SAUNDERS COMPANY
A Division of Harcourt Brace & Company
Philadelphia   London   Toronto   Montreal   Sydney   Tokyo

W.B. SAUNDERS COMPANY
A Division of
Harcourt Brace & Company

The Curtis Center
Independence Square West
Philadelphia, Pennsylvania 19106

Library of Congress Cataloging-in-Publication Data

Katzberg, Richard W.

Diagnosis of the temporomandibular joint / Richard W. Katzberg,
Per-Lennart Westesson.—1st ed.

   p.   cm.

ISBN 0–7216–2368–9

1. Temporomandibular joint—Diseases—Diagnosis.
   2. Temporomandibular joint—Imaging.   3. Diagnostic
   Imaging.   I. Westesson, Per-Lennart.   II. Title.

[DNLM: 1. Temporomandibular Joint—anatomy & histology.
2. Temporomandibular Joint—pathology.
3. Temporomandibular Joint Diseases—diagnosis.
WU 140 K19d 1994]

RK470.K38 1994

617.5′22—dc20

DNLM/DLC   93-20535

Diagnosis of the Temporomandibular Joint   ISBN 0–7216–2368–9

Printed in the United States of America.

Last digit is the print number: 9   8   7   6   5   4   3   2   1

This book is dedicated with deepest love and affection to my wife, Susan Ann Brimberry Katzberg, and to our children, Jenna Kempton, Kimberly, and Richard.

DWK

This book is dedicated with great love to my wife, Ann-Margaret, and to our children, Karin, 10; Oscar, 8; and Nils, 6.

P-LW

Contributors

Tore A. Larheim, DDS, PhD
Professor and Chairman, Department of Oral Radiology
Faculty of Dentistry
University of Oslo
Oslo, Norway

Ralph G. Merrill, DDS, MScD
Professor and Chairman,
Department of Oral and Maxillofacial Surgery
Oregon Health Sciences University
Portland, Oregon
Active Medical Staff, Oregon Health Sciences University Hospital
Legacy Health Systems Hospitals,
Portland, Oregon

Foreword

Those of us with an interest in the dysfunctions of the temporomandibular joint have long sought the development of improved ways and means to provide information about the conditions we see in this area.

More and more complicated technical procedures, especially for imaging, are now available. Some of these new diagnostic methods are based on progress in other specialty fields. Their results, therefore, to some degree must be explained and even confirmed by previous imaging techniques such as arthrography, with either single or double contrast, and by tomography.

Which methods to use and when to use them are problems with several ramifications, including economic factors, the natural preference for painless procedures, and least risk of radiation exposure. Selection of the most appropriate imaging technique is still difficult, even for experienced practitioners.

The full understanding of anatomic and functional disorders and the techniques for eliciting the optimal information for each situation are important preambles for good diagnosis and treatment.

The authors of this book have participated in and actively influenced the progress in this special field. With several years of practical experience, they have the ability to describe and evaluate the present state of knowledge and to discuss the many open questions that yet offer interesting problems for further research.

For those who wish to keep abreast of the latest achievements in and the considerations about practical and sensible choices for imaging the temporomandibular joint, this is the book of reference for today. Anyone considering working in this area as either a diagnostician or a therapist will find it no less than a "must."

FLEMMING NØRGAARD, MD, DSc (Med), DSc (Odont)
Gentofte, Denmark

Preface

The purpose of this textbook is to provide a comprehensive overview of the imaging techniques in the diagnosis of diseases of the temporomandibular joint (TMJ) with a special emphasis on internal derangement. *Internal derangement* is defined as an abnormal positional and functional relationship between the disk and the mandibular condyle and the articulating surface of the temporal bone, which is often associated with pain, clicking, and limitation of jaw opening. This condition frequently progresses to osteoarthrosis. In conjunction with mechanical and anatomic disk derangement, intrinsic alteration of the disk, per se, also develops. Included is a change in the configuration of the disk to include marked deformity and thickening. In turn, these abnormalities in disk configuration are also associated with alterations in disk histology. Recent studies have shown that inflammatory reactions with joint effusion and synovitis frequently accompany painful internal derangement. We now are approaching a better understanding of the mechanisms responsible for patients' pain symptoms.

The first section of this text provides a detailed description of both the normal and abnormal anatomy of the soft and hard tissues of the TMJ. This material is derived from our clinical experience and from fresh cadavers that graphically depict the findings commonly observed in the clinical setting. The spectrum of abnormality is outlined, beginning with the earliest of findings to severe, end-stage disease. The interrelationship between different abnormalities is also described.

The next section of this text emphasizes the imaging modalities that are commonly available and utilized for diagnosis. The relative advantages and disadvantages of these modalities are discussed in detail. These imaging tools have provided an immense knowledge base about anatomic and physiologic aspects of this joint. We have emphasized arthrography and magnetic resonance imaging (MRI) since these modalities have been the staples of routine diagnosis. Our experience with arthrography is summarized from over 10,000 arthrographic studies that emphasize the marked variability and remarkable spectrum of findings associated with internal derangement. Though relatively new, MRI has rapidly advanced our knowledge originally acquired from the invasive arthrographic technique.

Miscellaneous diagnostic techniques, such as computed tomography (CT), single photon emission computed tomography (SPECT), and acoustical analysis, provide somewhat limited yet unique insights that are valuable to appreciate better the full nature of the disorders of the TMJ. These techniques continue to be extremely useful in depicting the multifaceted characteristics of TMJ diseases.

Imaging techniques such as arthrography and MRI have significantly assisted in treatment planning and follow-up of patients undergoing different forms of surgical and nonsurgical treatment. For example, the arthrographic procedure is ideal for the initiation of certain types of splint therapy, whereas MRI is superior for accurate detection of morphologic alterations. Arthrography, but especially MRI, is extremely valuable in assessing patient outcomes following splint therapy or surgery. These imaging tools have established a very important role in the refinement of treatment options.

The third section of the text provides a comprehensive overview of conditions other than internal derangement that affect the TMJ. The spectrum of findings in rheumatoid arthritis is presented with an emphasis on MRI as a uniquely suited tool for analysis. This is an exciting new frontier for MRI, not only for the TMJ but also throughout medicine in the depiction of active rheumatologic diseases.

Trauma to the TMJ is common and can lead to severe anatomic and functional disorders. CT is an excellent modality for the assessment of osseous disorders of the TMJ following trauma and for the assessment of facial asymmetry as the result of trauma causing soft tissue or bony injury. The future role of MRI in trauma of the TMJ is yet to be fully established, but it has enormous potential for providing much-needed information on the staging and possible treatment options following intra-articular injury.

Unusual abnormalities of the TMJ include synovial abnormalities, intra-articular loose bodies, primary and secondary bone lesions, mandibular asymmetry, dislocation of the jaw, and infection. Although these conditions are relatively rare, they complete the overview of virtually all organic disorders that might be encountered.

Section IV describes the arthroscopic assessment of the TMJ as both a diagnostic and a therapeutic tool. Many conditions arising within the TMJ can be assessed accurately by this new and exciting modality. This complements the imaging aspects of the TMJ by providing a direct visualization of the articulating surfaces.

The final section is an organizational scheme for the diagnosis of patients presenting with suspected internal derangement. The intent of this discussion is to provide the optimal triage to diagnosis in order to initiate the optimal treatment plan. We offer a recommendation based on our own imaging capabilities and clinical environments. With such a variety of techniques, selection of the appropriate imaging modality for the condition to be evaluated is important. Our belief, however, is that imaging should always be viewed as a diagnostic aid and never as a substitute for thorough clinical evaluation and good clinical judgment.

RICHARD W. KATZBERG, MD
PER-LENNART WESTESSON, DDS, PhD

Acknowledgments

I have had the pleasure of maintaining two main academic careers, one as a genitourinary radiologist and one as a temporomandibular joint (TMJ) diagnostician. They are not related.

My interest in TMJ imaging began in 1977 during the first year following my residency program in radiology at the University of Rochester in Rochester, New York, while stationed at Wilford Hall USAF Medical Center in San Antonio, Texas. I was encouraged by Col. Dave Bales, DDS, to attempt arthrography in patients at the dental clinic who had pain and dysfunction, no specific diagnosis, and no known treatment regimen, since internal derangement was an unknown entity at that time. I owe a great deal of gratitude to Dr. Bales for that reason and also for introducing me to a young oral surgery faculty member at Wilford Hall, M. Franklin Dolwick, DMD, PhD. Frank and I were given the mission to figure out what was wrong with these TMJ patients. Fortunately, we were aware of the new concepts that were being introduced by Bill Farrar, DDS, Bill McCarty, DMD, and Clyde Wilkes, DDS, MD, PhD. We are all grateful for their pioneering insights.

Frank and I began doing arthrograms by trial and error since we were not familiar with the few reports on the technique. We were successful after several tries and rapidly developed a consistently successful technique. Clyde Helms, MD, was the skeletal radiologist at Wilford Hall and my office mate, and he quickly became a major contributor to our arthrographic techniques and diagnoses. I am grateful for his enthusiasm, encouragement, and subsequent contributions.

A small group of us began to communicate our experiences on imaging of internal derangement, and I owe a large amount of gratitude to their collaboration and insights. These other pioneers were Quentin Anderson, MD, William Murphy, MD, Paul Nance, MD, James V. Manzione, Jr., MD, DMD, and, of course, Per-Lennart Westesson, DDS, PhD. Since that time numerous other excellent radiologists have contributed innumerable studies in the literature that have provided a remarkable growth in our knowledge.

A major milestone in imaging of TMJ disorders occurred with the advent of magnetic resonance imaging. I owe extreme gratitude to the scientists at the NMR Research Facility in Schenectady, New York, who donated their time and truly remarkable scientific expertise to us in Rochester in 1985. These dedicated scientists are John Schenck, MD, Tom Foster, PhD, Howard Hart, PhD, and Chris Hardy, PhD.

TMJ clinicians who have been outstanding contributors to the clinical aspects of TMJ diagnosis and treatment include Ross Tallents, DDS, Don Macher, DMD, Russ Bessette, DDS, MD, Ed Sommers, DMD, Lars Eriksson, DDS, PhD, Christopher Roberts, DDS, and Steve Messing, DMD.

The ultimate pioneer and friend who planted the seed almost 50 years ago is of course Flemming Nørgaard, MD, PhD.

Edie Johnson, Lori Neville, Nancy Steers, and Lisette Bralow have provided outstanding encouragement, dedication, and editorial assistance, for which I am immensely grateful and indebted.

RICHARD W. KATZBERG, MD

Writing this book has been a highlight in my professional career. I have been involved in clinical and research work on TMJ imaging since 1977 and summarizing information from my work as well as the work of many others has been exciting. My professional career started in the Department of Oral and Maxillofacial Radiology at the School of Dentistry, University of Lund, Sweden, under the guidance of Karl-Åke Omnell, DDS, PhD. Dr. Omnell was a dynamic and stimulating leader, and he as well as my colleagues in the department, Arne Petersson, DDS, PhD, and Madeleine Rohlin, DDS, PhD, should be acknowledged for stimulation and guidance in my early professional career. In 1977 Dr. Omnell gave me the task of developing a technique for double-contrast arthrotomography of the TMJ. At the same time, Clyde Wilkes, DDS, MD, PhD, Bill Farrar, DDS, and Bill McCarty, DMD, initiated a rediscovery of internal derangement on the other side of the Atlantic. This had an immediate impact on my clinical work since TMJ arthrography now changed from a research tool to a technique that was clinically useful. A clinical demand to perform arthrography in order to identify different forms of internal derangement developed over the next few months.

Very stimulating visits with Drs. Clyde Wilkes, Bill Farrar, Bill McCarty, and Quentin N. Anderson in the early 1980s will always stand out as bright spots of my professional career. During these visits we were able to share experience and gain insight into how arthrography could be used for the planning of surgical treatment. Contact was established with Lars Eriksson, DDS, PhD, at the University Hospital of Lund, Sweden, and he was enthusiastic about the possibility of directing a surgical treatment team. In 1985 Lars Eriksson presented his PhD thesis on surgical treatment of TMJ disorders. Lars and I have had a stimulating collaboration that we have been able to continue even after I left Sweden and moved to Rochester.

Not every patient needs surgical treatment. Conservative treatment is a necessity for an efficiently functioning TMJ team. Håkan Lundh, DDS, PhD, at the University of Lund was willing to take on the responsibility for nonsurgical treatment. He was enthusiastic and developed precise skill in treatment modalities relative to internal derangement. In 1987 he presented his PhD thesis on the evaluation of nonsurgical treatment of TMJ internal derangement.

Stimulating contact with researchers from all over the world has accompanied the TMJ research. Individuals such as Sidney L. Bronstein, Denver, Colorado, USA; Annika Isberg, Stockholm, Sweden; Toshiro Kondoh, Yokohama, Japan; Kenichi Kurita, Nagoya, Japan; Jonas Liedberg, Malmö, Sweden; Daniel Paesani, Rosario, Argentina; and Sven-Erik Widmalm, Ann Arbor, Michigan, USA are now long-time friends and continue to be stimulating professional contacts. During the years I have had a fruitful collaboration with the pathology department at the University of Lund and I would like to mention Nils H. Sternby, MD, PhD, Mr. Thomas Cedergren, and Fritz Rank, MD, PhD as key persons in this exciting collaboration.

Another significant person who was a pleasure to meet was Flemming Nørgaard, MD, DSc (Med), DSc (Odont), who appeared at the defense of my PhD thesis in 1982. Dr. Nørgaard has continued to follow the development in the area of TMJ arthrography, which he pioneered during the 1940s. I also had the pleasure of meeting Karl Boman, MD, PhD. Dr. Brown was a general surgeon who developed an interest in TMJ treatment as early as 1939, after reading the classical articles by James B. Costen, MD. Dr. Boman presented his thesis on surgical treatment of TMJ disorders in 1947. Lars Eriksson and I were fortunate to be able to reevaluate his surgically treated patients at 30-year follow-up. Drs. Boman and Nørgaard should be acknowledged for being early pioneers who had to wait several decades before their work was appreciated.

Richard W. Katzberg, MD, and I worked parallel to one another for several years and knew of each other through the literature long before we met. In 1984 we met and started planning for collaborative research. Several research projects have been completed and this book is a documentation of our long and stimulating collaboration.

In 1986 I was offered a position at the University of Rochester as a maxillofacial radiologist, and I undertook this challenge with great enthusiasm. My colleagues in the neuroradiology section in the Department of Radiology at the University of Rochester School of Medicine and Dentistry and especially my chairman at that time, Robert E. O'Mara, MD, have been strong supporters of my professional development and should be acknowledged for creating a fruitful environment at the University of Rochester.

Significant TMJ clinicians should be acknowledged for their continuing efforts to develop better treatment modalities. These include Russell B. Bessette, DDS, MD; M. Frank Dolwick, DMD, PhD; Fred Emmings, DDS, PhD; Lars Eriksson, DDS, PhD; Vernon Loveless, DMD; Håkan Lundh, DDS, PhD; Donald Macher, DMD; and Ross H. Tallents, DDS, and many other highly skilled clinicans who I have had the privilege to work with.

I have had financial support for the research on which a significant part of this book is based from several institutions and foundations. I would especially mention the Torsten and Ragnar Söderberg Foundation, Stockholm, Sweden, which has been supportive of my research for nearly ten years.

Finally I would like to acknowledge Mrs. Lisette Bralow at the W.B. Saunders Company for encouragement and editorial assistance and my secretaries, Mr. Gregory W. Aspinall and Ms. Alyce Norder, for outstanding secretarial service.

PER-LENNART WESTESSON, DDS, PhD

Contents

PART ONE
OVERVIEW OF INTERNAL DERANGEMENTS

CHAPTER ONE
NORMAL ANATOMY 3

CHAPTER TWO
PATHOLOGY 25

PART TWO
IMAGING INTERNAL DERANGEMENTS

CHAPTER THREE
PLAIN FILM AND TOMOGRAPHY 73

CHAPTER FOUR
TEMPOROMANDIBULAR JOINT ARTHROGRAPHY 101

    SECTION I · SINGLE-CONTRAST ARTHROGRAPHY 101

    SECTION II · DOUBLE-CONTRAST ARTHROGRAPHY 143

CHAPTER FIVE
MAGNETIC RESONANCE IMAGING 167

CHAPTER SIX
MISCELLANEOUS MODALITIES: COMPUTED TOMOGRAPHY, SINGLE PHOTON
EMISSION COMPUTED TOMOGRAPHY, AND SOUND ANALYSIS 223

CHAPTER SEVEN
POST-TREATMENT IMAGING 251

PART THREE
IMAGING MISCELLANEOUS CONDITIONS

CHAPTER EIGHT
RHEUMATOID ARTHRITIS AND RELATED JOINT DISEASES 303
    Tore A. Larheim

CHAPTER NINE
TRAUMA 327

CHAPTER TEN
MISCELLANEOUS CONDITIONS 343

PART FOUR
ARTHROSCOPY

CHAPTER ELEVEN
ARTHROSCOPY OF THE TEMPOROMANDIBULAR JOINT 371
    Ralph G. Merrill

PART FIVE
PUTTING IT ALL TOGETHER

CHAPTER TWELVE
SELECTION OF DIAGNOSTIC TESTS 397

INDEX 405

PART ONE

Overview of Internal Derangements

CHAPTER ONE

Normal Anatomy

A brief description of the anatomy of the temporomandibular joint (TMJ) and associated structures is presented to provide a clear understanding of the rationale of various imaging techniques and their interpretation and an understanding of joint pathology. Comprehensive descriptions of TMJ anatomy have been previously published.[1-6] Emphasis here is on a correlation between anatomy and radiographic techniques and interpretation.

OSSEOUS COMPONENTS

The normal TMJ is a freely movable articulation between the condyle of the mandible and the squamous portion of the temporal bone at the base of the skull. The osseous components of this joint consist inferiorly of the mandibular condyle and superiorly of the glenoid fossa and articular eminence (Fig. 1–1; Table 1–1). The bilateral articulation of the mandible to the cranium implies that the left and right TMJs must function together. The term *craniomandibular articulation* is sometimes used to emphasize this bilateral function.[5]

Mandibular Condyle

Dimension and Form

The mandibular condyle is located on top of the mandibular neck (Fig. 1–2). It is elliptic in shape and resembles a large olive that is oriented horizontally. The lateral pole of the condyle is located about 1 to 1.5 cm beneath the skin and can, in most individuals, be located by palpation when the jaw is moving.[2] The distance between the midpoints of the left and right condyles is on the average 100 mm.[2,7] Each mandibular condyle measures on the average 20 mm mediolaterally and 10 mm anteroposteriorly.[8] These measurements are based on observations in autopsy specimens[8] and include the soft tissue cover of the condyle. The dimensions vary considerably among individuals, with a range of 13 to 25 mm for the mediolateral length and 5.5 to 16 mm for the anteroposterior dimension.[8]

Yale studied the shape of the condyle and classified the appearance in a frontal aspect into four major categories[9] (Fig. 1–3). The convex type was most frequent (58 per cent) followed by flat (25 per cent), angled (12 per cent), and rounded (3 per cent) types. These observations were confirmed by Öberg and

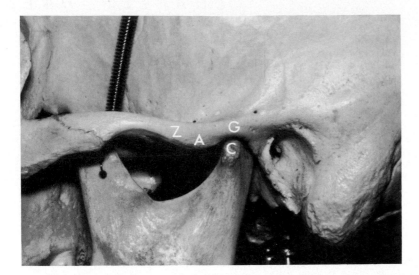

Figure 1–1
Osseous components. Lateral view of the TMJ in a dry skull. The mandibular condyle (C) is located in the glenoid fossa (G), and the articular eminence (A) at the posterior aspect of the zygomatic arch (Z) is well visualized.

Carlsson, who additionally pointed out that the condyle in children more often is rounded.[4] The different shapes of the mandibular condyle represent a variation of normal anatomy and are probably of no specific clinical significance. Discrete flattenings of the superior surface of the condyle or of the inferior aspect of the articular eminence have been observed radiographically in asymptomatic volunteers without internal derangement.[10] These are probably of no clinical significance and should not be regarded as indications of degenerative joint disease (see Chapters 2 and 3).

Spatial Orientation

An appreciation of the three-dimensional spatial orientation of the mandibular condyles is essential for an understanding of the principles of imaging the joint and for correct interpretation, since variations in condylar angulation influence both the radiographic projection and depiction of the joint. The horizontal long axes of the mandibular condyles usually converge in a posterior direction (see Fig. 1–2). The angle between the horizontal condylar long axis and the frontal plane has been investigated in a large series of dry skulls and found to vary between 0° and 30°, with mean values of about 15°.[11–13] The horizontal condylar angle (Fig. 1–2A) also has been measured in patients and

Table 1–1
GROSS ANATOMIC COMPONENTS OF THE TEMPOROMANDIBULAR JOINT

Osseous	Glenoid fossa
	Articular eminence (articular tubercle)
	Mandibular condyle
	Postglenoid tubercle
Soft Tissue	Disk
	Posterior disk attachment
	Joint capsule, articular soft tissue cover
	Synovia
	Lateral ligament
Other	Upper and lower joint spaces

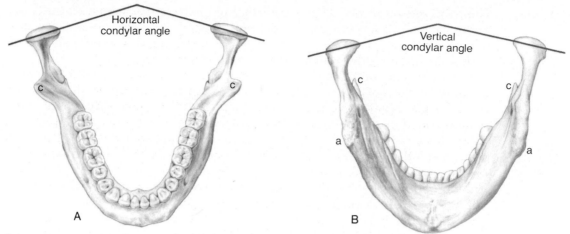

Figure 1–2
A, Axial aspect of the mandible, showing the horizontal condylar angle. The coronoid processes (c) are also indicated for orientation. B, The posterior aspect of the mandible. The vertical condylar angle is indicated. The coronoid processes on left and right sides are indicated for orientation as well as the angle of the mandible (a).

has a mean value of about 20°.[14–17] There appears to be a larger condylar angle in patients than in dry skulls.[18–24] This means that the lateral pole of the condyle is located more anteriorly in symptomatic patients than in individuals with normal TMJs.

Studies using arthrography and more recently magnetic resonance imaging have shown that there is a larger angle of the condyle in patients with internal derangement and degenerative joint disease, compared with normal joints.[23, 24] Furthermore, the condylar angle was larger in joints with advanced internal derangement and degenerative joint disease, compared with joints in earlier stages of disease.[23, 24] There is no immediate explanation for this finding. It

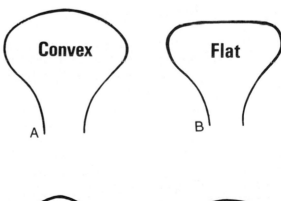

Figure 1–3
Frontal aspect of the mandibular condyles. The most frequent types of condylar shape are convex (A), flat (B), angled (C), and rounded (D).

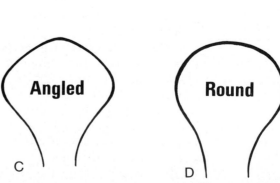

could be the result of congenital factors or the fact that joints with a larger angle have a greater tendency to develop internal derangement and degenerative joint disease than joints with a smaller condylar angle. Another explanation is that the large condylar angle is the result of remodeling.

An appreciation of the degree of condylar angulation is useful in clinical imaging of the TMJ, since optimal imaging can be obtained by directing the central x-ray beam along the condylar long axis.[25] Comparative studies have demonstrated that more information is obtained from a transcranial projection when the x-ray beam is directed along the horizontal condylar long axis than when a standard projection at 0° is used (see Chapter 3).[25] Analogous studies using tomography[26] also have confirmed the potential advantage of individualizing the projection through the long axis of the condyle. Studies of the importance of individualized projections in arthrotomography have not been published, but it is reasonable to assume that more precise information is gained if the projection is standardized with respect to the condylar long axis than if a projection that is not tailored to the individual variations in anatomy is used.

The long axis of the condyle also forms an angle with the horizontal plane. This angle is named the vertical condylar angle (Fig. 1–2*B*) and was reported by Moffet to average 8°, with the lateral pole being higher than the medial pole.[2] Our clinical experience is somewhat different: the lateral pole is frequently at the same level as or lower than the medial pole in patients with TMJ disorders. Most investigators do not specifically recommend correction for the vertical condylar angle in imaging of the joint. This is difficult to correct for, since the superior surface of the condyle is frequently rounded and usually does not form a flat surface (Fig. 1–3). Rosenberg and coworkers, however, advocate correction for the condylar angle when performing corrected sagittal tomography and have demonstrated high-quality tomograms using this technique[26, 27] (see Chapter 3).

Temporal Component

The temporal component of the TMJ consists of the concave glenoid (mandibular) fossa and the convex articular tubercle (see Fig. 1–1), both formed by the squamous part of the temporal bone. The temporal part of the joint measures about 23 mm, both in mediolateral width and in anteroposterior length,[2] measured using capsular attachments as the margins. The depth of the fossa was reported by Moffet to average 7 mm when measured from the highest point in the fossa to the lowest point of the articular eminence.[2] The inclination reported by Angel was about 40° when measured by the angle between the Frankfort plane and a line from the bottom of the fossa to the articular eminence.[28]

Many unsuccessful attempts have been made to correlate the slope and form of the articular eminence with specific features of the dentition. It seems reasonable to assume, however, that these two variables are not closely related, as was also pointed out by Moffet.[2] The osseous roof of the fossa is quite thin—in some individuals it can be paper thin—and appears translucent when a dried skull is held against light. An awareness of this anatomic feature of the TMJ is important, especially in arthroscopy, since one should avoid inserting a large needle or any other instrument forcefully in the direction of the superior part of the fossa, to avoid the risk of creating an intracranial communication. In arthroscopy the instruments are relatively thick (2 to 3 mm), and a comparatively large force must be used to penetrate the lateral capsule when an instrument is inserted into the joint.

Medially the fossa narrows considerably and is closed by an osseous plate that prevents the condyle from being displaced medially.

Posterior to the fossa is the postglenoid tubercle, with an average height or vertical dimension of about 5 mm.[2] The postglenoid tubercle also belongs to the squamous part of the temporal bone and forms the posterior border of the glenoid fossa. The fissure that separates the fossa from the tympanic portion of the temporal bone is called the petrotympanic fissure (squamotympanic fissure). The chorda tympani nerve and the anterior tympanic vessels pass through the lateral part of the petrotympanic fissure.

SOFT TISSUE COMPONENTS

Disk and Disk Attachments

The joint is divided by the interpositioned disk into upper and lower joint compartments (Figs. 1–4 and 1–5), which normally do not communicate. The disk is a flexible but firm plate of dense collagenous connective tissue that merges around its periphery with the surrounding capsule. Its central part is considerably thinner than its periphery, and its posterior band is considerably thicker. The underaspect of the disk is concave and fits on top of the rounded condyle. The anterior and posterior bands of the disk have been called leading edges. The form of the undersurface of the disk and the top of the condyle fit so well together that they can move in fresh cadaver specimens in a way very similar to the living function.

The peripheral attachment to the capsule binds the disk firmly to the lateral and medial poles of the condyle (Fig. 1–6). Anteriorly there is no direct connection between the disk and the mandibular condyle. Thus, the disk can rotate relatively freely over the condyle in an anteroposterior direction, but it can move relatively little in the mediolateral direction unless the attachments

Figure 1–4
Sagittal section through a normal TMJ. The disk (arrow) is located with its posterior thick part superior to the condyle. The articular soft tissue covers on the condyle and in the glenoid fossa are thin.

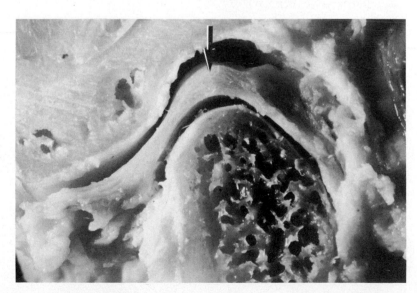

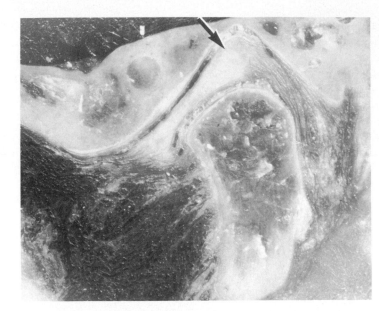

Figure 1–5
Sagittal section through the medial part of a normal TMJ. The disk (arrow) is biconcave and is located with its central thin zone apposing the anterior prominence of the condyle.

to the capsule and condyle have been torn or elongated. Anterior movement of the disk is limited by the length of the undersurface of the posterior disk attachment. This extends from the posterior band of the disk down to the back of the condyle and prevents the disk from moving anteriorly over the condyle.

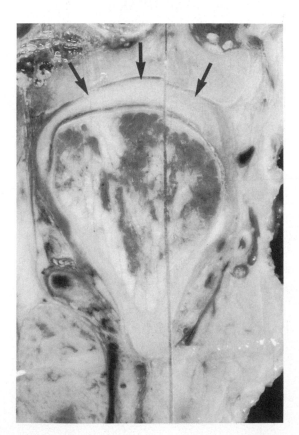

Figure 1–6
Coronal section through a normal TMJ shows the disk (arrows) superior to the condyle, merging to the capsule and condyle laterally and medially.

This surface consists of fibrous tissue. If it is damaged, the disk can translate anteriorly relative to the condyle, resulting in disk displacement. This has been shown in experimental study on fresh human autopsy material.[29]

In the sagittal plane, the disk is biconcave; that is, it is thickest anteriorly and posteriorly (see Fig. 1–5). The thickness of the disk is 1 mm in its central part, 3 mm posteriorly, and 2 mm anteriorly.[30] There is great variation in the configuration of the disk; generally its shape is well adapted to the shape of the condyle and the temporal component. In joints with a deep fossa, the posterior band is usually thick and pronounced (Fig. 1–5), whereas in joints with a flat or shallow fossa the disk is more even in thickness (see Fig. 1–4). Blood vessels and nerves are absent in the disk but are frequent in its peripheral attachment to the capsule.

Disk Position

The normal position of the disk has traditionally been described as a 12 o'clock relationship between the superior aspect of the condyle and the posterior band of the disk (see Figs. 1–4 and 1–5). An example of an "ideal" normal superior disk position is shown in Figure 1–7A. However, not all normal joints show an ideal superior disk position, and variation of normality has led us to suggest an alternative landmark for the determination of the position of the disk. When the posterior band is not in the perfect 12 o'clock position, the next step is to look for the relationship between the anterior prominence of the condyle and the central thin zone of the disk. We have found that this can be used as an additional criterion for normal disk position.[31] In the example shown in Figure 1–7B, the posterior band of the disk is anterior to the 12 o'clock position while the anterior prominence of the condyle opposes the central thin part of the disk. This is also considered a normal disk position since the function in these joints is smooth without irregularities or evidence of internal derangement. Separation of the anterior prominence of the condyle and the central thin zone of the disk is evidence of disk displacement (Fig. 1–7C).

An example of a joint with anterior disk displacement by both the 12 o'clock and the central thin zone criteria is shown in Figure 1–7C. The relationship of the posterior band to the condyle is not so very different in Figure 1–7B and C, but the disk is clearly anteriorly displaced in Figure 1–7C using the central thin zone criterion.

A second criterion for normal versus abnormal is joint function on jaw opening. The function on opening should be smooth, without hindrances. The disk rotates in the lower joint compartment, and the disk and condyle complex rotates and translates against the temporal component (Fig. 1–8). Anterior to the articular eminence at the end of jaw opening, the condyle opposes the anterior band of the disk and the central thin zone. The articular surfaces of the disk and condyle should not be separate from each other during opening. The anterior and posterior bands of the disk are the leading edges. On opening there is expansion of the posterior disk attachment (Fig. 1–9).

Joint Compartments

In the sagittal plane, the *upper joint compartment* extends from a margin several millimeters anterior to the most inferior prominence of the articular

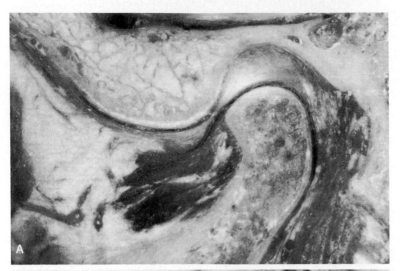

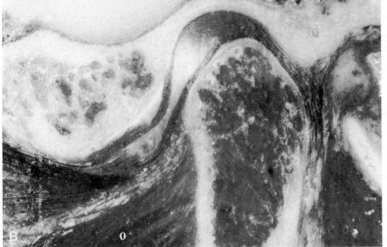

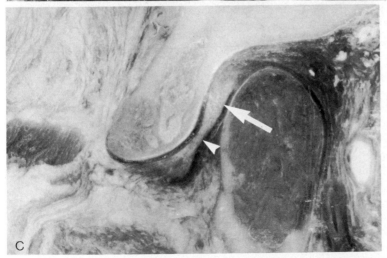

Figure 1–7
A, *Sagittal section through the central part of the joint showing an "ideal" normal position of the disk. The posterior band of the disk is located on top of the condyle, and the central thin zone of the disk is between the anterior prominence of the condyle and the posterior prominence of the articular tubercle. B, Sagittal section through the central part of the joint, showing the posterior band in an anterior relationship to the 12 o'clock position. However, the central thin zone of the disk and the anterior prominence of the condyle are located in a normal relationship. This joint should be interpreted as normal with respect to disk position. C, Sagittal section showing anterior displacement. The anterior prominence of the condyle is articulating against the posterior band of the disk (arrow) and not against the central thin zone. The central thin zone (arrowhead) is anterior and inferior to the prominence of the condyle, and this is interpreted as anterior disk displacement.*

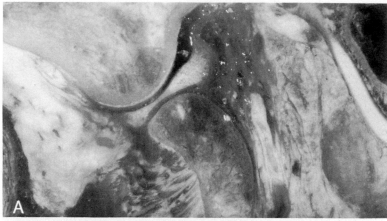

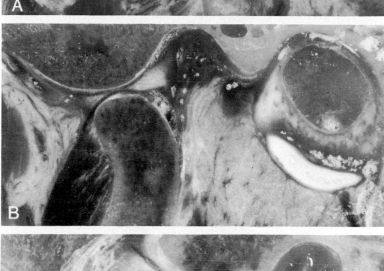

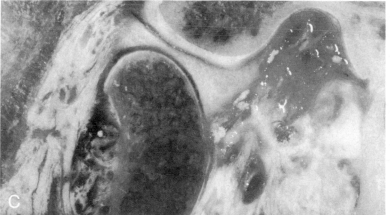

Figure 1–8
Opening sequence. A series of different degrees of jaw opening: half open (A), three-quarters open (B), and maximal opening (C). The relationship between the central thin zone of the disk and the anterior and superior prominence of the condyle remains the same in all open-mouth positions. The posterior disk attachment is expanded on opening, and vascular structures are filling the space behind the condyle.

tubercle to the posterior aspect of the roof of the fossa (see Figs. 1–4 and 1–5). From a frontal visual inspection, the upper joint compartment demonstrates a crescent configuration and has a medial recess and a lateral recess that encompass the disk and the lower joint compartment (see Fig. 1–6). Frequently the medial recess extends more inferiorly than the lateral recess.

The *lower joint compartment* extends in the sagittal plane over the condyle and has a posterior recess and an anterior recess. The posterior recess reaches more inferiorly than the anterior recess (see Figs. 1–4 and 1–5). The dimension of the anterior recess of the lower joint compartment varies between individuals,

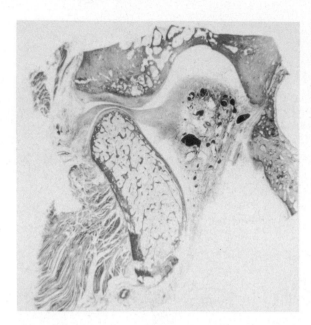

Figure 1-9
This open-mouth histologic section shows expansion of the posterior disk attachment and extensive vascularity of this area. (Courtesy of Dr. R. P. Scapino, Chicago, Illinois.)

and this can cause confusion in the interpretation of lower joint space arthrograms.[32, 33] Sagittal sections of autopsy specimens with superior disk position and arthrographic examinations of asymptomatic individuals[34, 35] have shown that the size of the anterior recess of the lower joint compartment can vary considerably even when the disk is located superiorly. Therefore the size of the anterior recess should not be used as the only diagnostic criterion for determining the position of the disk.

Articular Surfaces

The intra-articular osseous parts of the mandibular condyle and the temporal component are covered by a thin layer of dense collagenous connective tissue that can become cartilaginous.[4] The thickness of the articular soft tissue cover has been measured in postmortem studies of normal and pathologic joints and varies between 0.1 and 1 mm.[30] Thickening of the soft tissue cover on the articular eminence is frequently seen (Figs. 1–8C and 1–9). This probably represents part of a remodeling process. The total area of the articulating surface of the temporal compartment of the joint is two to three times greater than that of the mandibular condyle. This difference is to a large extent a function of the larger anterior recess of the upper joint compartment, which extends about 8 to 10 mm anterior to the apex of the articular tubercle. The large articular surface on the temporal component is necessary to accommodate the condyle when it translates anteriorly on jaw opening. In the lower joint space there is less translation and more rotation. The extensive articular surface in the lower joint space is on the back of the condyle. This surface is there to provide an articulating surface for the disk when the condyle rotates forward as the posterior band of the disk articulates against the posterior aspect of the condyle.

Joint Capsule

The TMJ capsule originates from the periphery of the articulating surface of the temporal bone. It extends inferiorly in the shape of a funnel, encloses the disk and condyle, and attaches to the lower part of the condyle and the upper part of the condylar neck. Medially and laterally the capsule is firm, to stabilize the mandible during movement. Anteriorly and posteriorly the capsule is loose, to allow for mandibular movements. The capsule consists of two layers: (1) the outer layers, called the stratum fibrosum, and (2) the inner layer that is adjacent to the joint spaces, called the stratum synoviale.[4] The synovial tissue functions to produce synovial fluid, which lowers friction between surfaces as a lubricant, removes degradation products from the joint space, and provides nutrition to the avascular regions of the articular surfaces and disk. The amount of synovial fluid in the TMJ is usually so small, however, that it cannot be aspirated. Thus, there is usually only a thin lining of synovial fluid on the articular surfaces. Larger amounts of joint fluid usually are associated with painful internal derangement.[36] The synovial fluid consists mainly of a plasma dialysate enriched with a polysaccharide-protein complex. Normal synovial fluid contains only a few cellular elements.[4]

Ligaments

Excessive displacement of the mandible is restricted by the joint capsule and ligaments. The ligaments associated with the mandible and TMJ are listed in Table 1 2. Closest to the joint is the temporomandibular joint ligament, which consists of a fibrous thickening in the lateral joint capsule. This ligament extends from the inferior surface of the posterior aspect of the zygomatic arch to the lateral part of the neck of the condyle. There is debate whether this ligament is clearly identifiable in all joints,[37] and it may be just a thickening of the joint capsule rather than a ligament in many cases. Medially the capsule is also strengthened by a thickening of the capsule, although this is not as pronounced as in the lateral ligament. Other ligaments that support the TMJ are the sphenomandibular and the stylomandibular.

MUSCLES

As mentioned by Moffet, an appreciation of the muscles acting on the TMJ is much more fundamental to an understanding of mandibular movements

Table 1–2
LIGAMENTS RELATED TO THE TEMPOROMANDIBULAR JOINT

Ligament	Location
Temporomandibular joint ligament	Lateral joint capsule as a thickening of the capsule
Sphenomandibular ligament	Greater wing of sphenoid to mandible
Stylomandibular ligament	From styloid process to mandible

Table 1–3
MUSCLES OF MASTICATION

Muscle	Location	Function	Innervation
Temporalis	From lateral surface of skull to coronoid process	Closing the jaw, maintaining rest position, and protrusion of jaw	Trigeminal nerve, V3
Masseter	From zygomatic arch to angle of mandible	Closing the jaw	Trigeminal nerve, V3
Lateral pterygoid, inferior belly	From lateral pterygoid plate to condyle	Protruding mandible	Trigeminal nerve, V3
Lateral pterygoid, superior belly	From base of skull on sphenoid bone to joint capsule, disk, and condyle	Stabilization of disk and condyle during closing; jaw opening	Trigeminal nerve, V3
Geniohyoid	From mental spine to hyoid	Jaw opening	Hypoglossal nerve and cervical plexus
Mylohyoid	Inside of mandible to hyoid	Jaw opening	Mylohyoid nerve from trigeminal nerve, V3
Digastric, anterior belly	Inside of mandible to hyoid	Jaw opening	Mylohyoid nerve from trigeminal nerve, V3

than are the contours of the joint components or the direction of the ligaments.[2] The muscles involved in mandibular movements are mainly the temporalis, the masseter, the medial and lateral pterygoids (Table 1–3; Figs. 1–10 and 1–11), and the suprahyoid; the latter constitute the geniohyoid, genioglossus, anterior bellies of the digastric, and the mylohyoid muscles.

Jaw Closing

The temporalis muscle, which functions to close the jaw, extends from the lateral fascia of the skull and inserts onto the coronoid process of the mandible,

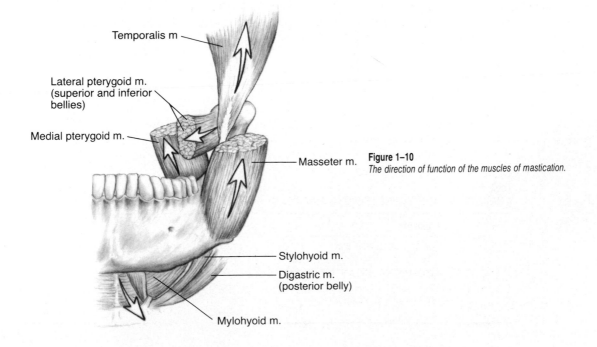

Figure 1–10
The direction of function of the muscles of mastication.

Temporalis m

Lateral pterygoid m. (superior and inferior bellies)

Medial pterygoid m.

Masseter m.

Stylohyoid m.

Digastric m. (posterior belly)

Mylohyoid m.

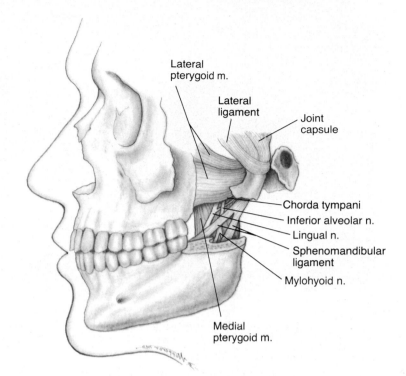

Figure 1–11
Deep muscles of mastication and other structures anterior and medial to the TMJ.

with an attachment extending inferiorly on the anterior and medial surfaces of the ramus. The other major muscle for jaw closing is the masseter, which arises from the zygomatic process of the maxilla and the zygomatic arch and inserts onto the lateral surface of the angle and ramus of the mandible. The superior aspect of the masseter actually consists of three layers that fuse inferiorly.[38] The medial pterygoid also has a jaw-closing function. It arises from the medial pterygoid plate in the pterygoid fossa and inserts onto the medial side of the angle and ramus of the mandible.

Jaw Opening

The muscles important in jaw opening are the suprahyoid muscle group and the inferior belly of the lateral pterygoid. The suprahyoid muscle group consists of the geniohyoid, genioglossus, anterior bellies of the digastric, and the mylohyoid muscles. The inferior belly of the lateral pterygoid muscle arises from the lateral pterygoid plate and inserts on the anterior part of the neck of the mandible.

Lateral Pterygoid

The superior belly of this muscle arises from the infratemporal crest of the greater wing of the sphenoid bone and passes through the anteromedial wall of the TMJ capsule. There has been debate about whether the superior belly of the lateral pterygoid muscle attaches to the disk or to the condyle.[39–46] One anatomic study has suggested that the upper belly of the lateral pterygoid

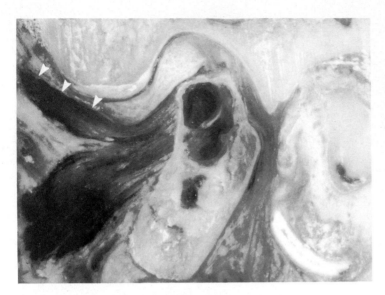

Figure 1–12
Upper head of the lateral pterygoid muscle attaching to the condyle. Sagittal section through a joint with a slightly anterior disk position, showing the upper belly of the lateral pterygoid muscle (arrowheads) attaching directly to the condyle. Note the different angles of action of the lower and upper heads of the lateral pterygoid muscle. There is thickening of the articular cartilage on the inferior part of the articular eminence. Some degenerative changes in the superior surface of the condyle are seen. The marrow space in the condylar head is prominent.

muscle attaches mainly to the fascia between the upper and lower bellies of this muscle.[47] This fascia then continues posteriorly and attaches to the condyle. An example of this is seen in Figure 1–12. Thus, the upper belly of the lateral pterygoid muscle would be regarded as functional mainly for movement of the condyle but not actually of the disk. These observations militate against the theory that spasm in the upper head of the lateral pterygoid muscle could be a direct cause of anterior displacement of the disk.[48]

The anatomy of the lateral pterygoid muscle, however, is variable in humans.[46] A study of human autopsy material showed that 65 per cent of specimens have two heads to this muscle while 20 per cent actually have three heads (Fig. 1–13) and 15 per cent have only a single head.[46] The same study showed that in about 30 per cent of specimens, the superior head of the lateral pterygoid muscle inserts into the disk,[46] as shown in Figure 1–14. Thus the anatomy of function of the lateral pterygoid muscle is probably quite variable in humans. The significance of this is unknown. From a review of the literature

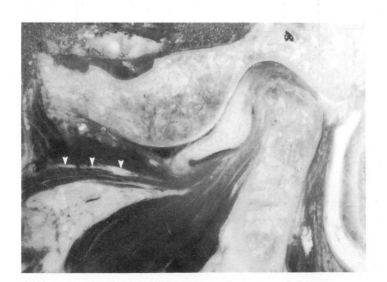

Figure 1–13
Sagittal section of a joint with two heads of the upper part of the lateral pterygoid muscle. Note how the upper head of this muscle is divided by a fat plane (arrowheads). Also, the upper head of the muscle is essentially inserting into the condyle and not into the disk. The disk is displaced.

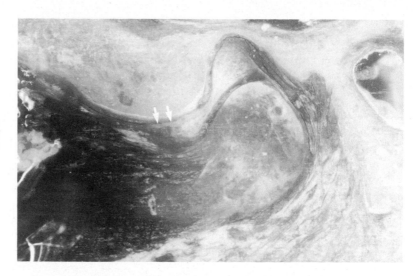

Figure 1–14
Sagittal section from the medial part of the joint, showing the upper head of the lateral pterygoid muscle inserting directly into the disk (arrows).

and our own experience with cadaver material, it seems reasonable to assume that the attachment of the lateral pterygoid muscle is not only to the condyle and not only to the disk but to both in some joints and to only one in other joints[42, 46] (Fig. 1–15).

The directions of action of the masticatory muscles are illustrated in Figure 1–12. The initial phase of jaw opening is thought to be a function of the suprahyoid muscles, whereas the lateral pterygoid muscle is active during the later part of the opening movement. Electromyographic studies of both animals and humans have indicated that the lower belly of the lateral pterygoid muscle is active during jaw opening.[49–52] The upper belly of the lateral pterygoid muscle is active during closing. Thus, the upper and lower bellies of this muscle have reciprocal functions.[51, 52] The upper belly has been considered to stabilize the mandible and the disk during closing. It is interesting that one study showed that the reciprocal function of the upper and lower bellies of the lateral pterygoid muscles was disturbed in patients with pain and dysfunction, so that the lower head of the pterygoid muscle, which normally is active only when protruding and deviating the mandible, also becomes active when closing and clenching in patients suffering pain.[52] This observation deserves further inves

Figure 1–15
Attachment of the upper and lower heads of the lateral pterygoid muscle. Numbers in the muscle heads indicate the number of joints in which the muscle attached this way. (Redrawn from Moritz T, Ewers R: The attachments of the lateral pterygoid muscle to the TMJ in humans. A histological study. Dtsch Zahnartz Zeitschr 1987;42:680–685.)

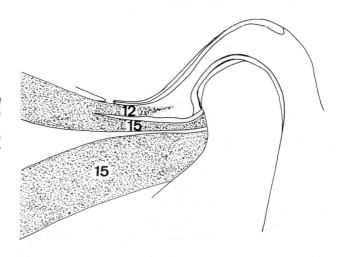

tigation with larger patient material, including patients with more specific diagnoses. A causal relationship between muscle dysfunction and joint abnormality has not been established. We do not know whether the joint abnormality causes the muscle dysfunction or the muscle dysfunction causes the joint abnormality. Further studies are needed.

BLOOD SUPPLY

The TMJ is supplied by the superficial temporal and maxillary arteries, which arise from the external carotid artery. The blood vessels surround the joint in a network of fine branches. Venous drainage is via the superficial temporal, the maxillary, and the pterygoid plexus of veins. The joint capsule and the attachments of the disk are richly vascularized during growth but are not vascularized in the adult.

INNERVATION OF THE JOINT

The TMJ and the masticatory muscles (temporalis, masseter, medial and lateral pterygoids) are innervated via the mandibular nerve, which is the third and largest branch of the trigeminal nerve (cranial nerve V). Thus, the medial, posterior, and lateral walls of the capsule of the temporomandibular joint are innervated from a large branch of the auriculotemporal nerve as it crosses posteriorly behind the neck of the mandible. The lateral half of the anterior wall of the capsule is also innervated from this nerve. The anterior region of the joint is innervated from the masseteric nerve and from the posterior deep temporal nerve. The posterior and lateral parts of the joint have considerably more innervations than the medial and anterior parts. Comprehensive descriptions of the innervation of the TMJ have been presented by several investigators.[53-59] The sensory innervation of the TMJ also seems to be via the fifth cranial nerve.[60]

The nerve fibers mainly follow the vascular supply and terminate as free nerve endings. Thus, the capsule, the subsynovial tissue, and the periphery of the disk are innervated. The articular cartilage and the central part of the disk contain no nerves. Both myelinated and nonmyelinated nerves are seen in the TMJ.

Polypeptide substance P has been suggested as an excitatory transmitter in certain primary sensory neurons, and it has been postulated that substance P has been involved in pain transmission. Studies have shown that substance P immunoreactive fibers are present in the normal monkey TMJ.[61] Further studies in this field would probably increase our understanding of the biologic background of TMJ pain.

MICROSCOPIC ANATOMY

The microscopic anatomy of the TMJ previously has been reviewed by Öberg and Carlsson[4] and Kreutziger and Mahan,[3] among others. The TMJ differs from most other synovial joints of the human body by having its articular covering made of fibrous connective tissue instead of hyaline cartilage. This fibrous connective tissue covers the osseous components of the joint and merges

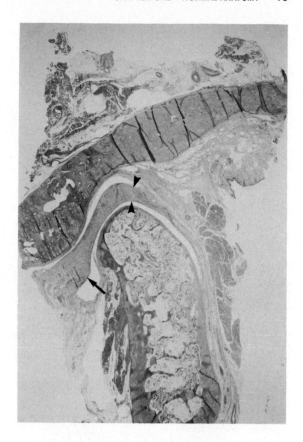

Figure 1–16
Microscopic sagittal histologic section of a normal TMJ, showing normal position and normal configuration of the disk. The distinction between the posterior band of the disk and the posterior disk attachment is clearly seen (arrowheads). There is slight prominence of the anterior band of the disk (arrow). (Courtesy of Dr. Bengt Lindahl, Ljungby, Sweden.)

with the periosteum at the periphery of the joint. The articular soft tissue cover is avascular. The soft tissue cover in the normal joint is usually thickest on the inferior and posterior regions of the articular tubercle, varying between 0.5 and 1.5 mm. In the mandibular fossa, the soft tissue cover is usually much thinner, being about 0.1 mm in thickness (Fig. 1–16).

The articular cartilage of synovial joints is composed predominantly of chondrocytes, collagen fibrils, proteoglycans, and water. The collagen fibers and the proteoglycans form the articular cartilage matrix.[62] The articular cartilage is avascular, alymphatic, and aneural tissue. The articular surface is not covered by a perichondrium. The synovial fluid covers the articular surface and is essential for lubrication, nutrition, and removal of debris. Fibrous cartilage has a higher content of collagen type I than hyaline cartilage, whereas hyaline cartilage has a higher content of collagen type II. Only a few cells in the cartilage are visible microscopically. The articular soft tissue cover in the TMJ can be divided into four zones. Starting from the surface, these are the articular, proliferative, fibrocartilage, and calcified cartilage zones.[63] Electron microscopic studies have shown that the articular surface is composed of closely packed collagen fibrils.[62]

Disk and Posterior Disk Attachment

The disk is composed of compact collagen of mainly type I, a system of small collagen elastic fibers, and glucose aminoglycans.[64–68] The collagen fibers of the disk have a characteristic organization. The fibers in the central thin

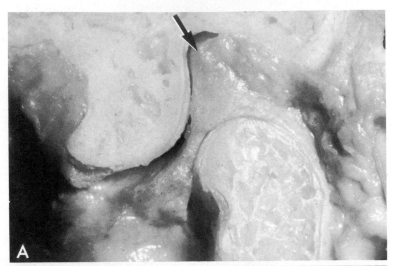

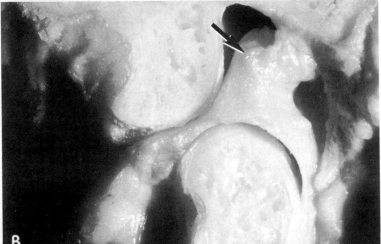

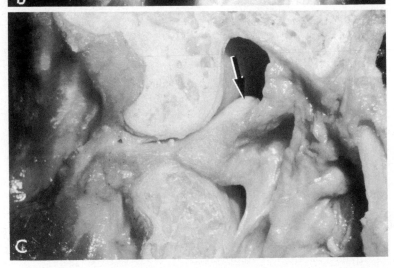

Figure 1–17
Normal opening sequence. A, Closed-mouth sagittal section through a normal joint, showing the biconcave disk with its posterior band (arrow) and central thin zone in a normal relationship to the condyle and temporal component. B, At quarter open, there is rotation and translation in the lower compartment, and the central thin zone remains between the two joint components. C, At nearly full open, the condyle is under the articular eminence, and the central thin zone is interposed between the two joint components. Note how the configuration of the joint compartment corresponds to what is seen in arthrography (see Chapter 4).

zone are predominantly oriented in an anteroposterior direction, with much interlacing superiorly and inferiorly and from side to side.[69]

The fibers flare out into the posterior band where they interface with the three-dimensional meshwork of fibers within the band. The disk is fibrocartilage in which fibers predominate. The disk continues posteriorly into the tissue of the posterior disk attachment, which also has been called the bilaminar zone,[1] retrodiskal pad,[6] or retroarticuläre plastische Polster.[70] We prefer using the term *posterior disk attachment*. This tissue is composed of a loosely organized network of collagen fibers intermixed with a branching system of large elastic fibers, fat, and numerous blood vessels and nerves.[69] The posterior disk attachment has been divided into temporal and condylar parts.[71] In contrast to the disk, which is firm, the posterior attachment is readily deformable, and when the mouth is opened widely it becomes substantially expanded (see Figs. 1–8 and 1–9).

FUNCTIONAL ANATOMY

Since joints are almost constantly moving, more emphasis should be placed on functional anatomy. Functional anatomy, however, has not attracted as much interest as static anatomy, partly because there have been few methods to study joint dynamics.

During the initial phase of jaw opening there is rotation in the lower joint space and mainly translation in the upper joint space (Fig. 1–17). This is the classic description of the function of the TMJ. Probably substantial variations occur within normal limits. The function of the normal and abnormal joint has not been extensively studied. It is not known what the clinical significance of different types of joint function is. Another relatively unknown area is the function of the disk and joint spaces during sideways movement. The amount of sideways movement of the disk relative to the condyle is not known.

The configuration of the joint compartments varies substantially at different jaw positions. The principal movements described for jaw opening vary considerably between individuals, and further study is needed before we can understand the relationships between shape of the joint components and movement patterns. The posterior disk attachment expands substantially on opening because of filling of venous structures.

References

1. Rees LA: The structure and function of the mandibular joint. Br Dent J 1954;*96*:125–133.
2. Moffet B: The temporomandibular joint. *In* Sharry JJ, ed: Complete Denture Prosthodontics. New York, McGraw-Hill, 1968, pp 56–104.
3. Kreutziger KL, Mahan PE: Temporomandibular degenerative joint disease. Part I: Anatomy, pathophysiology, and clinical description. Oral Surg Oral Med Oral Pathol 1975;*40*:165–182.
4. Öberg T, Carlsson GE: Macroscopic and microscopic anatomy of the temporomandibular joint. *In* Zarb GA, Carlsson GE, eds: Temporomandibular Joint Function and Dysfunction. Copenhagen, Munksgaard, 1979, pp 155–174.
5. Dolwick MF: The temporomandibular joint: Normal and abnormal anatomy. *In* Helms CA, Katzberg RW, eds: Internal Derangements of the Temporomandibular Joint. San Francisco, Radiology Research and Education Foundation, 1983, pp 1–14.
6. DuBrul EL: Sichers and DuBrul's Oral Anatomy. St. Louis, Tokyo, Ishiyaku EuroAmerica, 1988, pp 107–132.
7. Posselt U: Condyle-to-skin relationship and length of the intercondylar axis. Acta Morphol Neerl Scand 1959;*2*:276–279.

8. Öberg T, Carlsson GE, Fajers CM: The temporomandibular joint. A morphologic study on human autopsy material. Acta Odontol Scand 1971;*29*:349–384.
9. Yale SH, Allison BD, Hauptfuehrer JD: An epidemiological assessment of mandibular condyle morphology. Oral Surg Oral Med Oral Pathol 1966;*21*:169–177.
10. Brooks SC, Westesson P-L, Eriksson L, et al: Prevalence of osseous changes in the temporomandibular joint of asymptomatic persons without internal derangement. Oral Surg Oral Med Oral Pathol 1992;*73*:118–122.
11. Craddock FW: Radiography of the temporomandibular joint. J Dent Res 1953;*32*:302–321.
12. Berry DC: The relationship between some anatomical features of the human mandibular condyle and appearance on radiographs. Arch Oral Biol 1960;*2*:203–208.
13. Yale SH: Radiographic evaluation of the temporomandibular joint. J Am Dent Assoc 1969;*79*:102–107.
14. Lysell L, Petersson A: The submento-vertex projection in radiography of the temporomandibular joint. Dentomaxillofac Radiol 1980;*9*:11–17.
15. Amer A: Approach to surgical diagnosis of the temporomandibular articulation through basic studies of the normal. J Am Dent Assoc 1952;*45*:668–688.
16. Taylor RC, Ware WH, Fowler D, Kobayashi J: A study of temporomandibular joint morphology and its relationship to the dentition. Oral Surg Oral Med Oral Pathol 1972;*33*:1002–1013.
17. Williamson EH, Wilson CW: Use of a submentovertical-vertex analysis for producing quality temporomandibular joint laminagraphs. Am J Orthod 1976;*70*:200–207.
18. Hüls A, Schulte W, Voigt K: Neue Aspekte der Myoarthropathien durch die Computertomographie. Dtsch Zahnartzl Z 1981;*36*:776–786.
19. Hüls A, Schulte W, Voigt K, Ehrlich-Treuenstt V: Computed tomography of the temporomandibular joint—New diagnostic possibilities and initial clinical results. Electromedica 1983;*51*:14–19.
20. Hüls A, Walter E, Schulte W: Konventinelle Röntgendiagnostik und Computertomographie der Kiefergelenke bei Myoarthropathien. Radiologe 1984;*24*:360–368.
21. Hüls A, Walter E, Schulte W, Freesmayer WB: Computertomographiesche Stadieneiteilung des dysfunktionellen Gelenkkopfumbaus. Dtsch Zahnartzl Z 1985;*40*:37–51.
22. Hüls A, Walter E, Schulte W: Zur Darstellung des Discus articularis im Computertomogramm. Dtsch Zahnartzl Z 1985;*40*:326–331.
23. Westesson P-L, Bifano JA, Tallents RH, Hatala MP: Increased horizontal angle of the mandibular condyle in abnormal temporomandibular joints. A magnetic resonance imaging study. Oral Surg Oral Med Oral Pathol 1991;*72*:359–363.
24. Westesson P-L, Liedberg J: Horizontal condylar angle in relation to internal derangement of the temporomandibular joint. Oral Surg Oral Med Oral Pathol 1987;*64*:391–394.
25. Omnell K-Å, Petersson A: Radiography of the temporomandibular joint utilizing oblique lateral transcranial projections. Comparison of information obtained with standardized technique and individualized technique. Odontol Revy 1976;*26*:77–92.
26. Rosenberg HM, Graczyk RJ: Temporomandibular articulation tomography: A corrected anteroposterior and lateral cephalometric technique. Oral Surg Oral Med Oral Pathol 1986;*62*:198–204.
27. Rosenberg HM, Silha RE: TMJ radiography with emphasis on tomography. Dent Radiogr Photogr 1982;*55*:1–24.
28. Angel JL: Factors in temporomandibular joint form. Am J Anat 1948;*83*:223–246.
29. Eriksson L, Westesson P-L, Macher D, et al: Creation of disc displacement in human temporomandibular joint autopsy specimens. J Oral Maxillofac Surg 1992;*50*:869–873.
30. Hansson T, Öberg T, Carlsson GE, Kopp S: Thickness of the soft tissue layers and the articular disk in the temporomandibular joint. Acta Odontol Scand 1977;*35*:77–83.
31. Tasaki M, Westesson P-L: Temporomandibular joint: Diagnostic accuracy with sagittal and coronal MR imaging. Radiology, 1933;*186*:723–729.
32. Farrar WB: Arthrography of the TMJ (letter). J Am Dent Assoc 1980;*100*:655–656.
33. Kaplan PA, Tu KH, Sleder PR, et al: Inferior joint space arthography of normal temporomandibular joints: Reassessment of diagnostic criteria. Radiology 1986;*159*:585–589.
34. Westesson P-L, Bronstein SL, Liedberg JL: Internal derangement of the temporomandibular joint: Morphologic description with correlation to joint function. Oral Surg Oral Med Oral Pathol 1985;*59*:323–331.
35. Westesson P-L, Eriksson L, Kurita K: Temporomandibular joint: Variation of normal arthrographic anatomy. Oral Surg Oral Med Oral Pathol 1990;*69*:514–519.
36. Westesson P-L, Brooks SL: Temporomandibular joint: Relation between MR evidence of effusion and the presence of pain and disk displacement. AJR 1992;*159*:559–563.
37. Savalle WPM: Some aspects of the morphology of the human temporomandibular joint capsule. Acta Anat 1988;*131*:292–296.
38. McMinn RM, Hutchins RT, Logan BM: Color Atlas of Head and Neck Anatomy. London, Wolfe Medical Publication Ltd, 1991, pp 114–115.
39. Sumnig W, Bartolain G, Fanghanel J: Histological studies of the morphological relationship of the lateral pterygoid muscle to the articular disk in the human temporomandibular joint. Anat Anz 1991;*173*:279–286.
40. Wilkinson T, Chan EK: The anatomic relationship of the insertion of the superior lateral

pterygoid muscle to the articular disc in the temporomandibular joint of human cadavers. Aust Dent J 1989;*34*:315–322.

41. Ashworth GJ: The attachments of the temporomandibular joint meniscus in the human fetus. Br J Oral Maxillofac Surg 1990;*28*:246–250.

42. Moritz T, Ewers R: The attachments of the lateral pterygoid muscle to the TMJ in humans. A histological study. Dtsch Zahnartzl Z 1987;*42*:680–685.

43. Wong GB, Weinberg S, Symington JM: Morphology of the developing articular disc of the human temporomandibular joint. J Oral Maxillofac Surg 1985;*43*:565–569.

44. Carpentier P, Yung JP, Marguelles-Bonnet R, Meunissier M: Insertions of the lateral pterygoid muscle. An anatomic study of the human temporomandibular joint. J Oral Maxillofac Surg 1988;*46*:477–482.

45. Wilkinson TM: The relationship between the disk and the lateral pterygoid muscle in the human temporomandibular joint. J Prosthet Dent 1988;*60*:715–724.

46. Naohara H: The macroscopic and microscopic study of the human lateral ptyergoid muscle. Tsurumi Shigaku—Tsurumi U Dent J 1989;*15*:1–26.

47. Meyenberg K, Kubik S, Palla S: Relationship of the muscles of mastication to the articular disc of the temporomandibular joint. Schweiz Monatsschr Zahnmed 1986;*96*:816–834.

48. Farrar WB, McCarty WL Jr: Inferior joint space arthrography and characteristics of condylar paths in internal derangements of the TMJ. J Prosthet Dent 1979;*41*:548–555.

49. McNamara JA Jr: The independent functions of the two heads of the lateral pterygoid muscle. Am J Anat 1973;*138*:197–205.

50. Mahan PE, Wilkinson TM, Gibbs CH, et al: Superior and inferior bellies of lateral pterygoid muscle; EMG activity at basic jaw positions. Jaw Prosth Dent 1983;*50*:710–718.

51. Juniper RP: Electromyography of the two heads of external pterygoid muscle via the intra-oral route. Electromyogr Clin Neurophysiol 1983;*23*:21–33.

52. Juniper RP: Temporomandibular joint dysfunction: A theory based upon electromyographic studies of the lateral pterygoid muscle. Br J Oral Maxillofac Surg 1984;*22*:1–8.

53. Thilander B: Innervation of the temporomandibular joint capsule in man. An anatomic investigation and a neurophysiologic study of the perception of mandibular position (thesis). Trans R Dent Schools Dent, Stockholm and Umeå, Series 1961;*2*:7.

54. Ruedinger N: Gelenknerven des menschlichen Körpers. Erlanger, Verlag von Ferdinand Enke, 1857.

55. Baumann JA: Contribution á l'étude de l'innervation de l'articulation temporo-maxillaire. C R Assoc Anat 1951;*38*:120–122.

56. Hromada J: Die Innervation des Kiefergelenkes und einige anatomische-klinische Bemerkungen. Dtsch Zahn Mund Kieferheilkd 1960;*34*:19–28.

57. Thilander B: Innervation of the temporomandibular joint capsule in man. Publication of the Umeå Library, Sweden, 1961.

58. Schmid F: On the nerve distribution of the temporomandibular joint capsule. Oral Surg Oral Med Oral Pathol 1969;*28*:63–65.

59. Keller JM, Moffett BC: Nerve endings in the temporomandibular joint of the *Rhesus macaque*. Anat Rec 1968;*160*:587–594.

60. Widenfalk B, Wiberg M: Origin of sympathetic and sensory innervation of the temporomandibular joint. A retrograde axonal tracing study in the rat. Neurosci Lett 1990;*109*:30–35.

61. Johansson AS, Isacsson G, Isberg A, Granholm AC: Distribution of substance P-like immunoreactive nerve fibers in temporomandibular joint soft tissues of monkey. Scand J Dent Res 1986;*94*:225–232.

62. Bont LGM de, Haan P de, Boering G: Structuur en bouw van het kaakgewricht. Ned Tijdschr Tandheelkd 1985;*92*:184–189.

63. Bont LGM de, Boering G, Havinga P, Liem RSB: Spatial arrangement of collagen fibrils in the articular cartilage of the mandibular condyle: A light microscopic and scanning electron microscopic study. J Oral Maxillofac Surg 1984;*42*:306–313.

64. Bont LGM de, Liem RSB, Havinga P, Boering G: Fibrous component of the temporomandibular joint disc. J Craniomandib Pract 1985;*3*:368–373.

65. Hirschmann PN, Shuttleworth CA: The collagen composition of the mandibular joint of the foetal calf. Arch Oral Biol 1976;*21*:771–773.

66. Griffin CJ, Sharpe CJ: Distribution of elastic tissue in the human temporomandibular meniscus, especially in respect to "compression" areas. Aust Dent J 1962;*7*:72–78.

67. Griffin CJ, Hawthorn R, Harris R: Anatomy and histology of the human temporomandibular joint. Monogr Oral Sci 1975;*4*:1–26.

68. Kopp S: Topographical distribution of sulfate glycosaminoglycans in human temporomandibular joint disks: A histochemical study of autopsy material. J Oral Pathol 1976;*5*:265–276.

69. Scapino RP: Histopathology of the disk and posterior attachment in disk displacement internal derangements of the TMJ. *In* Palacios E, Valvassori GE, Shannon M, Reed CF, eds: Magnetic Resonance of the Temporomandibular Joint. New York, Thieme, 1990, pp 63–74.

70. Zenker W: Das retroarticuläre plastische Polster des Kiefergelenkes und seine mechanische Bedeutung. Z Anat Entwickl Gesch 1956;*119*:375–388.

71. Scapino RP: Histopathology associated with malposition of the temporomandibular joint disc. Oral Surg Oral Med Oral Pathol 1983;*55*:382–397.

CHAPTER TWO

Pathology

The normal anatomy of the temporomandibular joint (TMJ) and surrounding structures has been extensively reviewed in Chapter 1. The purpose of this chapter is to describe pathologic alterations that affect this joint, describe specific characteristics of these conditions, and show how they relate to each other. Since the TMJ is a synovial joint, the same diseases and disorders that affect other parts of the musculoskeletal system also affect the TMJ. Thus internal derangement, degenerative joint disease (arthrosis), inflammatory arthritis, and synovitis are all seen in the TMJ. When studying patients presenting with signs and symptoms of TMJ disorder, the most common findings are different forms of disk displacement causing internal derangement and degenerative joint disease. New imaging modalities such as magnetic resonance (MR) have also shown that inflammatory changes in the form of joint effusion and capsular thickening frequently accompany painful internal derangement.[1-3] In addition to the morphologic abnormalities of disk displacement, inflammatory arthritis, muscular disorders, and congenital anomalies will be briefly reviewed.

TERMINOLOGY

Basic terminology for describing patients with signs and symptoms of TMJ disorders has not been standardized over the years, and a multitude of terms have been used. Because of the lack of strict criteria for differential diagnosis, clinicians and researchers have used broader diagnostic categories, such as Costen's syndrome,[1, 5] mandibular dysfunction, temporomandibular joint syndrome, craniomandibular disorders, and, more recently, temporomandibular disorders. These are all loosely defined umbrella terms and include several entities that have a different etiology but may present with similar signs and symptoms. TMJ disorders and these terms are based on clinical examination findings and their reliability and validity have not been documented. One subgroup of any of these umbrella terms is disorders of the TMJ. This chapter will describe abnormalities within the joint and no attempt will be made to define or describe the total content of these umbrella terms.

TMJ disorders are defined as intra-articular morphologic abnormalities, such as different forms of disk displacement, degenerative joint disease (arthrosis), inflammatory arthritis, synovitis, and congenital and neoplastic anomalies. "Temporomandibular joint disorders" is a morphologic definition that may or may not be associated with clinical signs and symptoms.

DISK DISPLACEMENT

The most common abnormality encountered when imaging patients with signs and symptoms of TMJ disorders is different forms of disk displacement. There is convincing evidence in the medical and dental literature that disk displacement often but not always is responsible for the mechanical symptoms frequently seen in patients presenting with TMJ pain and dysfunction. These patients have a high prevalence of disk displacement,[6] but disk displacement also may be present in asymptomatic volunteers.[7-9] The etiology of pain related to internal derangement and disk displacement is not completely understood. The pain has several possible origins, such as tearing and laceration of the joint capsule, compression of the posterior disk attachment, impingement of the inside of the capsule by the displaced disk, synovitis, expansion of the joint spaces by inflammatory exudate, tension and stretching in the joint capsule due to peripheral adhesions, and nerve entrapment.[10] There is still a lot to be learned about the etiology of pain, its variation over time, and its relationship to morphologic alterations in the joint.

Definition

Anterior disk displacement is defined as an alteration of the position of the disk from its expected normal location on top of the condyle (see Chapter 1), a deviation from the relationship between the posterior band of the disk and the 12 o'clock location on top of the condyle (Fig. 2–1). Extensive experience with both patient and cadaver material has indicated some variation in this exact relationship. The disk located in a 12 o'clock position relative to the condyle is normal. Recent experiences with asymptomatic volunteers, however, have suggested that the relationship between the anterior prominence of the condyle and the inferior concavity of the disk under the central thin zone could be used as an ancillary criterion to differentiate abnormal from normal. When these two joint surfaces are in contact with each other, the disk should be regarded as being in normal position even when the posterior band of the disk may not be exactly at the 12 o'clock position (Fig. 2–2). Separation of these two joint surfaces can be interpreted as a criterion for disk displacement (Fig. 2–3). The definition of disk displacement is given in Table 2–1.

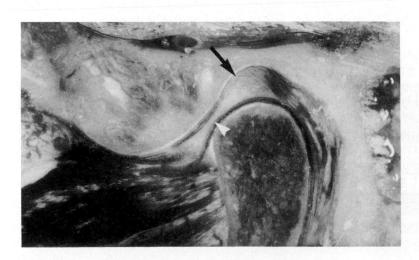

Figure 2–1
Sagittal section of normal TMJ. The posterior band of the disk (arrow) is located in an "ideal" normal superior position. The central thin zone (arrowhead) is opposing the anterior superior prominence of the condyle.

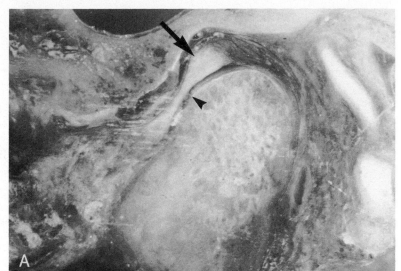

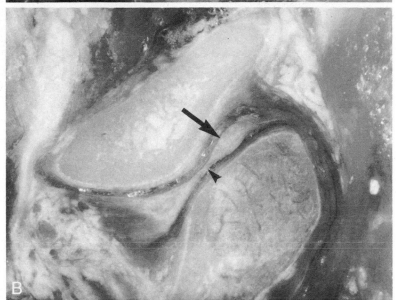

Figure 2–2

Anterior position of the posterior band. A, The posterior band (arrow) is located anterior to the 12 o'clock position, but the relationship between the central thin zone (arrowhead) of the disk and the anterior prominence of the condyle is normal. Based on this second criterion, the disk position should be regarded as normal. Arthrotic changes in the articular eminence are observed. B, Posterior band (arrow) located in the 10 o'clock position relative to the top of the condyle. The relationships among the anterior prominence of the condyle, the central thin zone (arrowhead) of the disk, and the posterior prominence of the articular tubercle are normal. The position of this disk is considered within normal limits.

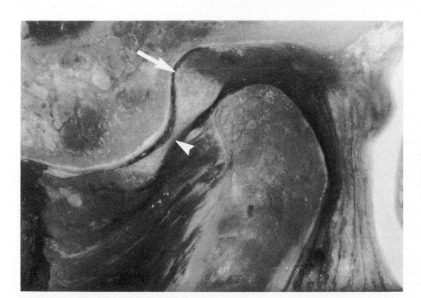

Figure 2–3

Anterior disk displacement. The posterior band of the disk (arrow) is located anterior to the 12 o'clock position. More important, however, is the relationship between the central thin zone (arrowhead) of the disk and the anterior prominence of the condyle, which confirms anterior disk displacement.

Table 2–1
DEFINITIONS OF DISK DISPLACEMENT

Term	Definition
Disk displacement	A displacement from the superior position of the disk over the condyle: evident as alteration in the 12 o'clock location of the posterior band over the condyle or separation of the anterior joint surface of the condyle and the inferior articular surface of the disk in the region of the central thin zone
Internal derangement	An abnormal positional and functional relationship between the disk, the mandibular condyle, and the articulating surfaces of the temporal bone
Disk deplacement with reduction	The disk is displaced in the closed-mouth position but assumes a normal position relative to the condyle with jaw opening
Disk displacement without reduction	The disk is displaced at all mandibular positions
Arthrosis	Deterioration of the articular soft tissue cover of the joint components with exposure of bone
Remodeling	Alterations in the form of the articular joint components with an intact articular soft tissue cover

Sideways and Rotational Displacement

Disk displacement can occur in any anatomic direction; the six general categories are listed in Table 2–2. The most common displacement is anterior (Fig. 2–4). Displacement may also occur in the lateral (Fig. 2–5), medial (Fig. 2–6), and, very rarely, posterior directions. A dramatic example of medial disk displacement associated with extensive degenerative joint disease is seen in Figure 2–7. Most frequently the medial and lateral displacements are associated with anterior displacement and are termed *rotational displacement* (Fig. 2–8). Occasionally, however, there may be simple lateral or simple medial displacement, termed *sideways displacement*.[11]

Partial and Complete Displacement

Displacement of the disk in any direction may also be complete or partial. Partial disk displacement implies that one part of the disk is still interposed between the condyle and the glenoid fossa while another part of the disk has been displaced out of its normal position. Complete disk displacement implies that the entire disk has been displaced out of its normal position. Commonly the simple lateral and simple medial displacements are a partial type of displacement, indicating that a part of the disk remains between the condyle and glenoid fossa. There are two forms of partial anterior disk displacement. In one, the disk is anteriorly displaced in the lateral part of the joint and in normal position in the medial part of the joint (Figs. 2–9 and 2–10). In the other, the disk is anteriorly displaced in the medial part of the joint and remains in a normal position in the lateral part of the joint (Fig. 2–11). The etiology of partial or total disk displacement is unknown but probably is related to stretching and elongation of the different parts of the attachment of the disk to the condyle and capsule.

Text continued on page 33

Table 2–2
CLASSIFICATION OF DISK DISPLACEMENT WITH RESPECT TO THE DIRECTION OF THE DISPLACEMENT

Anterior	Lateral
Anterior and lateral	Medial
Anterior and medial	Posterior

Figure 2–4
A, *Sagittal section showing anterior disk displacement. The condyle is articulating against the posterior disk attachment, and the posterior band (arrow) of the disk is clearly anterior to a normal position. B, Sagittal section showing the disk clearly anterior to a normal position. There is also some thickening of the posterior band (arrow).*

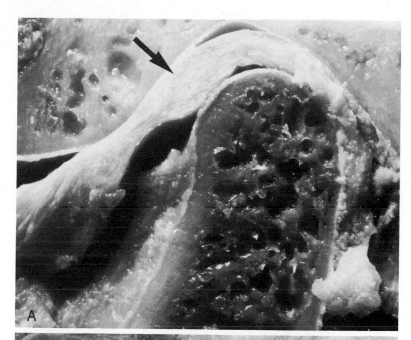

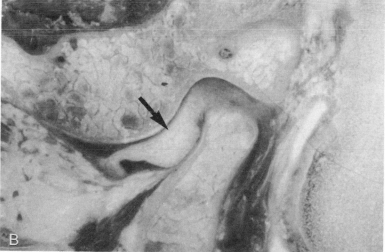

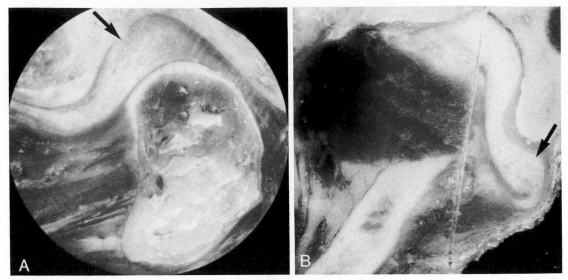

Figure 2–5
Lateral disk displacement. A, Sagittal cryosection shows normal superior disk position. The posterior band of the disk is indicated by an arrow. B, Coronal cryosection shows lateral disk displacement. The disk (arrow) is displaced laterally.

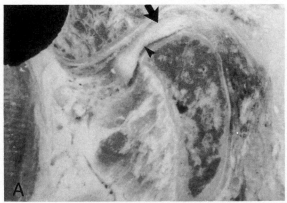

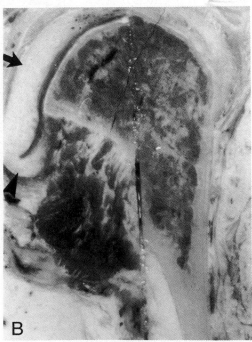

Figure 2–6
Medial displacement. A, Sagittal section showing normal superior disk position. The posterior band of the disk (arrow) and the central thin zone (arrowhead) are in normal position. B, Coronal section of the same joint showing medial disk displacement (arrow). The vertical line in the illustration represents the sagittal cryosection. Note that there is folding (arrowhead) of the disk in its inferior medial aspect.

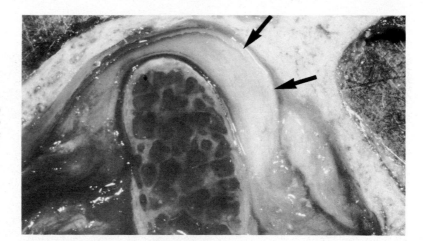

Figure 2–7
Posterior disk displacement. Sagittal section showing the disk (arrows) posterior to the condyle. This posterior disk position was confirmed histologically.

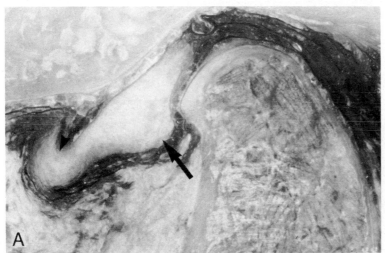

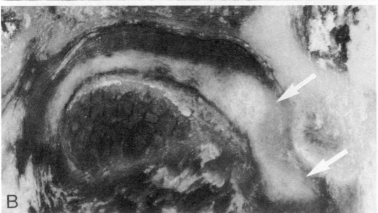

Figure 2–8
Anterior and lateral rotational disk displacement. A, Sagittal section showing anterior disk displacement, deformation, and folding (arrowhead) of the disk. The posterior band of the disk is indicated by an arrow. B, Coronal section shows lateral disk displacement. Disk is indicated by arrows. This specimen is from a different cadaver to show the anatomy optimally.

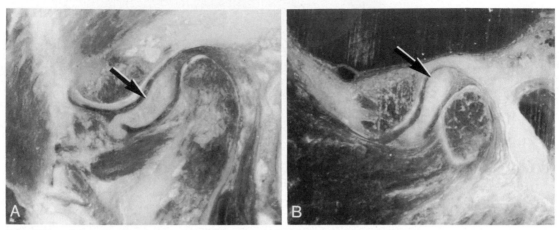

Figure 2–9
Partial anterior disk displacement in the lateral part of the joint. A, Sagittal section from the lateral part of the joint, showing anterior disk displacement. There is deformation of the disk, with substantial thickening and enlargement of the posterior band (arrow). Note that there is also some thickening of the articular soft tissue cover on the inferior aspect of the articular eminence. B, Sagittal section from the medial part of the same joint, showing normal position of disk (arrow). This constitutes partial anterior disk displacement.

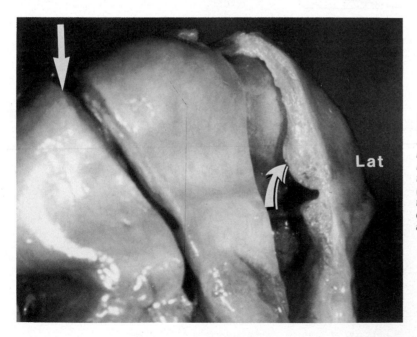

Figure 2–10
Partial anterior disk displacement. Frontal aspect of joint with anterior disk displacement in the lateral part of the joint (Lat) and normal superior position in the medial part of the joint. The posterior band of the disk (curved arrow) is anterior to the condyle in the lateral part of the joint but superior to the condyle in the medial part of the joint (straight arrow).

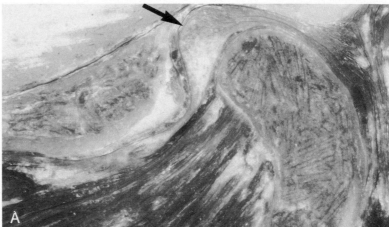

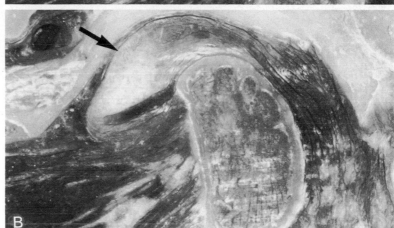

Figure 2–11
Partial anterior disk displacement in the medial part of the joint. A, Sagittal section from the central part of the joint, showing normal superior disk (arrow) position. B, Sagittal section from the medial part of the same joint, showing the disk (arrow) anterior to the condyle, suggesting partial anterior disk displacement in the medial part of the joint.

INTERNAL DERANGEMENT

Definition

In orthopedic terminology, internal derangement is defined as soft tissue between joint surfaces interfering with the smooth action of a joint[12] (see Table 2–1). The most common cause of internal derangement in the TMJ is disk displacement. Thus, if the disk is displaced from its normal position on top of the condyle and interferes with the smooth action of the joint, internal derangement ensues (Fig. 2–12). If, on the other hand, the disk is displaced but causes no interference with the function of the joint—no clicking, irregular movement or limitation of opening (Fig. 2–13)—no internal derangement is present, according to the general definition. TMJ disk displacement and internal derangement have been so closely associated that the two terms have been used interchangeably. A more precise use of terminology is desirable in order to communicate the exact nature of the disorder. Therefore, we advocate making a distinction between disk displacement and internal derangement,[9] since disk displacement may be present without irregular movements.[9] Also, there are other causes of internal derangement, such as adhesions, loose bodies, and degenerative and inflammatory joint diseases without an associated disk displacement.

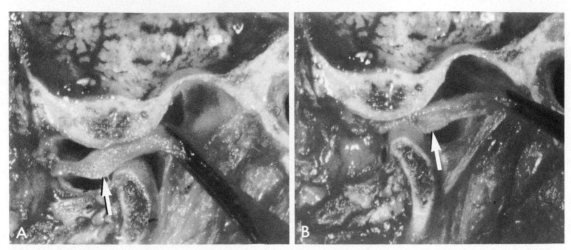

Figure 2–12
Disk displacement with reduction. A, Open-mouth position, with the disk anteriorly displaced and the posterior band (arrow) anterior to the condyle. A suture is applied in the posterior disk attachment for stabilizing. B, Open-mouth image after clicking. The disk is now located in a normal position. The posterior band (arrow) is located posterior to the condyle. At examination this joint demonstrated distinct reciprocal clicking.

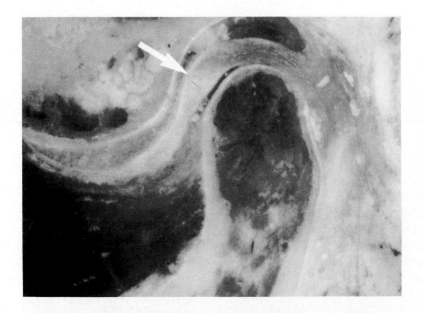

Figure 2–13
Anterior disk displacement without internal derangement. The disk (arrow) is anteriorly displaced, but there is no deformation and the joint functions normally without irregularity. This is an example of a slight disk displacement that does not cause internal derangement.

Functional Classification

To reflect the function of the disk in the joint with internal derangement caused by disk displacement, a functional classification is necessary (Fig. 2–14) (see Table 2–1). The two main categories of disk displacement are displacement with reduction (see Fig. 2–12) and displacement without reduction.

Disk Displacement with Reduction

Disk displacement with reduction (Figs. 2–12, 2–14, and 2–15) specifies that the displaced disk returns to a normal superior position relative to the condyle during jaw opening (see Table 2–1). This condition frequently is associated with clicking. During closing of the jaw the disk is again anteriorly displaced and this also is associated with a more subtle clicking or irregularity of movement. This type of double clicking has been termed *reciprocal clicking*, stressing the dependence of the closing click on the opening click.[13] A joint

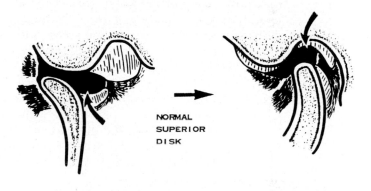

NORMAL
SUPERIOR
DISK

Figure 2–14
Classification of joint function. The posterior band of the disk is demonstrated by the curved arrow.

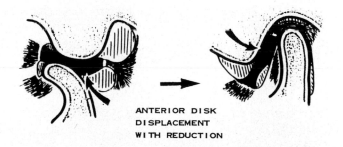

ANTERIOR DISK
DISPLACEMENT
WITH REDUCTION

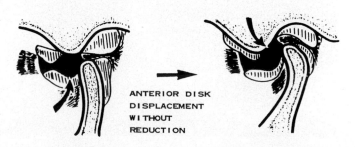

ANTERIOR DISK
DISPLACEMENT
WITHOUT
REDUCTION

with disk displacement with reduction, sectioned and photographed after reduction, is shown in Figure 2–15.

Disk displacement with reduction can be further subclassified into early, mid, or late reduction, as described in Chapter 4, Section 1. Early reduction implies that the disk position is normal while the condyle translates anteriorly within the glenoid fossa. Midreduction implies that the disk position is normal under the articular eminence. Late reduction implies that the disk position is normal while the condyle translates anterior to the articular eminence. Disk displacement with reduction does not always have to be associated with clicking or irregularity of movement. An example of a joint with anterior disk displacement with reduction but with no sound or irregularity of movement is shown in Figure 2–13.

Disk Displacement Without Reduction

Disk displacement without reduction (see Table 2–1) specifies that the disk remains in the displaced position during all mandibular movement (Fig. 2–14). This means that every attempt by the patient to manipulate the jaw so that the disk position is normal will be unsuccessful. Initially, during the late 1970s, this condition was termed *closed lock*,[14, 15] which is a more descriptive term. However, with time, the jaw opening can increase and eventually become relatively normal again in spite of the disk being anteriorly displaced. For that reason the term closed lock was later replaced by anterior disk displacement without reduction.[16]

The term *disk displacement with and without reduction* applies to all forms of disk displacement, not only displacement in the anterior direction. A lateral or medial displacement may be with or without reduction. Little is known about the relationship between the direction of the displacement and the prevalence of reduction. It is our impression from clinical treatment studies that medial and lateral disk displacement has a lower tendency to reduce than has pure anterior displacement.

Reduction of Partial Anterior Disk Displacement

Disk displacement with and without reduction also applies to the condition in which the disk is partially displaced. Here more information is available;

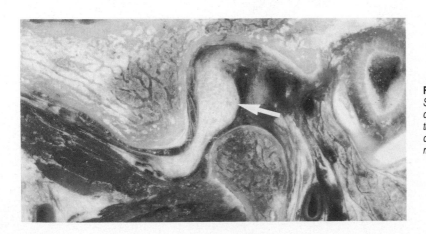

Figure 2–15
Sagittal section of a joint with anterior disk displacement with reduction. This cryosection was obtained after reduction. The condyle is in a normal relationship to the posterior band (arrow) of the disk.

several studies have shown a strong association between partial disk displacement and reduction on one hand and complete displacement and no reduction on the other hand.[17, 18] This is not surprising, since the vertical distance between the condyle and temporal component is maintained in the joint when only part of the disk is displaced. This allows the displaced part of the disk to reduce more easily than when the entire disk is displaced and the space between the condyle and temporal component is not maintained but instead is compressed owing to the softness of the posterior disk attachment.

Disk Displacement with Incomplete Reduction

Disk displacement with incomplete reduction specifies that the anteriorly displaced disk is only partially recaptured on opening. That part of the disk remains in the displaced position, whereas another part is in a normal position on opening. Figure 2–16 depicts a joint in which the medial part of the disk is normal on opening and there is anterior displacement without reduction in the

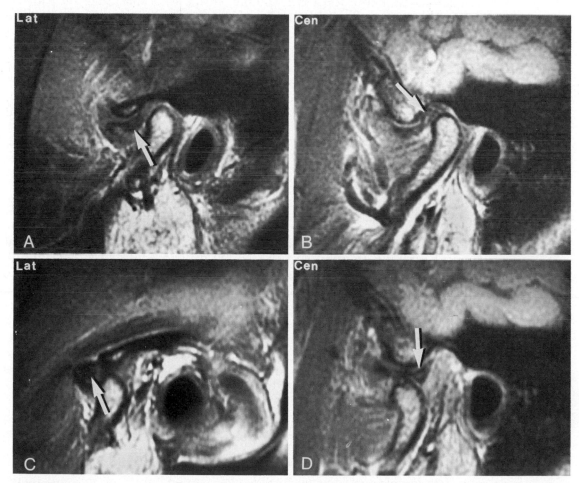

Figure 2–16
Partial anterior disk displacement with incomplete reduction. A, Closed-mouth MR image from the lateral (Lat) part of the joint, showing anterior disk displacement. The posterior band of the disk (arrow) is located anterior to the condyle. B, Closed-mouth MR image from the central (Cen) part of the same joint. The disk (arrow) is located in a slightly forward position. C, On opening the disk (arrow) in the lateral (Lat), part of the joint remains anterior to the condyle. D, In the medial part of the joint, the disk (arrow) position is normal.

lateral part of the joint. Incomplete reduction occurs with all forms of disk displacement but probably is more common with medial and lateral displacement. This is natural, since the condyle on jaw opening is moving in an anterior direction and thereby has a greater tendency to recapture an anteriorly displaced disk than a medially or laterally displaced disk.

Posterior Disk Displacement

Posterior displacement (see Fig. 2–7) is rare. The terminology of disk displacement with and without reduction does not apply to posterior displacements as it does to anterior displacements. The etiology of posterior disk displacement is unknown.

Clinical Staging of Internal Derangement

The preceding classifications for disk position and disk function are based on anatomic and functional aspects only. In the clinical setting, the patient's history, signs, and symptoms must be incorporated into the description of the stage of disease. A more global and clinically useful classification for TMJ disorders related to internal derangement is necessary. Several attempts have been made to develop such a classification, but we find the classification described by Wilkes (Table 2–3) to be the most useful and comprehensive.[19] This classification combines clinical, radiographic, and morphologic observations and categorizes internal derangement into five groups. This is discussed in greater depth in Chapter 11 (Arthroscopy).

Progression of Internal Derangement

TMJ internal derangement is generally a progressive disease. Thus nearly all patients in a late stage of internal derangement are thought to have had the symptoms of an earlier stage, yet there is relatively little documentation about the mechanism of progression. In a study of patients with clinical signs of disk displacement with reduction and relatively mild symptoms, 9 per cent of the patients developed clinical signs of disk displacement without reduction during the 3-year observation period.[20] In another study of patients with disk displacement with reduction and more severe clinical symptoms, 20 per cent developed disk displacement without reduction over a 6-month period.[21] Apparently joints with more advanced disk deformation have a greater tendency to progress to locking than those with mild deformation.[21] The progression of internal derangement has been presented by Wilkes in a large clinical study.[19]

EMINENCE INTERFERENCE

Clicking and irregularity of movement also can be caused by the condyle and disk complex moving in an irregular fashion under or in front of the articular eminence. In a normal individual, the condyle moves forward to the most inferior point of the articular eminence without irregularities or interference. In some individuals, however, clicking, irregularities, and even catching

Table 2–3
CLASSIFICATION OF INTERNAL DERANGEMENT ACCORDING TO WILKES

Early Stage
  Clinical — No significant mechanical symptoms, other than reciprocal clicking (early in opening movement, late in closing movement, and soft in intensity); no pain or limitation on opening motion
  Radiologic — Slight forward displacement, good anatomic contour of disk, normal tomograms
  Surgical — Normal anatomic form, slight anterior displacement, passive incoordination (clicking) demonstrable

Early/Intermediate Stage
  Clinical — First few episodes of pain, occasional joint tenderness and related temporal headaches, beginning major mechanical problems, increase in intensity of clicking sounds, joint sounds later in opening movement, and beginning transient subluxations or joint catching and locking
  Radiologic — Slight forward displacement, slight thickening of posterior edge or beginning anatomic deformity of disk, normal tomograms
  Surgical — Anterior displacement, early anatomic deformity (slight to mild thickening of posterior edge), and well-defined central articulating area

Intermediate Stage
  Clinical — Multiple episodes of pain, joint tenderness, temporal headaches, major mechanical symptoms—transient catching, locking, and sustained locking (closed locks), restriction of motion, and difficulty (pain) with function
  Radiologic — Anterior displacement with significant anatomic deformity/prolapse of disk (moderate to marked thickening of posterior edge), normal tomograms
  Surgical — Marked anatomic deformity with displacement, variable adhesions (anterior, lateral, and posterior recesses), no hard tissue changes

Intermediate/Late Stage
  Clinical — Characterized by chronicity with variable and episodic pain, headaches, variable restriction of motion, and undulating course
  Radiologic — Increase in severity over intermediate stage, abnormal tomograms, and early to moderate degenerative remodeling hard tissue changes
  Surgical — Increase in severity over intermediate stage, hard tissue degenerative remodeling changes of both bearing surfaces, osteophytic projections, multiple adhesions (lateral, anterior, and posterior recesses), and no perforation of disk or attachment

Late Stage
  Clinical — Characterized by crepitus on examination; scraping, grating, grinding symptoms; variable and episodic pain; chronic restriction of motion; and difficulty with function
  Radiologic — Anterior displacement, perforation with simultaneous filling of upper and lower compartments, filling defects, gross anatomic deformity of disk and hard tissues, abnormal tomograms, and essentially degenerative arthritic changes
  Surgical — Gross degenerative changes of disk and hard tissues, perforation of posterior attachments, erosions of bearing surfaces, and multiple adhesions equivalent to degenerative arthritis (sclerosis, flattening, and anvil-shaped condyle, osteophytic projections, and subcortical cystic formation)

may occur as a result of the condyle-disk complex moving in an irregular fashion under the articular eminence. This can frequently be mistaken for disk displacement with reduction. However, arthrography or MR imaging can demonstrate this entity clearly. Eminence interference may or may not be associated with disk displacement (see Chapter 4, Arthrography).

A more advanced form of eminence interference is the "open lock" or "dislocated jaw" (see Chapter 10, Miscellaneous Conditions). Classically this has been caused by the condyle being locked in front of the articular eminence, necessitating the patient seeking medical assistance to reduce the mandible from the locked position. Another cause of the open lock situation more recently documented is the condyle locked in front of the anterior band of the disk (see Chapter 5, Magnetic Resonance Imaging). Then the disk folds behind the condyle, preventing the condyle from moving posteriorly into the glenoid fossa. The condyle in this condition is usually located inferior or even posterior to the articular eminence. Thus, not the condyle but instead the disk is preventing the condyle from moving posteriorly. This is a different mechanism from the situation in which the condyle is locked in front of the articular eminence.

DISK DEFORMATION

Deformation of the disk appears to occur secondary to disk displacement. Deformation most commonly begins with thickening and enlargement of the posterior band of the disk (Fig. 2–17). Thus, the superoinferior thickness as well as the anteroposterior dimension of the posterior band gradually increases (Figs. 2–18 and 2–19). The thickening of the posterior band takes place essentially on the undersurface of the disk. The upper surface remains relatively flat (Fig. 2–20). At the same time the anterior one third of the disk merges with the anterior capsule and regresses in size. The central thin zone of the disk, which in this condition is nonfunctional, also gets smaller and sometimes folds on opening, ending with a biconvex configuration of the disk (Fig. 2–21). The end result is a bulged-up disk with a thickened posterior band.

In conjunction with disk deformation, the posterior disk attachment appears stretched and gets longer and thinner. This partially explains the increasing opening capacity of the jaw that many patients experience after initially suffering from limitation of opening with disk displacement without reduction. Loosening or tearing of the joint capsule, resolution of muscle spasm, and detachment or perforation of the posterior disk attachment probably are also responsible for the increased jaw mobility that frequently occurs over time.

Deformation of the disk is significant for treatment planning because it may no longer be possible to reposition the disk surgically or conservatively into a normal position between the convex articulating surfaces of the condyle and the temporal joint component. Surgical attempts to recontour or shave off the disk surface to eliminate the deformity and fit the disk into its normal position have met with variable success. An example of a surgically removed disk with significant deformation on the inferior surface in the lateral part of the disk is shown in Figure 2–22. There is a prominent bulge on the inferior

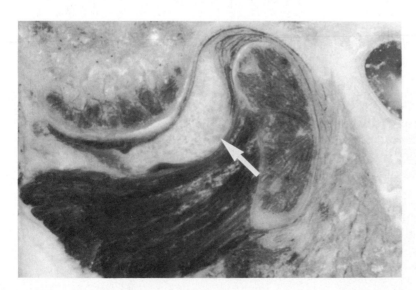

Figure 2–17
Sagittal cryosection showing thickening and enlargement of the posterior band (arrow) of the disk.

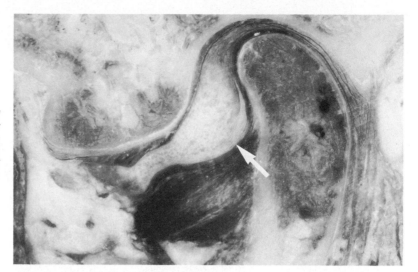

Figure 2–18
Sagittal cryosection showing advanced thickening and enlargement of the posterior band (arrow) of the disk. The form of the inferior surface of the posterior band creates the characteristic image of the enlargement of the lower joint space seen in arthrography.

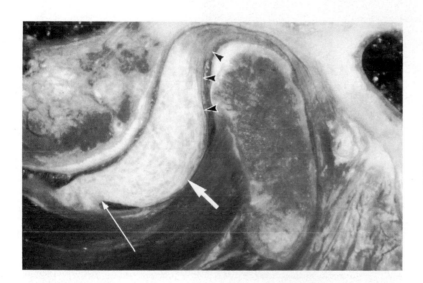

Figure 2–19
Enlargement and thickening of the posterior band (thick white arrow) and fibrosis of the anterior part of the posterior disk attachment (arrowheads). The central thin zone of the disk (thin arrow) and the anterior third of the disk are diminished.

Figure 2–20
Prominent bulge on the inferior surface of disk causing clicking. Sagittal cryosection showing marked prominence of the inferior aspect of the posterior band (arrow). This joint demonstrated reciprocal clicking on opening.

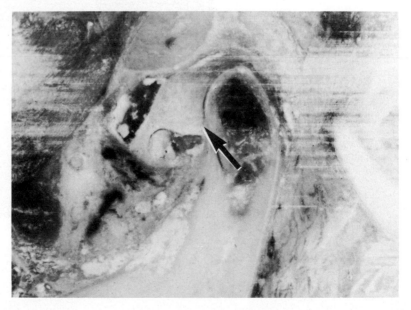

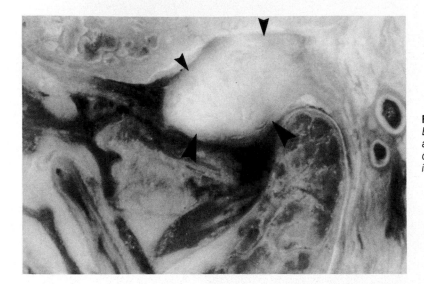

Figure 2–21
Biconvex disk. Sagittal cryosection showing a markedly deformed disk (arrowheads). The condyle is normal but the articular eminence is irregular.

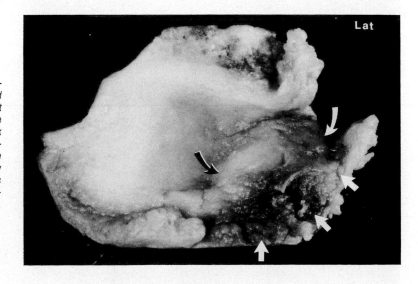

Figure 2–22
Deformed disk removed at surgery. Photograph of the undersurface of disk removed from a patient with painful disk displacement without reduction. There is a prominent bulge on the inferior lateral surface of the disk (curved arrows). The condyle has been articulating posteriorly to this bulge against the posterior disk attachment (area indicated by small arrows). The medial part of the disk is relatively normal in appearance and configuration. (Courtesy of Dr. Lars Eriksson, Lund, Sweden.)

lateral surface of the disk. The condyle has been articulating against the posterior disk attachment posterior to this bulge. The medial part of the disk is relatively normal in structure and configuration.

Deformation of the disk is rarely seen in joints with normal superior disk position. If a deformation occasionally is seen in such a joint on sagittal plane images (Fig. 2–23), the disk is usually displaced in a lateral or medial fashion, which should be evident on coronal plane images (see Chapter 5, MR Imaging). This type of deformation usually involves a flat-appearing disk on the side from which the disk is displaced. Thus, a medially displaced disk frequently appears flat in the lateral aspect. This is probably due to pulling of the capsule between the condyle and fossa, giving the appearance of a flattened (Fig. 2–24) or even perforated disk in the lateral part of the joint (Fig. 2–23).

HISTOLOGY

Disk

In the normal disk, the collagen fibers are transversely oriented in the anterior and posterior bands. The fibers in the central part of the normal disk have a predominantly anteroposterior course and are interlaced with the transversely oriented fibers of the anterior and posterior bands. Also, vertical collagen fibers in the posterior band of the disk are interlaced with the transverse fibers.[22] The disk is composed of a compact collection of type I collagen,[23] a system of small-caliber elastic fibers,[24, 25] and glycosaminoglycans.[26] The collagen fibers in the central thin zone of the disk flare out into the posterior band where they interlace with a three-dimensional meshwork of fibers within it.

Several types of pathologic changes occur in a displaced disk. Most of these are surface irregularities, including fissuring, fibrillation, and fraying, which are essentially seen in advanced derangement.[27–35] The chronically displaced disk often shows thickening of the posterior band (Fig. 2–25), as previously noted. Histologically, the deformed disk frequently shows layers of proliferating cells on the surface of the abnormally thickened posterior band (Fig. 2–26).

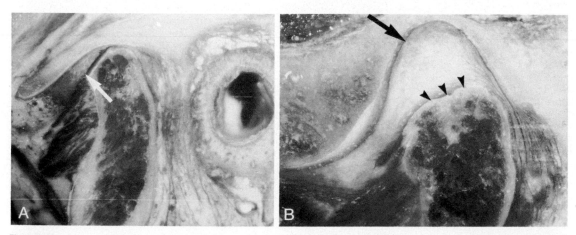

Figure 2–23
Deformation of normally positioned disk. A, Sagittal section from the lateral part of the joint, showing perforation and a small triangular part of the disk (arrow) remaining anterior to condyle. B, Sagittal section from the medial part of the same joint, showing the disk (arrow) in normal superior position and arthrotic changes in the superior aspect of the condyle (arrowheads).

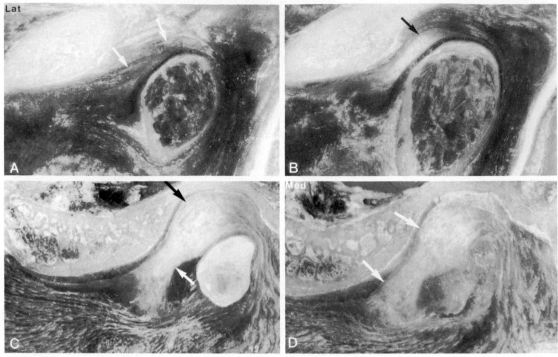

Figure 2–24
Flat configuration of disk with medial disk displacement. A, Sagittal cryosection from the lateral part of the joint, showing tissue (arrows) between the condyle and the glenoid fossa resembling a flat disk. This tissue represents capsular tissue that has been pulled in between the condyle and fossa. B, Sagittal cryosection from the central part of the joint, showing a flat disk (arrow) in normal position. C, Sagittal section from the medial part of the joint, showing the posterior band of the disk (black arrow) in normal relationship to the condyle. The central thin zone (white arrow) of the disk, however, is anteriorly displaced. Compare Figures 2–2 and 2–3. D, Section medial to the joint, showing medial displacement of the disk (arrows).

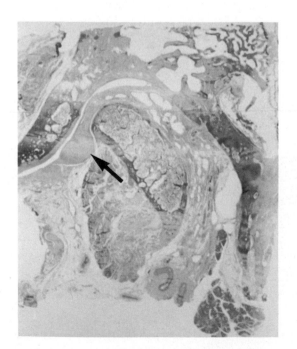

Figure 2–25
Anterior disk displacement with deformation. Histologic section shows anterior disk displacement and thickening of the posterior band (arrow). (Courtesy of Dr. Bengt Lindahl, Ljungby, Sweden.)

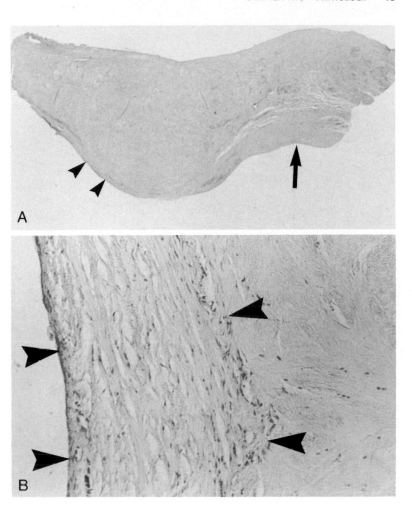

Figure 2–26
Thickening of the posterior band. A, Sagittal histologic section through a surgically removed disk, showing marked deformation. The condyle has been articulating against the posterior disk attachment, as indicated by the arrow. The posterior band is significantly thickened. The area shown in B is indicated by arrowheads on the anterior aspect of the posterior band. B, Magnified view of the anterior aspect of the posterior band, showing proliferative layers of tissue (between arrowheads).

Studies of surgically removed disks have also shown chondrocytes (Fig. 2–27), vessels in the disk (Fig. 2–28), and splitting of the disk and posterior disk attachment tissues (Fig. 2–29).[33]

When the posterior band becomes vertically thickened, increased numbers of transverse fibers are noted encroaching upon the central part of the disk. In addition to changes in fiber organization, tissue composition usually undergoes extensive alteration. A comparison of computed tomographic attenuation numbers in both patients and cadaver specimens with displaced disks correlated with remarkable histologic alterations, including hyalinization, calcification, and cartilaginous metaplasia of the disk.[36, 37]

Posterior Attachment

Changes in the posterior disk attachment are commonly observed in association with chronic disk displacement. The normal posterior attachment of the disk is composed of a superior stratum and an inferior stratum.[24, 38, 39] The superior stratum consists of a loosely organized meshwork of elastic and collagen fibers, fat, and blood vessels. The inferior stratum consists of compact, inelastic sheets of collagen fibers that attach to the posterior surface of the

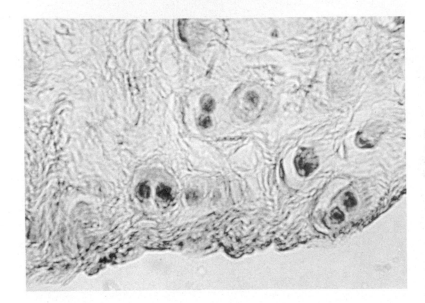

Figure 2–27
Chondrocytes in disk. A specimen from a surgically removed disk shows chondrocytes in the disk.

Figure 2–28
Histologic section shows vessels (arrowheads) in a normally avascular part of the disk.

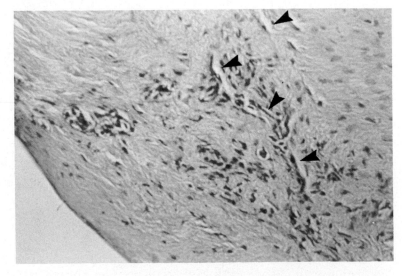

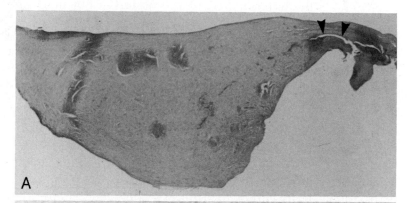

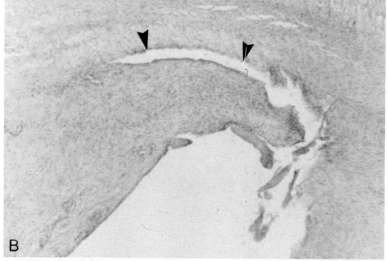

Figure 2–29
Splitting in the posterior disk attachment. A, Sagittal section of a surgically removed disk, showing substantial thickening of the posterior band. In the posterior disk attachment is an area of splitting (arrowheads). B, Higher magnification showing the area of splitting (arrowheads), starting from the inferior surface and extending horizontally into the posterior attachment. C, Higher magnification of the same area shows a layer of flat cells along the surface of the splitting. This documents that this is not a sectional artifact but degeneration of tissue.

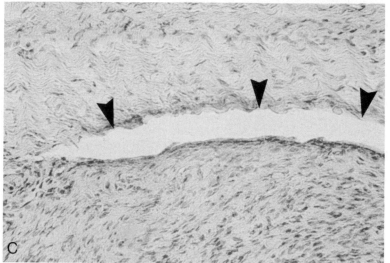

condyle below its posterior articular covering.[39] The union of the superior and inferior strata of the posterior attachment at the posterior band of the normal disk is fairly distinct. With chronic internal derangement, on the other hand, the anterior part of the posterior attachment near the posterior band of the disk develops a fibrotic character. The normal pattern of collagen fibers at the union of the posterior attachment and the posterior band is replaced by a compact mass of fibers that contains fewer or none of the small vessels normally present. When this fibrosis develops, the configuration of the posterior disk attachment sometimes also changes to resemble the posterior band of the disk (Fig. 2–30; see also Fig. 2–40). This has been likened to a "pseudodisk." The histologic composition of the posterior disk attachment developing to fibrosis has not been extensively documented, and the long-term clinical significance of the pseudodisk is not known.

Though some chronically displaced disks are associated with fibrosis of the anterior aspect of the posterior disk ligament, in other cases increased vascularity rather than fibrosis is noted.[40] Figure 2–31 depicts a disk with a highly vascularized posterior disk attachment, which was removed from a patient with painful anterior disk displacement without reduction. A cryosection of a cadaver joint with a similar type of high vascularity of the posterior disk attachment is shown in Figure 2–32. The clinical significance of this observation is not totally understood, but there are indications that this condition could be associated with severe TMJ pain.[40]

When the remodeling process is not adequate for the degree of anatomic and functional abnormalities, the tissues become irreversibly damaged and perforations of the posterior disk attachment may occur.

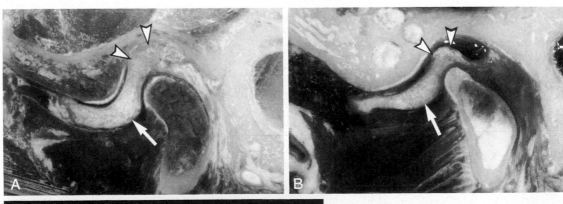

Figure 2–30
Fibrosis of the posterior disk attachment. A, Cryosection of a joint with anterior disk displacement and formation of a "pseudoposterior band" (arrowheads) posterior to the true posterior band (arrow) of the anteriorly displaced disk. B, Pseudoposterior band (arrowheads) in a joint with anterior disk (arrow) displacement and disk deformation. C, Surgically removed disk from a patient with mechanical dysfunction and painful disk displacement. The posterior disk attachment (arrowheads) appears fibrotic. The disk (arrow) is deformed. (Courtesy of Dr. Lars Eriksson, Lund, Sweden.)

Figure 2–31
Surgically removed disk showing high vascularity of the posterior disk attachment. Sagittal section through a surgically removed disk from a patient with painful disk displacement without reduction. The disk (arrow) is deformed. The posterior disk attachment (arrowheads) is highly vascularized and appears hyperplastic. (Courtesy of Dr. Lars Eriksson, Lund, Sweden.)

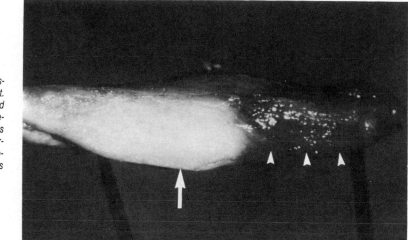

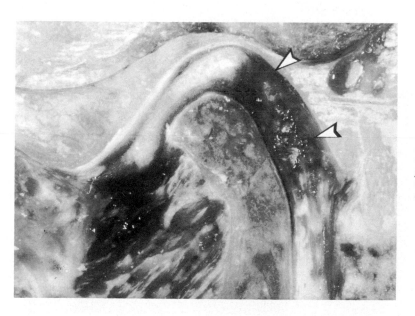

Figure 2–32
Hyperplastic, highly vascularized posterior disk attachment. Sagittal section through a joint with superior disk position. The posterior disk attachment (arrowheads) is highly vascularized and appears hyperplastic.

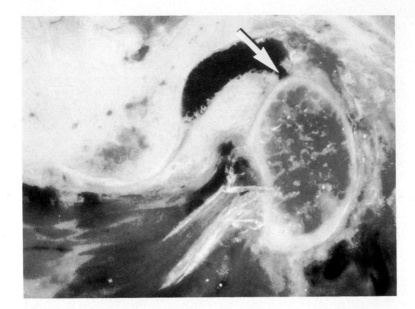

Figure 2–33
Sagittal section of a joint with anterior disk displacement and a small perforation (arrow) in the posterior disk attachment just posterior to the posterior band of the disk.

Perforations

Perforation (Figs. 2–33 and 2–34) is seen in approximately 5 to 15 per cent of joints with disk displacement. Perforations may occur both in the disk and the disk attachment. Perforations associated with disk displacement are more commonly seen in the attachment rather than in the disk itself[41] and in late stages are associated with arthrosis (Fig. 2–35). Perforation was the first pathologic entity of the soft tissue of the TMJ to be clearly recognized radiographically and surgically.[42]

Macroscopically, perforations frequently seem to start in the undersurface of the posterior attachment as a surface defect (Fig. 2–36) that gradually

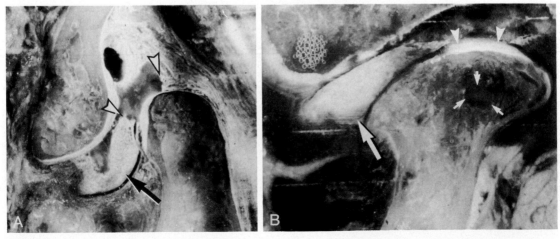

Figure 2–34
A, Sagittal cryosection of a joint with anterior disk (arrow) displacement and a large perforation (arrowheads) in the posterior disk attachment. Arthrotic changes in the condyle are also seen. B, Sagittal cryosection of a joint with anterior disk (arrow) displacement and perforation in the posterior disk attachment. There are significant arthrotic changes, with thickening of the articular soft tissue cover (arrowheads) on the condyle and cystic change in the condyle (small arrows).

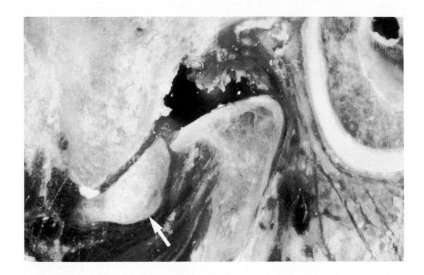

Figure 2–35
Sagittal cryosection of a joint with a large perforation, anterior disk displacement, and deformation (arthrosis). The disk (arrow) is biconvex.

deepens and eventually penetrates into the upper joint space, as in surgical cases in which small ruptures are frequently seen on the inferior surface of the disk. These have been termed partial perforations. Partial perforations were extensively described by Takaku in 1983.[43, 44] Infrequently these partial perforations start from the superior surface. Partial perforation found morphologically probably corresponds to the splitting seen histologically (see Fig. 2–29). Occasionally the partial perforation can be diagnosed with arthrography as a small peak of contrast sticking up into the tissue of the posterior disk attachment (see Fig. 4–45 in Chapter 4).

Perforation in the disk proper is also seen, especially in elderly individuals. These probably have a different etiology, such as a simple wearing down over

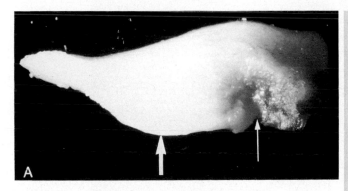

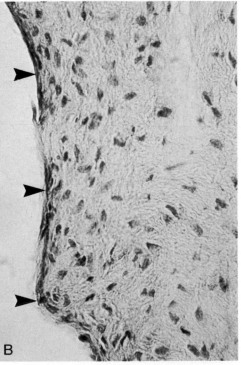

Figure 2–36
Partial perforation. A, Sagittal section of a disk removed from a patient with painful disk displacement. The disk (thick arrow) is deformed, with thickening of the posterior band. In the inferior aspect of the posterior attachment (thin arrow) a partial rupture suggestive of a partial perforation is seen. (Courtesy of Dr. Lars Eriksson, Lund, Sweden.) B, Histologic section of this area shows a lining of flat cells (arrowheads) indicating the degenerative nature of the process.

time, compared with perforation of the posterior disk attachment associated with disk displacement.

ETIOLOGY OF DISK DISPLACEMENT

The etiology of disk displacement is unknown in the majority of cases, although trauma has been suggested as one possible factor.[16, 45, 46] A recent study of patients referred to an oral and maxillofacial surgery clinic showed that a significant proportion of those with internal derangement had a history of trauma, including tonsillectomy and difficult tooth extraction.[47] From an anatomic point of view, the lateral part of the posterior disk attachment to the condyle has a slightly different architecture than the more central and medial parts.[48, 49] Experience from TMJ surgery has indicated that when the inferior layer of the posterior and lateral attachment between the disk and the condyle is damaged it loses its firmness and becomes more elastic, allowing the disk to displace anteriorly or anteromedially. The hypothesis is that superficial damage to the inferior layer of the posterior attachment between the disk and the condyle permits disk displacement.

A study has shown that it is possible to create anterior displacement of the disk in the human TMJ by making superficial incisions into the inferior layer of the posterior disk attachment and then pushing the condyle up into the glenoid fossa behind the disk[50] (Fig. 2–37). Normally the disk is firmly attached

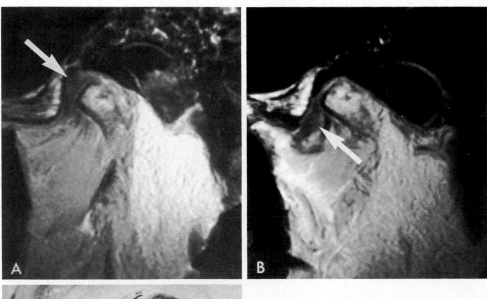

Figure 2–37
Creation of disk displacement. A, Sagittal MR image of a cadaver specimen before surgical intervention. The disk (arrow) is located with its posterior band superior to the condyle. B, Sagittal MR image after surgical intervention and creation of disk displacement. The disk (arrow) is displaced anterior to the condyle. C, Sagittal cryosection confirming disk displacement. The disk (arrow) is anterior to the condyle, and the posterior disk attachment is elongated.

to the condyle,[24] but after the superficial incisions (Fig. 2–38) were made, the posterior attachment became elastic and it was possible to move the disk forward manually. This observation suggests that weakness of the posterior attachment between the disk and the condyle might be one factor in the etiology of disk displacement. The study supports the hypothesis that disk displacement can be caused by trauma in some cases. The etiology of disk displacement, however, is unknown in the majority of patients.

Whether cervical musculoskeletal injury (whiplash) could cause TMJ internal derangement has been discussed.[46, 51–54] One study demonstrated arthrographic evidence of internal derangement in 88 per cent of patients in a series who sustained whiplash.[46] However, it is clear that this was not a representative group of those individuals sustaining whiplash; a more recent follow-up study of a larger sample of individuals sustaining whiplash injury showed that TMJ pain and clicking were extremely infrequent.[55] From a composite review of the literature and our experience, there is no convincing evidence that whiplash injury consistently or in a high frequency results in disk displacement.[55]

ARTHROSIS

Arthrosis, or degenerative joint disease, has been extensively described by Sokoloff.[56] This entity is defined as deterioration of the articular soft tissue cover and exposure of bone (Fig. 2–39). Degenerative joint disease of the TMJ is frequently associated with disk displacement without reduction and has been documented in more than 50 per cent of patients with this condition.[17, 57, 58] There are two forms of arthrosis: primary and secondary. Primary arthrosis is of unknown etiology. Secondary arthrosis is secondary to another disease, such as internal derangement or inflammatory arthritis.

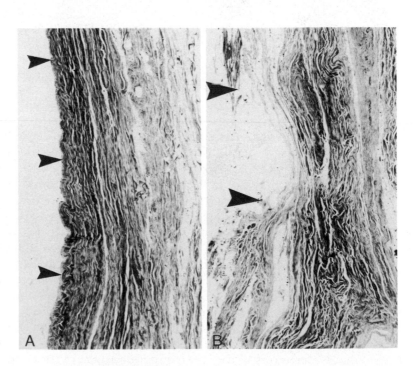

Figure 2–38
Histologic sections of the inferior surface of posterior disk attachment. A, Intact posterior disk attachment. The surface (arrowheads) of the attachment is intact. The collagen and the elastic fibers are organized in a relatively parallel fashion (elastic stain). B, Damaged inferior surface of the posterior disk attachment. The area of surgical intervention is indicated by arrowheads. The collagen and elastic fibers are disorganized (elastic stain).

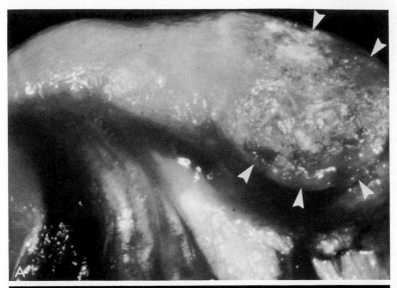

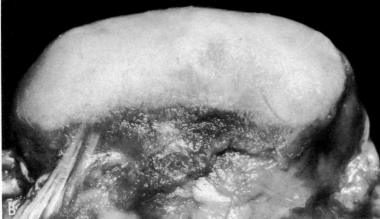

Figure 2–39
Condyle with arthrotic changes. A, Anterior aspect of a mandibular condyle with arthrotic changes (arrowheads) in the lateral third, including irregularities and exposure of bone. B, Anterior aspect of condyle with normal morphologic appearance shown for comparison.

Secondary Arthrosis

In younger age groups, secondary arthrosis is more common than primary arthrosis. Arthrosis is most frequently secondary to internal derangement caused by disk displacement. We have seen secondary arthrosis of the TMJ in individuals as young as 10 years. Primary arthrosis is seen in elderly individuals and may not be associated with internal derangement. It has been our experience that secondary arthrosis is much more common in the TMJ than is primary arthrosis. Examples of joints with advanced arthrosis and disk displacement are shown in Figures 2–40 and 2–41. Arthrosis is also characterized by erosive changes of the bone. Erosion of the mandibular condyle in a joint with degenerative joint disease is seen in Figure 2–42.

A recent experimental study on rabbits has shown that surgically created disk displacement can cause the development of TMJ arthrosis over a relatively short period of time.[59] This experimental study confirms speculation in multiple previous clinical studies that disk displacement can cause arthrosis. The arthrotic changes in the rabbit developed over a period of only 4 weeks and included erosions of the anterosuperior aspect of the condyle, breakdown of the articular

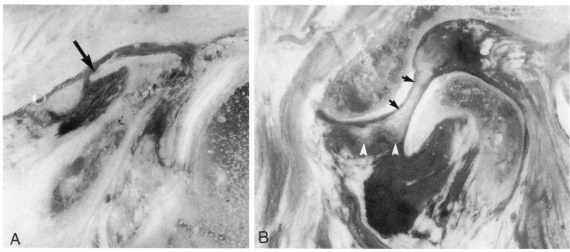

Figure 2–40

Advanced arthrosis with osteophytosis. A, Sagittal cryosection showing flattening of condyle and temporal component, osteophyte (arrow) of the condyle, and anterior disk displacement with deformation of the disk. B, Sagittal cryosection showing a significant osteophyte on the condyle anteriorly. The disk (arrowheads) is anteriorly displaced. There is formation of a pseudodisk (arrows) between the osteophyte of the condyle and the posterior slope of the articular eminence. This is an example of the dramatic adaptive changes.

Figure 2–41

Extensive arthrosis with disk displacement. A, Sagittal section of a joint with a biconvex folded disk (arrow) and a large perforation in the posterior disk attachment. There are arthrotic changes of the condyle and an osteophyte. B, Coronal section, showing arthrotic changes of the condyle (arrows) and a medially displaced disk (arrowheads).

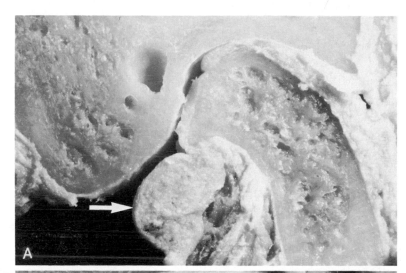

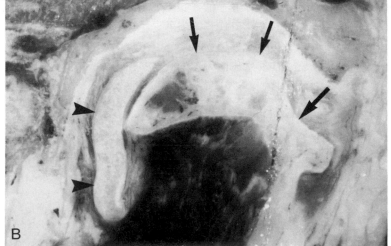

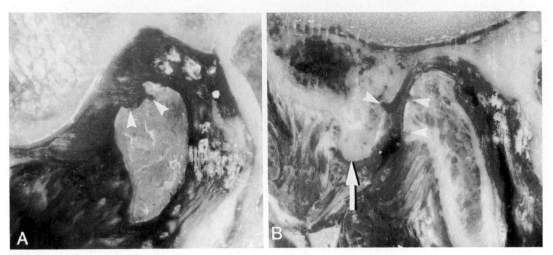

Figure 2–42
Erosions. A, Sagittal cryosection showing erosive changes (arrowheads) of the condyle. B, Sagittal cryosection showing erosive changes in the articular eminence and condyle (arrowheads). The arrow indicates an inferiorly directed osteophyte on the articular eminence.

soft tissue cover, and disruption of the subchondral layer of cartilage cells.[59] An unoperated joint and a joint that developed arthrosis after the disk was surgically displaced are seen in Figures 2–43 and 2–44.

Primary Arthrosis

Arthrosis is rarely seen in joints with normal superior disk position. This may occur, however, especially in elderly individuals, and is frequently related to perforation of the disk. Arthrosis in a joint with superior disk position but with a perforation of the lateral pole of the condyle is shown in Figure 2–45. Arthrosis is sometimes seen in joints with partial disk displacement but is more frequent in those with complete disk displacement. In the joints with partial disk displacement, the arthrosis is usually seen in the part of the joint where the disk is displaced. In such a case it should be termed secondary arthrosis rather than primary arthrosis. A joint with a medial disk displacement and arthrosis in the lateral aspect of the joint, evident as erosive changes of the superior surface of the condyle, is seen in Figure 2–46. This is also an example of secondary arthrosis. However, arthrosis occurs also under a normally positioned disk (Fig. 2–47; see also Fig. 2–2A). The joint shown in Figure 1–12 in Chapter 1 is another example of degenerative joint disease in the condyle under a relatively normally positioned disk.

REMODELING

The articular soft tissue cover on the condyle and on the temporal joint component has a capacity to proliferate sufficiently to alter the contours of the joint. This allows the contours to adapt morphologically to various mechanical stresses.[60] Remodeling is defined as changes in the form of the articular tissues with a remaining intact soft tissue cover (Fig. 2–48). Extensive changes in the form of the articular components are possible, but as long as the soft tissue cover is intact the joint does not qualify for the diagnosis of arthrosis.

Text continued on page 61

Figure 2–43
Normal mandibular condyle from nonoperated control rabbit. A, Lateral radiograph showing the smooth contour of the condyle, without erosions. B, Histologic section showing intact articular soft tissue cover (arrowheads) and a normal layer of subchondral cartilage cells.

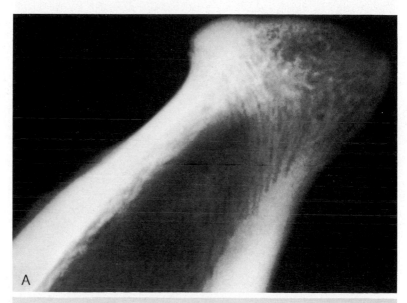

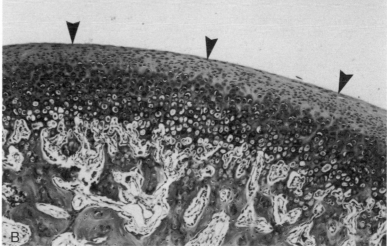

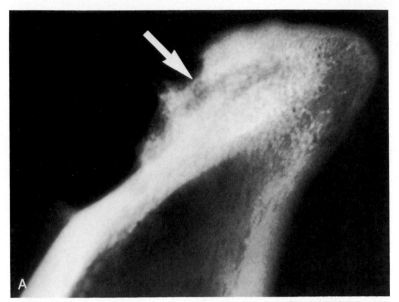

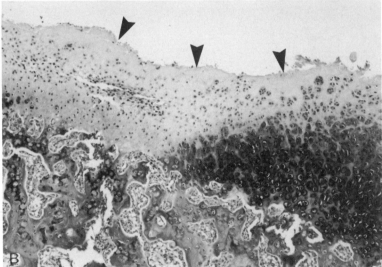

Figure 2–44

Mandibular condyle with arthrosis after a surgically created disk displacement in a rabbit. A, Lateral radiographs showing erosive change of the anterior surface (arrow) of the condyle. This corresponds to the area where the surgically displaced disk was located. B, Histologic section showing deterioration of the articular soft tissue cover (arrowheads) and irregularities of the subchondral cartilage cells.

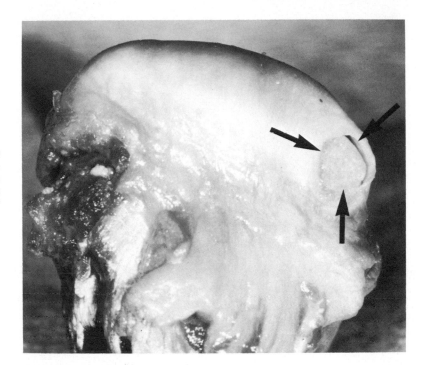

Figure 2–45
Perforation of disk. Anterior lateral aspect of a condyle with attached disk showing perforation (arrows) over the lateral pole of the condyle. The disk is in normal position. There are irregularities of the condyle at the site of the perforation.

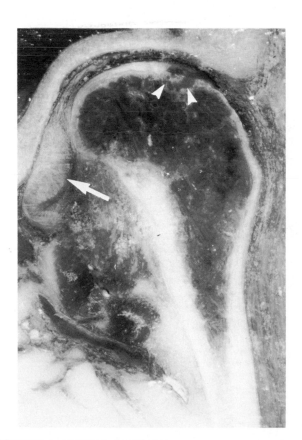

Figure 2–46
Medial disk displacement and arthrosis. Coronal cryosection showing medial displacement of the disk (arrow). Erosive changes (arrowheads) are seen in the lateral superior aspect of the condyle.

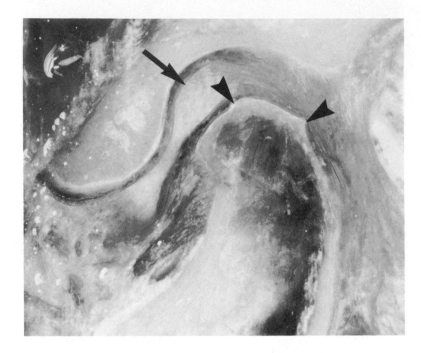

Figure 2–47
Osseous changes in a joint with normal disk position. Sagittal cryosection showing the disk (arrow) in normal position. The cortical irregularities and thickening of the condyle (arrowheads) could represent early arthrosis.

Figure 2–48
Sagittal cryosection showing advanced remodeling of the condyle and temporal joint components. The intact articular soft tissue cover on the condyle (arrowheads) indicates remodeling instead of arthrosis.

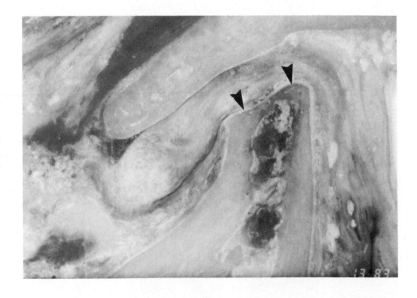

Remodeling was classified by Johnson into three categories: progressive, regressive, and circumferential.[61] Progressive remodeling implies proliferation and deposition of new cartilage with subsequent conversion to subchondral bone at a rate that is sufficient to add length to the end of the bone. Regressive remodeling results in shortening of the length of the bone and is recognized by the presence of remnants of calcified cartilage in the upper layers of the intact articular soft tissue cover. For the TMJ, the regressive remodeling is generally seen as a small condyle and a low condylar neck. Circumferential or peripheral remodeling results in an increased diameter of the joint. This usually takes place at the margin of the articular cartilage through a combination of progressive remodeling, periosteal elevation, and metaplastic chondrification followed by ossification of the capsular, ligamentous, and tendinous attachments. Remodeling should be differentiated from arthrosis, which represents changes associated with breakdown of the articular soft tissue cover, fibrillation, fissuring eburnation, and cystic alterations.

INFLAMMATORY ARTHRITIS

Inflammatory arthritis is a pathologic entity related to an autoimmune reaction, with proliferation of the synovial tissue, inflammatory reactions, and secondary breakdown of the articular surfaces. Inflammatory arthritis occurs in rheumatoid arthritis, juvenile rheumatoid arthritis, psoriatic arthritis, ankylosing spondylitis, and other inflammatory arthritides. A more detailed account of inflammatory arthritis and its effect on the TMJ is given in Chapter 8 (Rheumatoid Arthritis). An example of a mandibular condyle from a patient with rheumatoid arthritis is seen in Figure 2–49.

Although extremely unusual, the TMJ is also affected by gout.[62] The symptoms include pain, swelling, tenderness, and limitation of motion. Also unusual, the TMJ can be affected by chondrocalcinosis or calcium pyrophosphate deposition disease (pseudogout).[63–65] The symptoms are pain, tenderness, and possibly swelling and limitation of opening. The diagnosis is based on the presence of calcium pyrophosphate crystals in the synovial fluid or radiographic

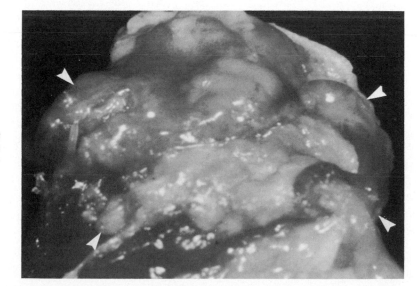

Figure 2–49
Anterior aspect of the condyle from a patient with rheumatoid arthritis. There are extensive proliferative changes on the condyle (arrowheads).

evidence of calcification in and around the joint space. However, so few cases have been reported that it still has to be regarded as unique.

MASTICATORY MUSCLE DISORDERS

Myofascial Pain–Dysfunction Syndrome

Masticatory muscle disorders and painful muscles are frequently associated with disk displacement, but these have not been extensively documented with objective techniques. Pain in the muscles of mastication has been described as part of a syndrome called myofascial pain–dysfunction syndrome,[66–69] also called primary masticatory myalgia.[70] This syndrome is characterized by four cardinal symptoms: pain of unilateral origin, masticatory muscle tenderness, limitation of mandibular movement, and clicking or popping sounds. The occurrence of joint sound alone is not sufficient to make a diagnosis of myofascial pain–dysfunction syndrome; there must be accompanying symptoms of myofascial pain and tenderness unrelated to muscle splinting. Patients usually have no clinical, radiographic, or biochemical evidence of organic changes in the TMJ.[66, 70] Muscular pain–dysfunction syndrome is a functional muscular disorder that ultimately can lead to degenerative changes in the joint as well as to internal derangement.[70] Its most common cause is believed to be muscle fatigue produced by chronic oral habits, such as clenching or grinding of the teeth;[66] muscle spasm and muscle injury may also have a role.[71]

Morphologic Alterations in Muscle

Recently more objective documentation of morphologic changes in the muscles of mastication related to TMJ disorders has been described using high-field magnetic resonance imaging.[72] These changes include muscle hypertrophy, muscle atrophy, inflammatory disorders, post-traumatic musculoskeletal deformities, and reflex sympathetic dystrophy. Atrophy, fatty replacement, fibrosis, and contracture of selected muscles of mastication sometimes accompany internal derangement of the TMJ. These muscular changes were thought to be secondary to internal derangement and TMJ injuries, in contrast to the situation with muscular pain–dysfunction syndrome in which the joint changes are thought to be secondary to the muscular disorder. An example of a patient with atrophic changes in the lateral pterygoid muscle after a condylar fracture is seen in Figure 2–50. MR studies of the muscles of mastication after orthognathic surgery with vertical ramus osteotomy have shown a high prevalence of atrophic changes of the muscles attaching to the ramus[73] (Fig. 2–51). The clinical significance of these alterations is not fully understood.

ASEPTIC NECROSIS

Aseptic necrosis, avascular necrosis, and ischemic necrosis are different terms for the same pathologic entity. This condition is most frequent in the femoral condyle, but there are intimations in the medical literature that aseptic necrosis may also occur in the TMJ.[74–76] This entity, however, has not been systematically documented at the histologic level, and it is still an open question

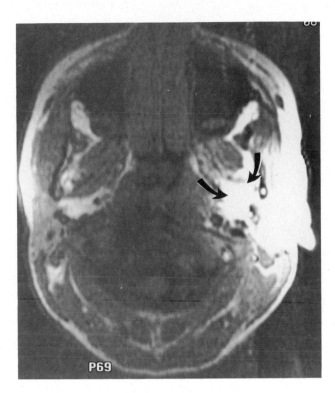

Figure 2–50
Atrophic changes of muscles of mastication. Axial MR scan of a patient with a history of a left condylar fracture, showing atrophic changes and fatty degeneration of the pterygoid (arrows) and masseter muscles on the left.

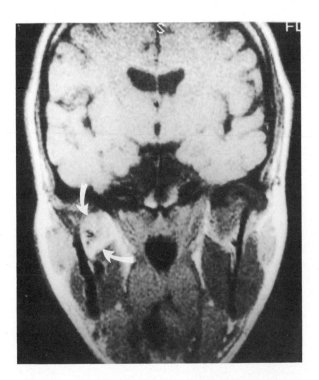

Figure 2–51
Coronal MR image showing atrophic changes of the medial pterygoid (arrows) and masseter muscles on the right side following orthognathic surgery with a vertical ramus osteotomy.

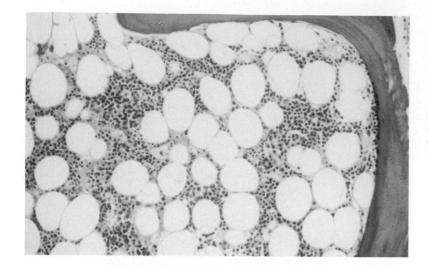

Figure 2–52
Histologic section showing normal bone marrow of a femoral condyle. (Courtesy of Dr. David Hicks, Rochester, New York.)

as to how frequently it occurs in the TMJ. The MR imaging characteristics of this entity have been described for the femoral head with pathologic correlation, but this is not available in the peer-reviewed literature for the TMJ.

In the femoral condyle, aseptic necrosis is due to avascular infarction. Frequently this condition is associated with other diseases, conditions, or treatment regimens, such as sickle cell disease, corticosteroid therapy, alcoholism, Gaucher's disease, dysbaric disorders, pregnancy, collagen vascular disorders, renal transplantation, and chemotherapy. However, aseptic necrosis in the TMJ is thought to be secondary to joint inflammation and synovitis.[75, 76] For comparison, an example of a normal bone marrow from a femoral head is shown in Figure 2–52. Histologically proved avascular necrosis of the femoral head is shown in Figure 2–53.

CONGENITAL AND DEVELOPMENTAL ANOMALIES

A broad variety of congenital and developmental anomalies affect the TMJ. These have been divided into malformations, deformations, disruptions,

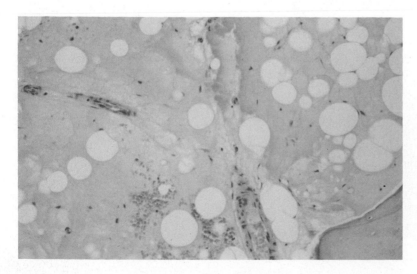

Figure 2–53
Histologic section showing avascular necrosis in bone marrow of a femoral condyle. (Courtesy of Dr. David Hicks, Rochester, New York.)

and dysplasias.[77] The malformations include, among others, facial microsomia, oculoauriculovertebral dysplasia, and Treacher Collins syndrome. These all result in a small or absent mandibular condyle and different degrees of underdevelopment of the mandibular ramus. Frequently there are other associated anomalies of the temporal bone. The deformations include Pierre Robin anomaly, which was explained by Poswillo as the loss of amniotic fluid causing the lower border of the mandible to be compressed against the sternum.[78] Typically in congenital anomalies the condyle and especially the temporal joint component are underdeveloped. Figure 2–54 shows an example of a TMJ in a patient with a congenital anomaly involving a hypoplastic temporal bone. The condyle is hypoplastic. The disk is located in a normal position. The hypoplasia of the temporal bone involves agenesis of the articular eminence, the middle ear, and the mastoid. The mastoid is filled with fat instead of the normal air that is characteristic of congenital anomaly of the temporal bone. The patient was diagnosed as having a form of hemifacial microsomia.

Disruption includes the bifid condyle, which is a relatively rare anomaly.[79–82] Clinically the patient demonstrates duplication of the condyle following fracture or dislocation, with a new condyle having developed on the long side of the displaced original condyle.[78, 83, 84] Double condyles have also been noted in dry skulls.[85] Poswillo has shown that a bifid condyle can occur following condylectomy in monkeys.[86]

Dysplasia may involve the entire mandible or the condyle only, and these are exceedingly rare conditions. Hypoplasia of the condyle has an unknown etiology. Condylar hypertrophy has been discussed elsewhere.

CONDYLAR HYPERPLASIA

This entity involves spontaneous growth of the condyle, leading to mandibular asymmetry. The etiology is unknown. A more detailed discussion is

Figure 2–54
Congenital hypoplasia of the TMJ. Sagittal MR scan shows hypoplasia of the TMJ. The disk is located normally. The articular eminence is absent. The middle ear and mastoid are absent. The mastoid is replaced by fat. The patient had a form of hemifacial microsomia.

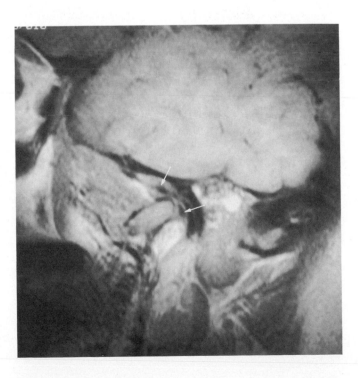

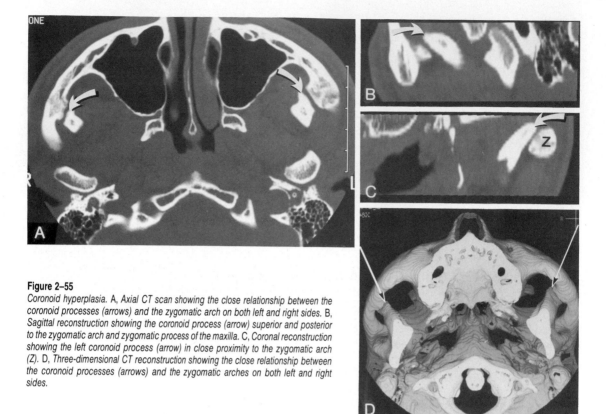

Figure 2–55
Coronoid hyperplasia. A, Axial CT scan showing the close relationship between the coronoid processes (arrows) and the zygomatic arch on both left and right sides. B, Sagittal reconstruction showing the coronoid process (arrow) superior and posterior to the zygomatic arch and zygomatic process of the maxilla. C, Coronal reconstruction showing the left coronoid process (arrow) in close proximity to the zygomatic arch (Z). D, Three-dimensional CT reconstruction showing the close relationship between the coronoid processes (arrows) and the zygomatic arches on both left and right sides.

available in Chapter 10, Miscellaneous Conditions. This entity must be differentiated from neoplasm of the condyle, such as osteochondroma.

ANKYLOSIS

Ankylosis can be divided into fibrous and bony ankylosis. This is most frequently secondary to middle ear infections and previous trauma; in recent years the most frequent cause of ankylosis has been failed TMJ surgery. Fibrous ankylosis can be clearly diagnosed with MR imaging. Bony ankylosis is best diagnosed with computed tomography (CT) scans in the direct sagittal or coronal plane. A further discussion is available in Chapter 10 under Miscellaneous Conditions.

CORONOID HYPERPLASIA

Hyperplasia of the coronoid process has an unknown cause. It occurs uncommonly and may present with signs and symptoms similar to those of disk displacement without reduction. The patient may have had and may also present with clicking and is usually unable to open the jaw wide at examination. Coronoid hyperplasia most frequently occurs in young males and should be considered in the differential diagnosis when there is limitation of opening that cannot be explained by the intra-articular observations.[87–89] An example of a 20-year-old patient with bilateral coronoid hyperplasia is shown in Figure 2–55.

Summary

A wide variety of abnormalities and anomalies affect the TMJ. Accurate information about these disorders forms the basis for treatment planning and evaluation of prognosis.[90-95] Imaging is an accurate method for assessing the status of the joint. The following chapters will review imaging techniques applied to the TMJ.

References

1. Schellhas KP, Wilkes CH: Temporomandibular joint inflammation: Comparison of MR fast scanning with T1- and T2-weighted imaging techniques. AJNR 1989;*10*:589–594.
2. Schellhas KP, Wilkes CH, Baker CC: Facial pain, headache, and temporomandibular joint inflammation. Headache 1989;*29*:228–231.
3. Westesson P-L, Brooks SL: Temporomandibular joint: Relation between MR evidence of effusion and the presence of pain and disk displacement. AJR 1992;*159*:559–563.
4. Costen JB: A syndrome of ear and sinus symptoms dependent upon disturbed function of the temporomandibular joint. Ann Otol Rhinol Laryngol 1934;*43*:1–15.
5. Costen JB: Neuralgias and ear symptoms involved in general diagnosis due to mandibular joint pathology. J Kansas Med Soc 1935;*36*:315–321.
6. Paesani D, Westesson P-L, Hatala M, Tallents RH, Kurita K: Prevalence of internal derangement in patients with craniomandibular disorders Am J Orthod Dentofacial Orthop 1992;*101*:41–47.
7. Kircos LT, Ortendahl DA, Mark AS, Arakawa MS: Magnetic resonance imaging of the TMJ disk in asymptomatic volunteers. J Oral Maxillofac Surg 1987;*45*:852–854.
8. Kaplan PA, Tu HK, Williams SM, Lydiatt DD: The normal temporomandibular joint: MR and arthrographic correlation. Radiology 1987;*165*:177–178.
9. Westesson P-L, Eriksson L, Kurita K: Reliability of a negative clinical temporomandibular joint examination—prevalence of disk displacement in asymptomatic temporomandibular joints. Oral Surg Oral Med Oral Pathol 1989;*68*:551–554.
10. Johansson A-S, Isberg A, Isacsson G: Radiographic and histologic study of the topographic relations in the TMJ region: Implication for nerve entrapment mechanism. J Oral Maxillofac Surg 1990;*48*:953–961.
11. Katzberg RW, Westesson P-L, Tallents RH, Anderson R, Kurita K, Manzione JV, Totterman S: Temporomandibular joint: MR assessment of rotational and sideways disk displacements. Radiology 1988;*169*:741–748.
12. Adams JC: Outline of Orthopaedics. 9th ed. London, Churchill Livingstone, 1981, pp 70–71.
13. Farrar WB: Characteristics of the condylar path in internal derangement of the TMJ. J Prosthet Dent 1978;*39*:319–323.
14. Wilkes CH: Arthrography of the temporomandibular joint in patients with the TMJ pain–dysfunction syndrome. Minn Med 1978;*61*:645–652.
15. Wilkes CH: Structural and functional alterations of the temporomandibular joint. Northwest Dent 1978;*57*:287–294.
16. Katzberg RW, Dolwick MF, Helms CA, Hopens T, Bales DJ, Coggs GC: Arthrotomography of the temporomandibular joint. AJR 1980;*134*:995–1003.
17. Eriksson L, Westesson P-L: Clinical and radiological study of patients with anterior disk displacement of the temporomandibular joint. Swed Dent J 1983;*7*:55–64.
18. Westesson P-L: Double-contrast arthrotomography of the temporomandibular joint: Introduction of an arthrographic technique for visualization of the disk and articular surface. J Oral Maxillofac Surg 1983;*41*:163–172.
19. Wilkes CH: Internal derangement of the temporomandibular joint. Pathological variations. Arch Otolaryngol Head Neck Surg 1989;*115*:469–477.
20. Lundh H, Westesson P-L, Kopp S: A three-year follow-up of patients with reciprocal temporomandibular joint clicking. Oral Surg Oral Med Oral Pathol 1987;*63*:530–533.
21. Westesson P-L, Lund H: Arthrographic and clinical characteristics of patients with disk displacement who progressed to closed lock during a six month period. Oral Surg Oral Med Oral Pathol 1989;*67*:654–657.
22. Scapino RP: Histopathology associated with malposition of the human temporomandibular joint disk. Oral Surg Oral Med Oral Pathol 1983;*55*:382–397.
23. Hirschmann PN, Shuttleworth CA: The collagen composition of the mandibular joint of the foetal calf. Arch Oral Biol 1976;*21*:771–773.
24. Griffin CJ, Sharpe CJ: Distribution of elastic tissue in the human temporomandibular meniscus especially in respect to "compression" areas. Aust Dent J 1962;*7*:72–78.
25. Griffin CJ, Hawthorn R, Harris R: Anatomy and histology of the human temporomandibular joint. *In* The Temporomandibular Joint Syndrome. Basel, Karger, 1975 (Oral Science; Vol 4).

26. Kopp S: Topographical distribution of sulfated glycosaminoglycans in human temporomandibular joint disks: A histochemical study of autopsy material. J Oral Pathol 1976;5:265–276.
27. Axhausen G: Das Kiefergelenkknacken und seine Behandlung. Dtsch Z Chir 1931;232:238–272.
28. Dufourmentel L: Chirurgie de l'articulation temporomaxillaire. Paris, Masson, 1929.
29. Konjetzny GE: Die operative Behandlung der habituellen Unterkieferluxation (Eine neue Operationsmethoide). Verh Dtsch Ges Chir 1921;2:207–218.
30. Konjetzny GE: Die Behandlung der habituellen Luxation, der sogenannten habituellen Subluxation des Unterkieferss und des Kiefergelenkknackens. Zentralbl Chir 1929;56:3018–3123.
31. Lanz O: Diskitis mandibularis. Zentralbl Chir 1909;36:289–291.
32. Scapino RP: Histopathology of the disk and posterior attachment in disk displacement internal derangements of the TMJ. *In* Palacios E, Valvassori GE, Shannon M, Reed CF, eds: Magnetic Resonance of the Temporomandibular Joint. New York, Thieme, 1990, pp 63–74.
33. Kurita K, Westesson P-L, Sternby NH, Eriksson L, Carlsson L-E, Lundh H, Toremalm NG: Histologic features of the temporomandibular joint disk and posterior disk attachment: Comparison of symptom-free persons with normally positioned disks and patients with internal derangement. Oral Surg Oral Med Oral Pathol 1989;67:635–643.
34. Isberg A, Isacsson G: Tissue reactions associated with internal derangement of the temporomandibular joint. A radiographic, cryomorphologic, and histologic study. Acta Odontol Scand 1986;44:160–164.
35. Isacsson G, Isberg A, Johansson AS, Larson O: Internal derangement of the temporomandibular joint: Radiographic and histologic changes associated with severe pain. J Oral Maxillofac Surg 1986;44:771–778.
36. Paz ME, Katzberg RW, Tallents RH, Westesson P-L, Proskin HM, Murphy WC: Computed tomographic evaluation of the density of the temporomandibular joint meniscus. Oral Surg Oral Med Oral Pathol 1988;66:519–524.
37. Paz ME, Carter LC, Westesson P-L, Katzberg RW, Tallents R, Subtelny JD, Goldin B: CT density of the temporomandibular joint disk. Correlation with histologic observations of hyalinization, metaplastic cartilage and calcification in autopsy specimens. Am J Orthod Dentofac Orthop 1990;98:354–357.
38. Öberg T, Carlsson GE: Macroscopic and microscopic anatomy of the temporomandibular joint. *In* Zarb GA, Carlsson GE, eds: Temporomandibular Joint: Function and Dysfunction. Copenhagen, Munksgaard, 1979, pp 101–118.
39. Rees LA: The structure and function of the mandibular joint. Br Dent J 1954;96:125–133.
40. Isberg A, Isacsson G, Johansson AS, Larson O: Hyperplastic soft-tissue formation in the temporomandibular joint associated with internal derangement. A radiographic and histologic study. Oral Surg Oral Med Oral Pathol 1986;61:32–38.
41. Westesson P-L, Bronstein SL, Liedberg JL: Internal derangement of the temporomandibular joint: Morphologic description with correlation to joint function. Oral Surg Oral Med Oral Pathol 1985;59:323–331.
42. Nørgaard F: Artrografi af kaebeleddet. Preliminary report. Acta Radiol 1944;25:679–685.
43. Takaku S: Surgical treatment of diskopathy of the temporomandibular joint. Jpn J Oral Maxillofac Surg 1983;29:78–93.
44. Takaku S: Temporomandibular Joint Disease. Tokyo, Shorin, 1986, pp 59–69.
45. Harkins SJ, Marteney JL: Extrinsic trauma: A significant precipitating factor in temporomandibular dysfunction. J Prosthet Dent 1985;54:271–272.
46. Weinberg S, Lapointe H: Cervical extension-flexion injury (whiplash) and internal derangement of the temporomandibular joint. J Oral Maxillofac Surg 1987;45:653–656.
47. Ishigaki S, Bessette RW, Mauruyama T: The distribution of internal derangement in patients with temporomandibular joint dysfunction—Prevalence, diagnosis, and treatments. Cranio 1992;10:289–296.
48. Scapino RP: The posterior attachment: Its structure, function, and appearance in TMJ imaging studies. Part 1. J Craniomandib Disord Fac Oral Pain 1991;5:83–95.
49. Scapino RP: The posterior attachment: Its structure, function, and appearance in TMJ imaging studies. Part 2. J Craniomandib Disord Fac Oral Pain 1991;5:155–166.
50. Eriksson L, Westesson P-L, Macher D, Hicks D, Tallents RH: Creation of disk displacement in human temporomandibular joint autopsy specimens. J Oral Maxillofac Surg 1992;50:869–873.
51. Schneider K, Zernicke RF, Clark G: Modeling of jaw-head-neck dynamics during whiplash. J Dent Res 1989;68:1360–1365.
52. Burgess J: Symptom characteristics in TMD patients reporting blunt trauma and/or whiplash injury. J Craniomandib Disord 1991;5:251–257.
53. Howard RP, Benedict JV, Raddin JH Jr, Smith HL: Assessing neck extension-flexion as a basis for temporomandibular joint dysfunction. J Oral Maxillofac Surg 1991;49:1210–1213.
54. Epstein JB: Temporomandibular disorders, facial pain and headache following motor vehicle accidents. Can Dent Assoc J 1992;58:488–489.
55. Heise AP, Laskin DM, Gervin AS: Incidence of temporomandibular joint symptoms following whiplash injury. J Oral Maxillofac Surg 1992;50:825–828.
56. Sokoloff L: The Biology of Degenerative Joint Disease. Chicago, The University of Chicago Press, 1969, p 2.

57. Katzberg RW, Keith DA, Guralnick WC, Manzione JV, Ten Eick WR: Internal derangement and arthritis of the temporomandibular joint. Radiology 1983;*146:*107–112.
58. Westesson P-L: Structural hard tissue changes in temporomandibular joints with internal derangement. Oral Surg Oral Med Oral Pathol 1985;*59:*220–224.
59. Macher DJ, Westesson P-L, Brooks SL, Hicks DG, Tallents RH: Temporomandibular joint: Surgically created disc displacement causes arthrosis in the rabbit. Oral Surg Oral Med Oral Pathol 1992;*73:*645–649.
60. Moffett PB, Johnson LC, McCabe JB, Askew HC: Articular remodeling in the adult human temporomandibular joint. Am J Anat 1964;*115:*119–142.
61. Johnson LC: Joint remodeling as the basis for osteoarthritis. JAMA 1962;*141:*1237–1241.
62. Chun HH: Temporomandibular joint gout (letter). JAMA 1973;*226:*353.
63. Good AE, Upton LG: Acute temporomandibular arthritis in a patient with bruxism and calcium pyrophosphate deposition disease. Arthritis Rheum 1982;*25:*353–355.
64. Hutton CW, Doherty M, Dieppe PA: Acute pseudogout of the temporomandibular joint: A report of three cases and review of the literature. Br J Rheumatol 1987;*26:*51–52.
65. Magno WB, Lee SH, Schmidt J: Chondrocalcinosis of the temporomandibular joint: An external ear canal pseudotumor. Oral Surg Oral Med Oral Pathol 1992;*73:*262–265.
66. Laskin DM: Etiology of the pain-dysfunction syndrome. J Am Dent Assoc 1969;*79:*147–153.
67. Laskin DM, Block S: Diagnosis and treatment of myofascial pain–dysfunction (MPD) syndrome. J Prosthet Dent 1986;*56:*75–84.
68. Greene CS, Laskin DM: Long-term evaluation of treatment for myofascial pain–dysfunction syndrome: A comparative analysis. J Am Dent Assoc 1983;*107:*235–238.
69. Laskin DM: Etiology of the pain-dysfunction syndrome. Information Dentaire 1977;*59:*21–32.
70. Laskin DM: Temporomandibular disorders: Diagnosis and etiology. *In* Sarnat BG, Laskin DM, eds: The Temporomandibular Joint: A Biological Basis for Clinical Practice. 4th ed. Philadelphia, W. B. Saunders, 1992, pp 316–328.
71. Yemm R: Pathophysiology of the masticatory muscles. *In* Sarnat BG, Laskin DM, eds: The Temporomandibular Joint: A Biological Basis for Clinical Practice. 4th ed. Philadelphia, W. B. Saunders, 1992, pp 143–149.
72. Schellhas KP: MR imaging of muscles of mastication. AJR 1989;*153:*847–855.
73. Westesson P-L, Dahlberg G, Hansson L-G, Eriksson L, Ketonen L: Osseous and muscular changes after vertical ramus osteotomy. A magnetic resonance imaging study. Oral Surg Oral Med Oral Pathol 1991;*72:*139–145.
74. Reiskin AB: Aseptic necrosis of the mandibular condyle: A common problem? Quint Int 1979;*2:*85–89.
75. Schellhas KP, Wilkes CH, Fritts HM, Omlie HM, Lagrotteria LB: MR of osteochondritis dissecans and avascular necrosis of the mandibular condyle. AJR 1989;*152:*551–560.
76. Schellhas KP, Piper MA, Omlie MR: Facial skeleton remodeling due to temporomandibular joint degeneration: An imaging study of 100 patients. AJNR 1990;*11:*541–551.
77. Poswillo D, Robinson P: Congenital and developmental anomalies. *In* Sarnat BG, Laskin DM, eds: The Temporomandibular Joint: A Biological Basis for Clinical Practice. Philadelphia, WB Saunders, 1992, pp 183–206.
78. Poswillo DE: Foetal posture and causal mechanisms of deformity of the palate, jaws and limbs. J Dent Res 1966;*45:*584–596.
79. Balciunas BA: Bifid mandibular condyle. J Oral Maxillofac Surg 1986;*44:*324–325.
80. Gundlach JKH, Fuhrmann A, Beckmann-van der Ven G: The double headed mandibular condyle. Oral Surg Oral Med Oral Pathol 1987;*64:*249–253.
81. McCormick SU, McCormick SA, Graves RW, et al: Bilateral bifid mandibular condyles. Report of three cases. Oral Surg Oral Med Oral Pathol 1989;*68:*555–557.
82. Loh FC, Yeo JF: Bifid mandibular condyle. Oral Surg Oral Med Oral Pathol 1990;*69:*24–27.
83. Thomason JM, Yusuf H: Traumatically induced bifid mandibular condyle: A report of two cases. Br Dent J 1986;*161:*291–293.
84. Stadnicki G: Congenital double condyle of the mandible causing temporomandibular joint ankylosis: Report of a case. J Oral Surg 1971;*29:*208–211.
85. Moffett B: The morphogenesis of the temporomandibular joint. Am J Orthod 1966;*52:*401–415.
86. Poswillo DE: The late effects of mandibular condylectomy. Oral Surg 1972;*33:*500–512.
87. Isberg A, Isacsson G, Nah KS: Mandibular coronoid process locking: A prospective study of frequency and association with internal derangement of the temporomandibular joint. Oral Surg Oral Med Oral Pathol 1987;*63:*275–279.
88. Munk PL, Helms CA: Coronoid process hyperplasia: CT studies. Radiology 1989;*171:*783–784.
89. Blanchard P, Henry JF, Souchere B, Breton P, Freidel M: Permanent constriction of the jaw due to idiopathic bilateral hyperplasia of the coronoid process. Rev Stomatol Chir Maxillofac 1992;*93:*46–50.
90. Roberts CA, Tallents RH, Espeland MA, Handelman SL, Katzberg RW: Mandibular range of motion versus arthrographic diagnosis of the temporomandibular joint. Oral Surg Oral Med Oral Pathol 1985;*60:*244–251.

91. Roberts CA, Tallents RH, Katzberg RW, Sanchez-Woodworth RE, Manzione JV, Espeland MA, Handelman SL: Clinical and arthrographic evaluation of the temporomandibular joint. Oral Surg Oral Med Oral Pathol 1986;*62*:373–376.
92. Roberts CA, Tallents RH, Katzberg RW, Sandchez-Woodworth RE, Espeland MA, Handelman SL: Comparison of arthrographic findings of the temporomandibular joint with palpation of the muscles of mastication. Oral Surg Oral Med Oral Pathol 1987;*64*:275–277.
93. Roberts CA, Tallents RH, Katzberg RW, Sandchez-Woodworth RE, Espeland MA, Handelman SL: Comparison of internal derangements of the TMJ with occlusal findings. Oral Surg Oral Med Oral Pathol 1987;*63*:645–650.
94. Roberts CA, Tallents RH, Katzberg RW, Sandchez-Woodworth RE, Espeland MA, Handelman SL: Clinical and arthrographic evaluation of the location of temporomandibular joint pain. Oral Surg Oral Med Oral Pathol 1987;*64*:6–8.
95. Paesani D, Westesson P-L, Hatala MP, Tallents R, Brooks SL: Accuracy of clinical diagnosis for temporomandibular joint internal derangement and arthrosis. Oral Surg Oral Med Oral Pathol 1992;*73*:360–363.

PART TWO

Imaging Internal Derangements

CHAPTER THREE

Plain Film and Tomography

Plain film and tomography have been the most frequently used methods to image the temporomandibular joint (TMJ). For plain film imaging, as well as for tomography, a multitude of projections and techniques have been described over the years. This chapter reviews the most frequently used techniques, describes how the images are obtained, identifies anatomic landmarks, describes pathologic changes, and, based on our experience with the different techniques, recommends an approach to plain film and tomographic examination of the TMJ that can be practical and cost-effective in different clinical settings.

The purpose of the plain film and tomographic examinations is to demonstrate the relationship between the mandibular condyle and the glenoid fossa and to diagnose osseous changes, such as remodeling and arthrosis. Plain films and tomograms are also routinely obtained in patients with jaw and facial anomalies and jaw and facial fractures.

PLAIN FILM

Technique

The location of the TMJ close to the base of the skull makes it difficult to produce clear radiographs of the joint. It is, therefore, not surprising that a multitude of projections have been advocated over the years. Excellent reviews of various plain film techniques have been presented by Lindblom,[1] Clements-chitsch,[2] Omnell,[3] and Petersson.[4]

The basic principle of plain film examination of the TMJ is to have at least two projections of the joint at different angles. The most commonly used technique is the transcranial projection. This is obtained at an angle to the horizontal plane to avoid superimposition of the osseous structures of the base of the skull. This radiograph will depict only the cortical bone that is oriented parallel to the x-ray beam, and so only a small part of the joint will be visualized. The plain film assessment of the TMJ, therefore, should include a second projection at a different angle in order to appreciate the three-dimensional size, shape, and structure of the joint components. The second view could be an anteroposterior projection or a transmaxillary view. Third, the plain film evaluation of the TMJ should include an open-mouth view to assess range of condylar motion, a functional aspect of the examination. Thus, the basic plain film evaluation of the TMJ involves lateral transcranial projections at closed-

Table 3–1
PLAIN FILM EXAMINATION OF THE TMJ

1. Submentovertical projection
2. Lateral oblique transcranial projection at closed-mouth position
3. Lateral oblique transcranial projection at maximal mouth opening
4. Transmaxillary projection at maximal mouth opening

and open-mouth positions and an anteroposterior projection (Table 3–1). The many variations for obtaining these projections will be described in this chapter.

Submentovertical Projection

The axial or submentovertical projection is usually the first image obtained if individualized transcranial projections or sagittal tomography is to be done. Patient positioning and the resulting radiograph are seen in Figures 3–1 to 3–3. The submentovertical projection is used to identify the orientation of the mandibular condyles in the horizontal plane (Fig. 3–3). This information is a guide for patient positioning and orientation of the x-ray beam for tomography or the lateral transcranial projection. The submentovertical projection is not intended primarily for diagnostic purposes, although the image has some value in patients with fractures and hyper- or hypoplasia of the condyle and mandibular ramus. We have placed small lead markers in the external auditory canals (Figs. 3–2 and 3–3) to identify a baseline against which the angulation of the condyle can be measured (Fig. 3–3).

Orientation of the condyle in the horizontal plane varies greatly, and angles between the horizontal long axis of the condyle and the transverse plane have been measured from about −5° up to +50°.[5-7] A mean value of 20° has been found in normal joints.[6, 7] Several studies have shown that a larger condylar angle is seen in patients with abnormal joints than in those with normal joints.[5]

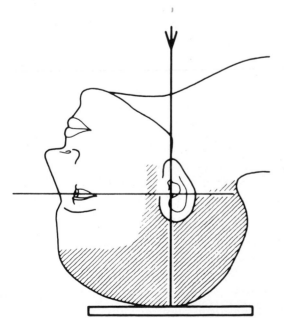

Figure 3–1
The principle of obtaining a submentovertical projection. Frequently the patients are not able to bend the neck as far back as in this drawing, and angulation of the x-ray tube is necessary to compensate for the lack of extension. (Reproduced with permission from Omnell K-Å, Lysell L: Röntgendiagnostik. In Krogh-Poulsen W, ed: Patofunktion. Bidfunktion bettfysiologi. Vol 2, 2nd ed. Copenhagen, Munksgaard Int. Publ. Ltd., 1979, Chapter 10.)

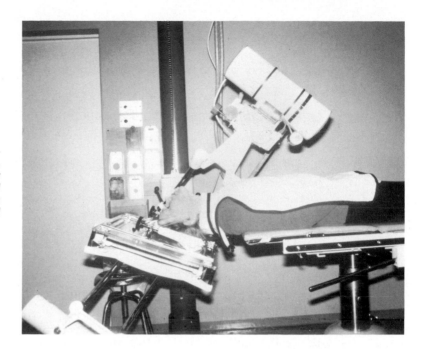

Figure 3–2
Submentovertical projection—patient positioning. The patient is lying flat on the table, and the head is tilted backward. The x-ray tube is angled in order to obtain a true axial projection of the mandibular condyle. An earplug with a lead marker has been placed in the external auditory canal.

Also, it appears that joints with more advanced internal derangement have a larger condylar angle than do joints with earlier stages of internal derangement.[5-7] The assessment of condylar angle does not have diagnostic value by itself but is primarily intended for patient positioning and optimal orientation of the x-ray beam.

The submentovertical projection is obtained with the x-ray source under the chin and the film at the top of the patient's head (Fig. 3–1). Thus a part of

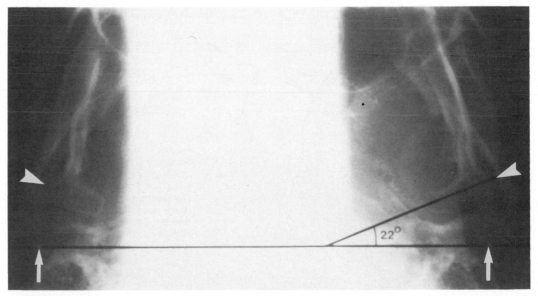

Figure 3–3
Submentovertical projection with centrally placed lead shield. The lead markers (arrows) in the external auditory canals are connected to form the baseline. The lateral poles of the condyles are indicated by arrowheads for orientation. The long axis of the condyle on the left is measured to 22°.

the thyroid gland is exposed to the x-ray beam as it passes through the neck. A relatively high radiation dose to the thyroid gland has been measured.[8] To reduce the radiation to the thyroid gland without losing important information, use of a centrally placed lead shield has been recommended (Fig. 3–3).[8]

Lateral Oblique Transcranial Projection

The lateral oblique transcranial projection is the most common method of imaging the TMJ. Numerous vertical and horizontal beam angulations have been described. Several manufacturers have introduced different types of devices to facilitate and standardize this projection.

The x-ray beam is angled from above, between 10° and 25°, to project the joint free of the osseous structures of the base of the skull (Fig. 3–4). The x-ray beam is usually also angled slightly from behind, so that the long axis of the mandibular condyle to be examined is parallel to the x-ray beam (Fig. 3–5). The degree of the horizontal angulation can be determined from the previously obtained submentovertical projection or by the use of fluoroscopy.[9]

Patient positioning by means of a cephalostat is shown in Figure 3–6. Several workers have pointed out the value of directing the x-ray beam along the horizontal long axis of the condyle instead of using a standard angle. Our awareness of the great variation in horizontal condylar angle leads us to endorse this recommendation. Examples of transcranial films obtained with the central x-ray beam along the horizontal long axis of the condyle and at the standard angle are shown in Figure 3–7. The improved image quality resulting from the individualized projection is obvious. An excellent study systematically compared the diagnostic information from standardized lateral projections with that obtained from an individualized technique based on submentovertical films: the individualized projection provided more diagnostic information than the standard projection (Fig. 3–8).[10] This agrees with our experience, and we recommend this technique.

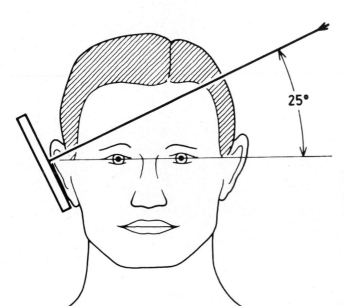

Figure 3–4
Transcranial projection—schematic drawing. The central x-ray beam is angled from above. This angle can vary between 10° and 25° and is necessary to avoid structures of the base of the skull. (Reproduced with permission from Omnell K-Å, Lysell L: Röntgendiagnostik. In Krogh-Poulsen W, ed: Patofunktion. Bidfunktion bettfysiologi. Vol 2, 2nd ed. Copenhagen, Munksgaard Int. Publ. Ltd., 1979, Chapter 10.)

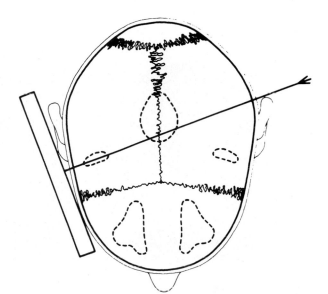

Figure 3–5
Transcranial projection—schematic drawing. The x-ray beam is oriented so that it coincides with the horizontal long axis of the condyle. (Reproduced with permission from Omnell K-Å, Lysell L: Röntgendiagnostik. In Krogh-Poulsen W, ed: Patofunktion. Bidfunktion bettfysiologi. Vol 2, 2nd ed. Copenhagen, Munksgaard Int. Publ. Ltd., 1979, Chapter 10.)

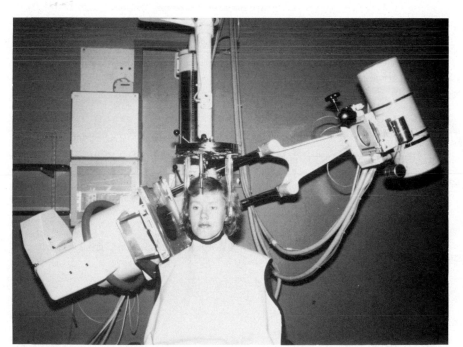

Figure 3–6
Transcranial projection—patient positioning. The patient's head is oriented with the aid of a cephalostat. The central x-ray beam is angled 25° from above when obtaining this transcranial projection.

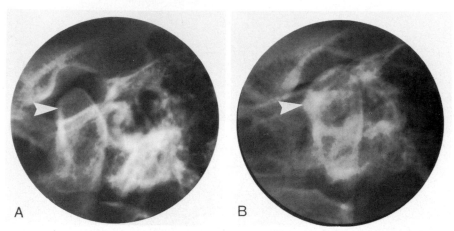

Figure 3–7
Transcranial projections, obtained with the x-ray beam parallel to the horizontal long axis of the condyle (A) and at a standard 10° angle (B). The improved image quality by individualized projection is obvious in A. The anterior aspect of the condyle is indicated by arrowheads for orientation.

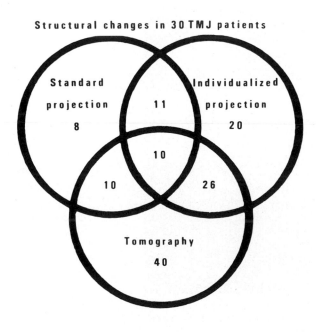

Figure 3–8
Comparison of standard and individualized projection. The number of structural hard tissue changes in 30 TMJ patients detected by standardized, individualized transcranial projection and with tomography. Tomography appeared to have the highest sensitivity for osseous changes. (Numbers derived from Omnell K-Å, Petersson A: Radiography of the temporomandibular joint utilizing oblique lateral transcranial projections. Odontol Review 1976;27:77–92.)

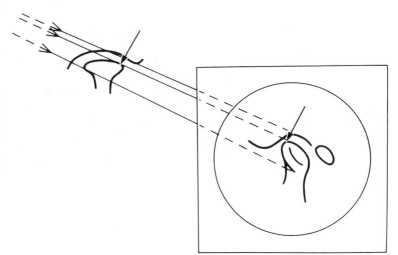

Figure 3–9
Transcranial projection—schematic drawing. The radiograph is a depiction of the lateral cortex. Essentially no good image can be obtained of the medial part of the joint. (Reproduced with permission from Omnell K-Å, Lysell L: Röntgendiagnostik. In Krogh-Poulsen W, ed: Patofunktion. Bidfunktion bettfysiologi. Vol 2, 2nd ed. Copenhagen, Munksgaard Int. Publ. Ltd., 1979, Chapter 10.)

It is desirable to have a similar technique when the radiographic examination is repeated after treatment or after follow-up. Many different methods of standardizing the radiographic imaging technique have been described.[11, 12] Essentially, these techniques include the orientation of the patient's head and the x-ray beam and film positioning in a standardized way, using a cephalometric device (see Figure 3–6). An alternative technique includes orientation based on light beam indicators. A number of commercially available devices can be used to overcome projectional alterations and improve the reproducibility of plain film imaging of the TMJ.

The transcranial projection depicts only the cortex of the lateral aspect of the joint components (Fig. 3–9). At first the transcranial image may resemble a true lateral projection of the joint (Fig. 3–10), but this is a misinterpretation. The angulation of the x-ray beam from above results only in an image of the lateral aspect of the joint (Fig. 3–9).

Functional Examination—Open-Mouth View

Plain film examination should include an open-mouth view to study how much the condyle translates anteriorly at maximal mouth opening (Fig. 3–10).

Figure 3–10
Transcranial projection. Obtained at the closed mouth position (A) and maximal mouth opening (B) of a TMJ with normal osseous components.

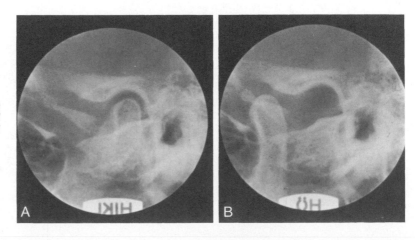

This is the most cost-effective way to obtain this information. However, attempts have also been made to use an image intensifier coupled to the tape recorder for the functional examination. A relatively good impression of condylar translation can be obtained by this technique, but it has not been shown clearly that a video recording of joint function is diagnostically more significant than just one single exposure at maximal mouth opening. By widening the aperture, some investigators have included both left and right joints on the same fluoroscopic image.[13] In this way they were able to correlate movement of the left and right joints and improve diagnosis of irregular movement. The technique of using videofluoroscopy of one or both joints during functioning has not gained wide clinical acceptance.

Posteroanterior Projection

The limitation of the transcranial projection to the depiction only of the lateral part of the joint has led to the need for an additional projection at a different angle. Many different anteroposterior projections are described for visualization of the TMJ. The transmaxillary projection, which has also been called the oblique infraorbital or transantral projection, is one of the most common ones.[19] Patient positioning and the direction of the x-ray beam for a transmaxillary projection are shown in Figures 3–11 through 3–13. The projection has to be obtained at maximal mouth opening. The condyle must be able to maintain a position inferior to the articular eminence in order to maximize the image quality. If the condyle is behind the articular tubercle, a clear depiction of the superior surface of the condyle cannot be achieved and the diagnostic gain from this projection will be limited. A device to stabilize the mouth in the open-mouth position during exposure (Fig. 3–14) helps reduce

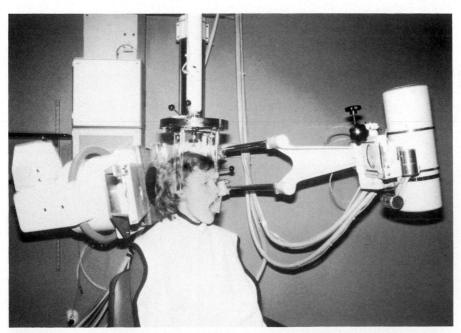

Figure 3–11
Transmaxillary projection—patient positioning. The patient's head is oriented by the aid of a cephalostat. The central x-ray beam is directed 10° from above.

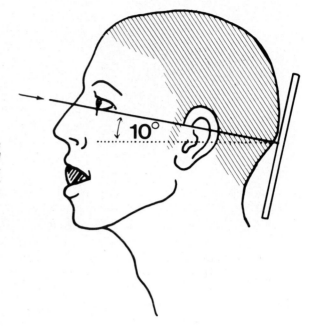

Figure 3–12
Transmaxillary projection—schematic drawing. The central x-ray beam is directed from 10° above the horizontal plane. The patient's mouth should be open. (Reproduced with permission from Omnell K-Å, Lysell L: Röntgendiagnostik. In Krogh-Poulsen W, ed: Patofunktion. Bidfunktion bettfysiologi. Vol 2, 2nd ed. Copenhagen, Munksgaard Int. Publ. Ltd., 1979, Chapter 10.)

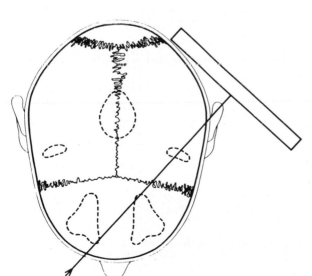

Figure 3–13
Transmaxillary projection—schematic drawing. The angulation of the x-ray beam in the horizontal plane is shown. (Reproduced with permission from Omnell K-Å, Lysell L: Röntgendiagnostik. In Krogh-Poulsen W, ed: Patofunktion. Bidfunktion bettfysiologi. Vol 2, 2nd ed. Copenhagen, Munksgaard Int. Publ. Ltd., 1979, Chapter 10.)

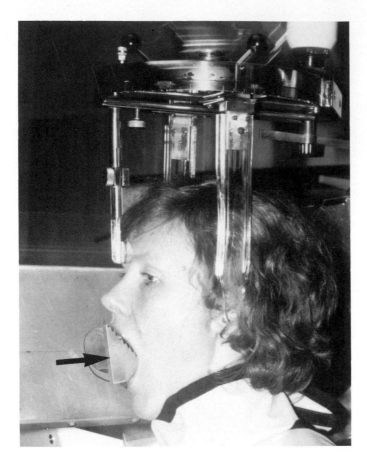

Figure 3–14
Open mouth device. Patient positioning in the cephalostat for an open mouth image. An aluminum stair is placed between the upper and lower teeth to stabilize the jaw during exposure.

motion artifact and ensure correct jaw position. Figure 3–15 shows a transmaxillary projection with clear visualization of the upper part of the condyle.

Comparison of the diagnostic information from the transcranial and the transmaxillary projections has been reported. The transmaxillary projection was superior for detection of erosive changes of the condyle, but the transcranial projection was better for delineation of osteophytes and sclerosis.[20] This is not surprising, since osteophytes usually develop on the anterior surface of the condyle and would not be depicted in an anteroposterior projection. For the temporal joint component, several studies have shown that the transcranial projection provides more diagnostic information than the transmaxillary pro-

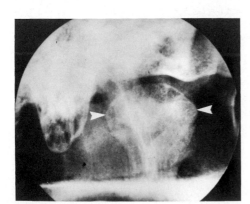

Figure 3–15
Transmaxillary projection. The mandibular condyle is clearly shown under the articular eminence. The cortical outline of the condyle is clearly seen. The inferior aspect of the articular eminence and the mastoid process also are identified. The lateral and medial poles of the condyle are indicated by arrowheads for orientation.

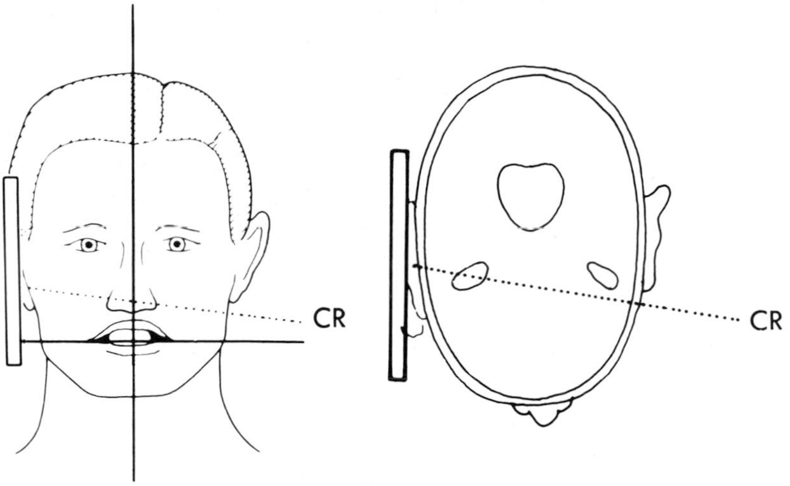

Figure 3-16
Transpharyngeal projection—schematic drawing. The central x-ray beam (CR) is directed from slightly below the horizontal plane and through the sigmoid notch on the opposite side to create an image of the condyle close to the film. (Reproduced with permission from Omnell K-Å: Radiology of the temporomandibular joint. In Irby WB: Current Advances in Oral Surgery. Vol III. St Louis, CV Mosby, 1980, pp 196–226.)

jection.[17, 20, 21] It is interesting that in these studies several of the findings were seen only with one projection. That means that findings seen in the transcranial projection were not seen in the transmaxillary projection and vice versa, which indicates that the two projections may be complementary.

Transpharyngeal Projection

A transpharyngeal projection could be an alternative to the transcranial projection, since it essentially produces a lateral image of the mandibular condyle. Schematic drawings of how this projection is obtained are shown in Figure 3–16. The image is obtained in the open-mouth position and shows essentially the mandibular condyle (Fig. 3–17). The image of the temporal component is usually not of diagnostic quality. The x-ray source is on the contralateral side; the central x-ray beam goes through the sigmoid notch, and the condyle of the opposite side is visualized under the articular eminence in the maximal mouth-open position (Fig. 3–16). The transpharyngeal projection can be successfully obtained only if the patient is able to open the mouth

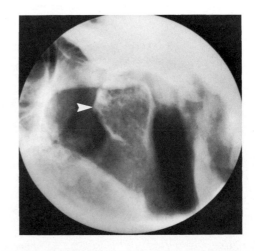

Figure 3-17
Transpharyngeal projection. The condyle is shown with good osseous details. There is a minimal osteophyte anteriorly (arrowhead). (Courtesy of Dr. Arne Petersson, Malmö, Sweden.)

sufficiently. If the condyle remains within the glenoid fossa, the transpharyngeal projection will not be successful.

The transpharyngeal projection has been used extensively to study degenerative changes of the condyle.[13–16] The greatest advantage of this projection is that it can be obtained with a dental x-ray machine, so there is no immediate need for expensive medical x-ray equipment. Obviously the image quality will improve with increasing film-focus distance and the use of a smaller focal spot, as with medical x-ray equipment, but the advantage of the transpharyngeal projection is its ready availability in the dental office. We do not recommend this technique unless the logistics of obtaining higher-quality radiographs is overwhelming. A study comparing diagnostic findings with respect to structure and tissue changes of the joint showed that more information was gained through the use of a transcranial projection than from the transpharyngeal projection.[17] However, some suggest that the transpharyngeal projection is especially useful to study small erosive changes of the condyle.[18]

Osseous changes diagnosed with the transpharyngeal projection have been compared with the transmaxillary projection: the latter provided more information about the articular eminence than did the transpharyngeal projection (Fig. 3–18).[17]

Panoramic Views

A standard panoramic radiographic unit can produce images of the TMJ (Fig. 3–19). The diagnostic value is mainly for large processes of the mandible but views extend up into the condylar neck and joint regions. It is now possible to obtain a specific view of the mandibular condyle and ramus using modern panoramic x-ray machines (Fig. 3–20). These panoramic images are especially valuable for diagnosis of fractures of the ramus and possibly for assessment of mandibular asymmetry due to changes in vertical ramus height. With these techniques, the mandibular component of the joint can be visualized as in the transpharyngeal projection but with superior image quality because of the tomographic technique incorporated in panoramic machines. The temporal bone component cannot be visualized with any degree of certainty. A few advanced panoramic radiographic units can produce linear tomographic images of the joint.

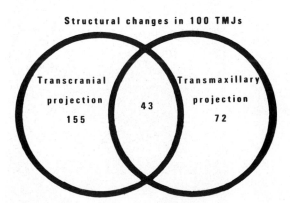

Figure 3–18
Comparison of transcranial and transmaxillary projection. Structural hard tissue changes in 100 TMJs as detected with transcranial and transmaxillary projection. The majority of the osseous changes were seen with only one of the two projections. Therefore the projections are complementary. (Numbers derived from Hansson L-G, Petersson A: Radiography of the temporomandibular joint using the transpharyngeal projection. Dentomaxillofac Radiol 1978;7:69–78.)

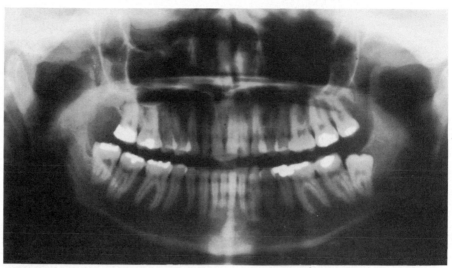

Figure 3–19
Panoramic radiograph. The maxilla and mandible are shown, as well as a relatively good image of the mandibular condyles.

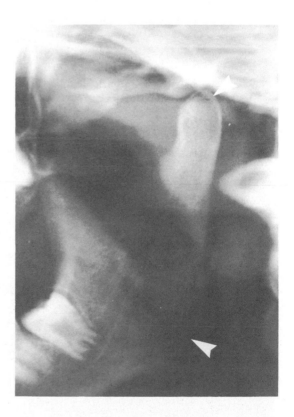

Figure 3–20
This panoramic view of the mandibular condyle and ramus was obtained with the Siemens Orthophos Panoramic X-Ray machine. It produces a tomographic section through the ramus and through the mandibular condyle. The mandibular condyle and the angle of the mandible are indicated by arrowheads for orientation.

TOMOGRAPHY

A more sophisticated imaging technique is linear or multidirectional tomography. Tomography implies sectional radiography in which a single section of the body is imaged, with structures on both sides of the tomographic section being blurred by a controlled simultaneous motion of the film and the x-ray source during exposure. The technique thereby eliminates obscuring superimpositions and depicts correct anatomic relationships between objects located in the tomographic plane, such as the mandibular condyle and glenoid fossa. Disadvantages of tomography are its higher cost and higher radiation dose. Several workers have assessed the value of tomography for imaging the TMJ.[10, 22–27]

The principle of tomography is that a predetermined tissue layer, the tomographic plane, is reproduced with constant magnification and with minimized tomographic unsharpness. Dense osseous structures outside the tomographic plane should be blurred but may give rise to ghost images in the tomograph image. This phenomenon frequently occurs with structures like the base of the skull and the temporal bone. These ghost images usually do not present a problem for interpretation when one knows anatomy and is experienced in tomographic imaging.

Many x-ray film-tube tomographic motions are available, such as linear, circular, ellipsoid, hypocycloidal, and tri-spiral. The hypocycloidal and tri-spiral movements are optimal for imaging the TMJ.[28] Upright patient positioning is aided by a cephalostat attached to a Philips polytome U (Philips Massiot, Paris, France), as shown in Figure 3–21. The cephalostat (Fig. 3–22) can rotate around its vertical axis: the patient's head can be positioned so that the horizontal long axis of the condyle of the joint being examined will be parallel to the central x-ray beam. This means that the tomographic plane will be perpendicular to the long axis of the condyle.

Tomography has been available for many years; Petrilli and Gurley presented high-quality tomograms of the TMJ as early as 1939.[29] Another pioneer in TMJ tomography was Ricketts, who used tomography on a series of normal

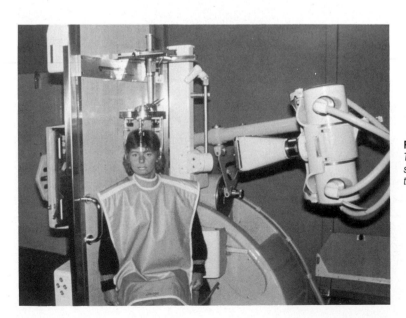

Figure 3–21
Tomography—patient positioning. The cephalostat is used for accurate orientation of the patient's head.

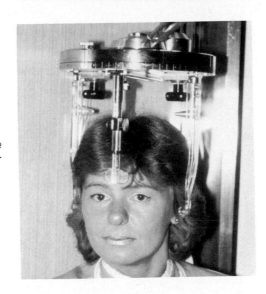

Figure 3–22
A cephalostat is used for orientation of the patient during tomography. It can be adjusted every fifth degree in order to have the sagittal tomographic sections perpendicular to the horizontal long axis of the mandibular condyle.

individuals to characterize the tomographic appearance of a normal joint.[30, 31] Ricketts oriented the patient's head so that the horizontal long axis of the condyle was perpendicular to the tomographic plane and called this form of TMJ tomography cephalometric laminagraphy.[30] Extensive use of TMJ tomography was described by Yale and others during the 1960s and 1970s.[25, 32–35] Several investigators have pointed out the value of tomography to determine the true relationship between the mandibular condyle and the glenoid fossa. However, controversy exists about the clinical significance of the position of the condyle in the glenoid fossa, since similar variations are noted in normal as well as abnormal subjects. Stanson and Baker showed that the diagnostic yield increased substantially for tomography compared with regular transcranial films.[25]

Simultaneous Tomography

Simultaneous tomography is a technique in which multiple films are exposed at the same time. By building a "book cassette" (Fig. 3–23) with three, five, or even seven films, and having a distance of approximately 2 to 3 mm between each film, it is possible to image several tomographic layers with one exposure.[36] Simultaneous tomography has been used extensively for TMJ imaging. Its two advantages are increased speed and decreased radiation dose. However, note that the decreased radiation dose is not proportional to the number of slices in one exposure, because the intensifying screens used in simultaneous tomography cannot be as efficient as single films. As a rule of thumb, the reduction of the radiation dose by the use of simultaneous tomography is somewhere around 50 per cent, compared with the same number of single exposures.

Thickness of Tomographic Layer

The optimal thickness of a tomographic layer using hypercycloidal motion is approximately 3 to 4 mm for imaging of the TMJ. This is an empirical

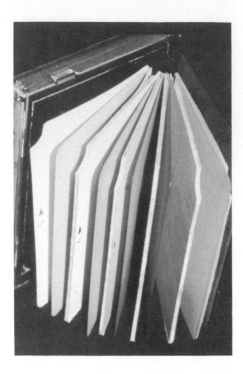

Figure 3–23
Cassette for simultaneous tomography. Five films and five pairs of intensifying screens are available.

estimate, because theoretically only an infinitesimal layer is optimally sharp, and then the unsharpness increases on each side. Eventually, the unsharpness becomes so pronounced that no anatomic structures can be identified, and this is the principle of tomography. For these reasons it is not possible to give a number for the thickness of the tomographic layer, unless the degree of unsharpness is also mathematically defined. The thickness of the tomographic layer obviously varies with the motion pattern but also with the morphology of the object being imaged. Tomography can be performed in the sagittal,[19] coronal,[26] and axial planes,[37] and the same principle with regard to tomographic thickness applies to all planes.

Individualized Sagittal Tomography

Several workers have recommended that the plane of tomographic sectioning should be perpendicular to the long axis of the mandibular condyle for lateral or sagittal tomography.[10, 26, 27, 38] Patient orientation can be determined by the submentovertical projection. To achieve individualized sagittal tomography, we have used a cephalometric device attached to the tomographic unit (Figs. 3–21 and 3–22). The patient's head can be oriented, based on measurements in the submentovertical projection, so that the horizontal long axis of the mandibular condyle becomes perpendicular to the tomographic plane for sagittal tomography and parallel to this plane for coronal or frontal tomography. One group of clinicians has also recommended that head positioning in a sideways orientation be corrected for the angulation of the condyle in the frontal plane.[26] Tomographic images obtained with the head position corrected in both the horizontal and frontal planes have been called corrected lateral tomography or cephalometrically corrected lateral tomography. The images can be of high quality, but no definitive study has demonstrated a significant difference in diagnostic accuracy between straight sagittal and oblique sagittal tomography. Eckerdal showed that there was an impressive degree of correspondence between lateral tomography and corresponding anatomic sections, even if the tomographic layer was not perfectly perpendicular to the long axis of the condyle.[34]

Lateral tomography, even when performed with correction for the angulation of the condyle, depicts only the central two thirds of the joint.[34] This means that approximately 3 mm of the lateral part of the joint and another 3 mm of the most medial part of the joint will not be imaged with tomography. This is a disadvantage since it has been shown that hard tissue pathology is frequently located in the most lateral aspect of the condyle and temporal bony components.[39]

A sagittal tomogram of an asymptomatic volunteer with a normal joint is shown in Figure 3–24. Frontal tomography also can be performed on the TMJ (Fig. 3–25), although this technique has not been as extensively used as sagittal tomography. Due to limited resolution, frontal or anteroposterior tomography is essentially diagnostic for osseous changes in the condyle. Anteroposterior or frontal tomography is probably of greatest value for diagnosis of subtle osseous changes of the condyle not seen on plain films.

FINDINGS IN PLAIN FILM AND TOMOGRAPHY

Condyle Position in the Glenoid Fossa

The radiographic anatomy in the lateral oblique transcranial projection has been extensively described.[10, 40] There are different opinions regarding the reliability of the transcranial projection to show the position of the condyle relative to the glenoid fossa. One group of investigators suggests that the standardized transcranial projection can demonstrate the relative joint space with accuracy[40, 41] and that the transcranial projection with the aid of fluoroscopy

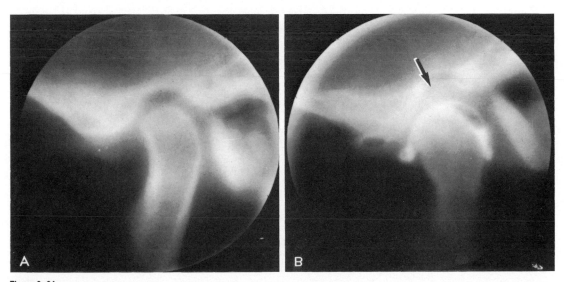

Figure 3–24
Sagittal tomogram and corresponding double-contrast arthrotomogram of an asymptomatic volunteer with a normal joint. The tomogram (A) shows a normal osseous component. The dual space double-contrast arthrotomogram (B) shows the disk in normal position. The posterior band (arrow) is located superior to the condyle.

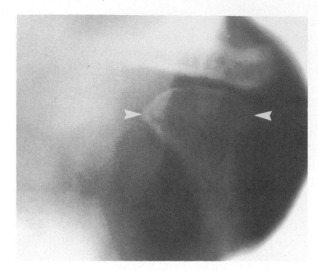

Figure 3–25
Frontal tomogram showing normal osseous structures. Arrowheads identify medial and lateral poles of the condyle. (Courtesy of Dr. Arne Petersson, Malmö, Sweden.)

provides the most accurate depiction of the true condylar position.[42, 43] Another opinion is that the joint space dimension cannot be accurately demonstrated by the transcranial projection.[10, 22, 23, 44, 45] A study comparing the condylar position using transcranial projection and tomography found that there is concordance in only 60 per cent of cases.[45] It is clear from the literature that the condylar position cannot be reliably determined using a transcranial projection;[4] a tomographic examination is necessary.

As noted, tomography is the method of choice if there is a clinical need to determine the position of the mandibular condyle in the glenoid fossa. This question may have relevance for patients undergoing orthognathic surgery or extensive orthodontic treatment and patients with dual bite undergoing extensive restorative dental work.

Multiple mediolateral sections must be obtained, since frequently there is variation of the condyle position within the same joint (Fig. 3–26). One study

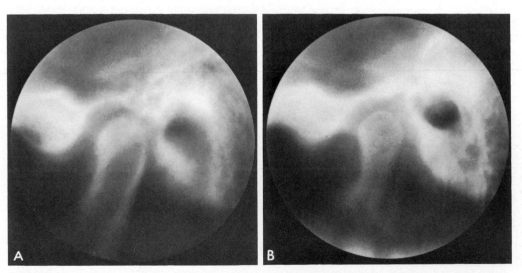

Figure 3–26
Difference in condylar position. Tomograms from the lateral (A) and medial (B) aspects of a TMJ. In the lateral part of the joint (A), the condyle is located posteriorly in the glenoid fossa. In the medial part the condyle is located in a central position. The two images were obtained in the same exposure, using the cassette for simultaneous tomography. (Courtesy of Dr. Arne Petersson, Malmö, Sweden.)

showed that the condyle position varied from medial to lateral within the same patient in 55 per cent of the subjects.[10] A similar study on normal subjects showed the same variation in 18 per cent.[45] This has also been demonstrated by computed tomography.[46] Thus, multiple tomographic images are necessary to determine the condyle position in the glenoid fossa.

Another important question is the significance of "abnormal condylar position." Katzberg and associates showed no correlation of condyle position in patients with or without internal derangement studied by arthrography.[47] Using tomography only, Pullinger and colleagues[48] showed that the condyle was radiographically concentric in the center of the glenoid fossa in only 50 to 65 per cent in the asymptomatic population, with a large degree of variability.[49] The same group showed that posterior condylar position is more frequent in patients than in normal individuals.[49] However, normal subjects still have a 22 per cent prevalence of the posterior condylar position.[49] Other studies also have demonstrated a slightly higher prevalence of the posterior condylar position in patients with disk displacement than in normal subjects.[50] On the other hand, in the same study, 42 per cent of the patients with a normal disk and absence of arthrosis also showed posterior condyle disk position in the glenoid fossa.

Based on the large variation of condyle position in tomographic studies, both in asymptomatic and symptomatic individuals, it is our opinion that the condyle-fossa relationship is only of very limited value for diagnosis. It could be valuable in patients undergoing orthognathic surgery or extensive orthodontic treatment, or after trauma. However, for the usual patient with signs and symptoms of TMJ disorders, the position of the condyle seems to be of relatively little clinical significance.

If there is a strong clinical need for determining the position of the condyle in the glenoid fossa, tomography should be used.[30, 32, 51-54] A transcranial projection is not reliable for determining the condylar position.

Condylar Translation at Maximal Mouth Opening

In normal joints, the condyle will translate to the most inferior aspect of the articular eminence or more anteriorly (Figs. 3–10 and 3–27). Restriction of anterior condylar translation at maximal mouth opening implies that the condyle does not translate all the way to the most inferior aspect of the articular eminence. This is an unspecific sign of abnormality. Based on the finding of limited condylar translation, the etiology of the restricted range of motion cannot be determined from plain films or tomograms in most instances.

Occasionally it can be seen that the distance between the mandibular condyle and the posterior slope of the articular eminence increases on opening in a joint with restricted range of motion (Fig. 3–28). This is an indication that soft tissue is interposed between the joint components, which may indicate disk displacement without reduction (Fig. 3–28) but is not pathognomonic.

The motion pattern of the mandible on opening has traditionally been described as a combination of rotation and translation. Rotation occurs in the beginning, and during the last phase of opening there is more translation. In clinical work we have recognized several different patterns of jaw motion on opening. However, the significance of the different motion patterns is unknown.

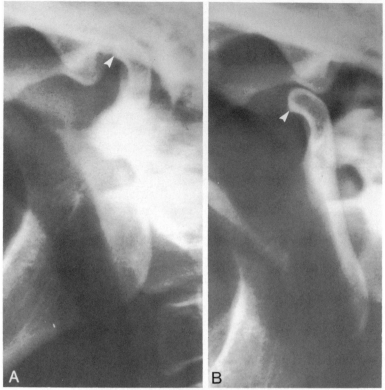

Figure 3–27
Normal range of motion. Panoramic views of a mandibular condyle and ramus obtained at closed mouth position (A) and at maximal mouth opening (B), showing the normal range of motion. There are mild remodeling changes of the condyle. The anterior aspect of the condyle is indicated by arrowheads for orientation.

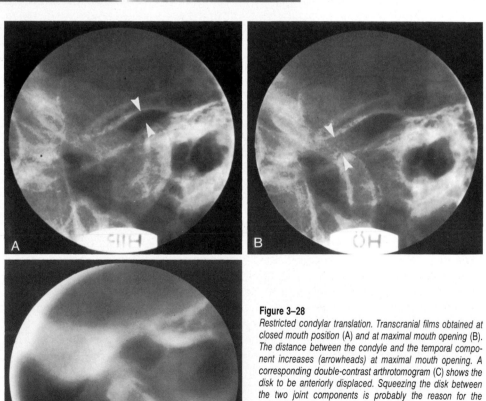

Figure 3–28
Restricted condylar translation. Transcranial films obtained at closed mouth position (A) and at maximal mouth opening (B). The distance between the condyle and the temporal component increases (arrowheads) at maximal mouth opening. A corresponding double-contrast arthrotomogram (C) shows the disk to be anteriorly displaced. Squeezing the disk between the two joint components is probably the reason for the increased distance between the condyle and the temporal component at maximal mouth opening.

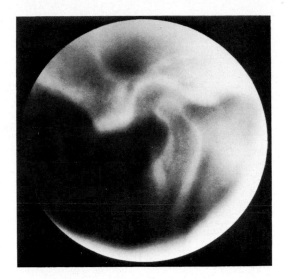

Figure 3-29
Tomogram of joint with advanced remodeling of the condyle. There are no erosive changes, and the condyle is marginated by cortical bone. This indicates remodeling. There is some sclerosis in the articular eminence.

Osseous Changes

The mildest forms of osseous changes have been described as deviations in form or remodeling (Fig. 3–27). An example of a joint with relatively advanced remodeling of the mandibular condyle is shown in Figure 3–29. Remodeling implies changes in the form of the osseous components of the joint, with an intact cortex and without erosions.

More advanced osseous changes include flattening (Fig. 3–30), osteophytosis (Fig. 3–31), sclerosis (Fig. 3–32), and erosion. All these can be diagnosed by plain film or tomography. Comparisons of the different techniques indicate that tomography is superior to plain film (see Figure 3–8).[10, 22]

Two separate studies in patients with suspected internal derangement showed that extensive changes were seen essentially only in joints with advanced internal derangement (Fig. 3–30).[55, 56] Osseous changes were rarely seen in normal joints or in joints with earlier stages of disk displacement with reduction.

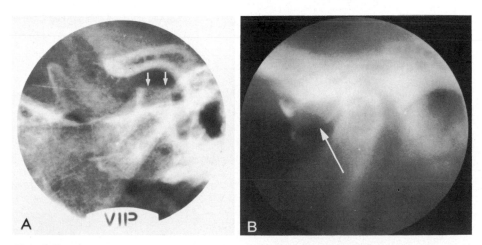

Figure 3-30
Transcranial projection (A) showing flattening (small arrows) of the condyle. Dual space double-contrast arthrotomogram (B) of the same joint, showing anterior displacement and deformation of disk. The posterior band of the disk is indicated by an arrow in B.

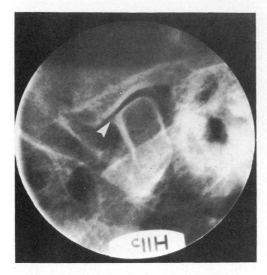

Figure 3–31
Anterior osteophytosis. Transcranial projection showing flattening of condyle and temporal component and an anterior osteophyte of the condyle (arrowhead).

Minimal flattening of the condyle or articular tubercle may be seen in asymptomatic volunteers without internal derangements (Fig. 3–33) and should not be interpreted as abnormal or a sign of arthrosis.[59] These flattenings were all discrete, well-marginated with cortical bone, and not associated with other osseous changes.

Studies of cadaver material have shown that changes in the condyle are more easily detected with radiographic methods than are those in the temporal component.[57, 58] Dissection studies, however, reveal that more changes actually occur in the temporal joint component than in the condyle. The overrepresentation of changes in the condyle in radiographic studies is probably a result of the technique.

Plain film imaging is essential when examining patients with inflammatory arthritis: rheumatoid arthritis,[60] psoriatic arthritis,[61] and ankylosing spondylitis.[62] Modern imaging techniques in the patient with inflammatory arthritis are extensively reviewed in Chapter 8.

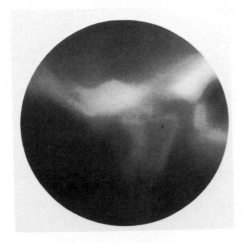

Figure 3–32
Extensive sclerosis in the articular tubercle. There are also extensive flattenings and osteophytosis of the condyle in this patient with inflammatory arthritis. (Courtesy of Dr. Arne Petersson, Malmö, Sweden.)

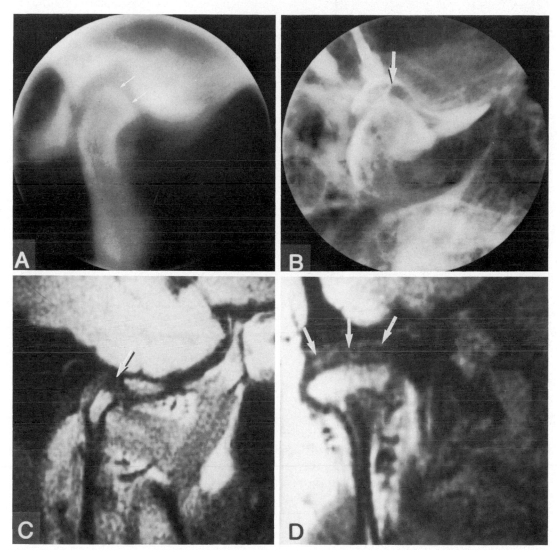

Figure 3–33
Minimal flattening of the condyle (arrows in A) in a joint of an asymptomatic volunteer without internal derangement. A double-contrast arthrogram (B) shows the disk (arrow) in normal superior position. Sagittal (C) and coronal (D) MR scans show the disk (arrows) in a normal location.

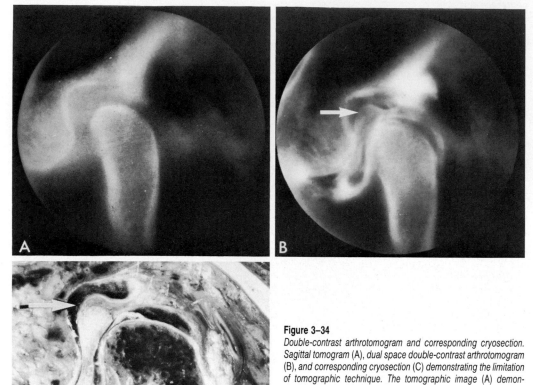

Figure 3–34
Double-contrast arthrotomogram and corresponding cryosection. Sagittal tomogram (A), dual space double-contrast arthrotomogram (B), and corresponding cryosection (C) demonstrating the limitation of tomographic technique. The tomographic image (A) demonstrates only the osseous parts of the joint. The posterior band of the disk is identified by the arrow.

Correlation with Soft Tissue Anatomy

Tomography, double-contrast arthrotomograms, and their corresponding cryosections are shown in Figure 3–34. These illustrate that even with the best possible technique only the osseous components of the joints are demonstrated with tomography. The more important soft tissue components of the joint are not accessible to diagnosis with plain film or tomography.

RADIATION DOSE

The radiation dose from plain film imaging and tomography has been found to be low. The average dose from one transcranial exposure to the parotid glands was 0.41 mGy. The average dose from one tomographic exposure with simultaneous cassette for five films was 0.13 mGy for the site toward the tube.[8] If anteroposterior tomography is used, the dose to the eye can be reduced significantly by the use of protective lead glasses. The energy imparted for a complete plain film examination, including submentovertical, four exposures of transcranial lateral oblique, two exposures of transmaxillary, and lateral tomography of both left and right joints, was 3.4 mGy.

CONCLUSION

Plain film and tomographic examinations are useful screening modalities. They are valuable for determining the presence of osseous changes and traumatic injury to the osseous components of the joint. Determination of condyle position can be valuable in patients undergoing orthognathic surgery, extensive orthodontic work, or prosthodontic work, as well as following trauma. It is our opinion that the position of the condyle in the glenoid fossa is not reliable as a diagnostic finding by itself. Findings of arthrosis on plain films or tomograms are valuable but nonspecific. Negative plain films are most frequent but do not provide information regarding the presence or absence of soft tissue disease.

References

1. Lindblom G: On the anatomy and function of the temporomandibular joint. Acta Odontol Scand 1960;(Suppl 28):17.
2. Clementschitsch F: Die Röntgendarstellung der Kiefergelenke. Röntgendiagnostik des Schädels. II. *In* Diethelm L, Strand F, eds: Handbuch der medizinischen Radiologie VII/2. Berlin, Springer-Verlag, 1963.
3. Omnell K-Å: Radiology of the TMJ. *In* Irby WB, ed: Current Advances in Oral Surgery. Vol III. St. Louis, CV Mosby, 1990, pp 196–226.
4. Petersson A: Plain film imaging and tomography. *In* Westesson P-L, Katzberg RW, eds: Imaging of the Temporomandibular Joint. Cranio Clinics International. Baltimore, Williams & Wilkins, 1991, pp 1–16.
5. Lysell L, Petersson A: The submento-vertex projection in radiography of the temporomandibular joint. Dentomaxillofac Radiol 1980;9:11–17.
6. Westesson P-L, Bifano JA, Tallents RH, Hatala MP: Increased horizontal angle of the mandibular condyle in abnormal temporomandibular joints. A magnetic resonance imaging study. Oral Surg Oral Med Oral Pathol 1991;72:359–363.
7. Westesson P-L, Liedberg J: Horizontal condylar angle in relation to internal derangement of the temporomandibular joint. Oral Surg Oral Med Oral Pathol 1987;64:391–394.
8. Borglin K, Petersson A, Rohlin M, Thapper K: Radiation dosimetry in radiology of the temporomandibular joint. Br J Radiol 1984;57:997–1007.
9. Palla S: Eine Mittelwertprojektion für Kiefergelenkaufnahmen in schräglateraler Projektion. Schweiz Mschr Zahnheilk 1976;86:1207–1226.
10. Omnell K-Å, Petersson A: Radiography of the temporomandibular joint utilizing oblique lateral transcranial projections. Comparison of information obtained with standardized technique and individualized technique. Odontol Review 1976;27:77–92.
11. Petersson A: Reproducibility of temporomandibular joint radiographs utilizing transmaxillary projection and oblique lateral transcranial projection with individualized technique. Dentomaxillofac Radiol 1975;4:85–88.
12. Kundert M: Limits of perceptibility of condyle displacements on temporomandibular joint radiographs. J Oral Rehabil 1979;6:375–383.
13. Isberg-Holm A, Ivarsson R: The movement pattern of mandibular condyles in individuals with and without clicking. Dentomaxillofac Radiol 1980;9:55–65.
14. Boering G: Arthrosis deformans van het kaakgewricht. Thesis, Rijksuniversiteit te Groningen, 1966.
15. Toller RA: The transpharyngeal radiography for arthritis of the mandibular condyle. Br J Oral Surg 1969;7:47–54.
16. Rasmussen OC: Longitudinal study of transpharyngeal radiography in temporomandibular arthropathy. Scand J Dent Res 1980;88:257–268.
17. Hansson L-G, Petersson A: Radiography of the temporomandibular joint using the transpharyngeal projection. A comparison study of information obtained with different radiographic techniques. Dentomaxillofac Radiol 1978;7:69–78.
18. Larheim TA, Johannessen S: Transpharyngeal radiography of mandibular condyle. Comparison with other conventional methods. Acta Radiol Diagn 1985;26:167–171.
19. McCabe JB, Keller SE, Moffett BC: A new radiographic technique for diagnosing temporomandibular joint disorders. J Dent Res 1959;38:663–673.
20. Petersson A, Nanthaviroj S: Radiography of the temporomandibular joint utilizing the transmaxillary projection. A comparison of the information obtained with the oblique lateral transcranial projection versus the transmaxillary projection. Dentomaxillofac Radiol 1975;4:76–83.

21. Larheim TA, Tveito L, Dale K, Ruud AF: Temporomandibular joint abnormalities in rheumatoid arthritis. Comparison of different radiographic methods. Acta Radiol Diagn 1981;*22*:703–707.
22. Klein IE, Blatterfein L, Miglino JC: Comparison of the fidelity of radiographs of mandibular condyles made by different techniques. J Prosthet Dent 1970;*24*:419–452.
23. Eckerdal O, Lundberg M: Temporomandibular joint relations as revealed by conventional radiographic techniques. A comparison with the morphology and tomographic images. Dentomaxillofac Radiol 1979;*8*:65–70.
24. Eckerdal O: Tomography of the temporomandibular joint. Correlation between tomographic image and histologic sections in a three-dimensional system. [Dissertation.] Acta Radiol Suppl 1973;*324*:107.
25. Stanson AW, Baker HL Jr: Routine tomography of the temporomandibular joint. Radiol Clin North Am 1976;*14*:105–127.
26. Rosenberg HM, Graczyk RJ: Temporomandibular articulation tomography: A corrected anteroposterior and lateral cephalometric technique. Oral Surg Oral Med Oral Pathol 1986;*62*:198–204.
27. Heffez L, Jordan S, Rosenberg H, Miescke K: Accuracy of temporomandibular joint space measurements using corrected hypocycloidal tomography. J Oral Maxillofac Surg 1987;*45*:137–142.
28. Eckerdal O: Tomography of the temporomandibular joint. Medica Mundi 1971;*16*:144.
29. Petrilli A, Gurley JF: Tomography of the temporomandibular joint. J Am Dent Assoc 1939;*26*:218–224.
30. Ricketts RM: Variations of the temporomandibular joint as revealed by cephalometric laminagraphy. Am J Orthod 1950;*36*:877–898.
31. Ricketts RM: Laminagraphy in the diagnosis of temporomandibular joint disorders. J Am Dent Assoc 1953;*46*:620–648.
32. Yale SH: Radiographic evaluation of the temporomandibular joint. J Am Dent Assoc 1969;*79*:102–107.
33. Yale SH, Rosenberg HM, Cellabos M, Hauptfuehrer JD: Laminagraphic cephalometry in the analysis of mandibular condyle morphology: A preliminary report. Oral Surg Oral Med Oral Pathol 1961;*14*:793–805.
34. Eckerdal O: Tomography of the temporomandibular joint: Correlation between tomographic image and histologic sections in a three-dimensional system. Acta Radiol Diagn (Stockh) 1973; Suppl 329:196.
35. Williamson EH, Wilson CW: Use of a submentovertical analysis for producing quality temporomandibular joint laminagraphs. Am J Orthod 1976;*70*:200–207.
36. Petersson AR, Gratt BM: A rare-earth screen multisection cassette for temporomandibular joint tomography: A technical report. Dentomaxillofac Radiol 1985;*14*:31–36.
37. Faivovoch G, Omnell K-Å, Svensson A: Precision technique for positioning the head during tomography. AJR 1979;*132*:477–479.
38. Omnell K-Å: Radiology of the TMJ. *In* Irby WB, ed: Current Advances in Oral Surgery. Vol III. St. Louis, CV Mosby, 1980, pp 196–226.
39. Öberg T, Carlsson GE, Fajers CM: The temporomandibular joint: A morphologic study on human autopsy material. Acta Odontol Scand 1971;*29*:349–384.
40. Weinberg LA: What we really see in a TMJ radiograph. J Prosthet Dent 1973;*30*:898–913.
41. Mongini F: The importance of radiography in the diagnosis of the TMJ dysfunctions. A comparative evaluation of transcranial radiographs and serial tomography. J Prosthet Dent 1981;*45*:186–198.
42. Preti G, Fava C: Lateral transcranial radiography of temporomandibular joints. I. Validity in skulls and patients. J Prosthet Dent 1988;*59*:85–93.
43. Fava C, Preti G: Lateral transcranial radiography of temporomandibular joints. II. Image formation studied with computerized tomography. J Prosthet Dent 1988;*59*:218–227.
44. Aquilino SA, Matteson SR, Holland GA, Phillips C: Evaluation of condylar positions from temporomandibular joint radiographs. J Prosthet Dent 1985;*53*:88–97.
45. Pullinger AG, Hollender L, Solberg WK, Petersson A: A tomographic study of mandibular condyle position in an asymptomatic population. J Prosthet Dent 1985;*53*:706–713.
46. Christiansen EL, Thompson JR, Zimmerman G, et al: Computed tomography of condylar and articular disk positions within the temporomandibular joint. Oral Surg Oral Med Oral Pathol 1987;*64*:757–767.
47. Katzberg RW, Keith DA, Ten Eick WR, Gurolnick WC: Internal derangements of the temporomandibular joint: An assessment of condylar position in centric occlusion. J Prosthet Dent 1983;*49*:250–254.
48. Pullinger AG, Solberg WK, Hollender L, Guichet D: Tomographic analysis of mandibular condyle position in diagnostic subgroups of temporomandibular disorders. J Prosthet Dent 1986;*55*:723–729.
49. Pullinger A, Hollender L: Assessment of mandibular condyle position: A comparison of transcranial radiographs and linear tomograms. Oral Surg Oral Med Oral Pathol 1985;*60*:329–334.

50. Brand JW, Whinery JG Jr, Anderson QN, Keenan KM: The effects of temporomandibular joint internal derangement and degenerative joint disease on tomographic and arthrotomographic images. Oral Surg Oral Med Oral Pathol 1989;67:220–223.
51. Rosenberg HM: Laminagraphy: Methods and application in oral diagnosis. J Am Dent Assoc 1967;74:88–96.
52. Lundberg M, Welander U: The articular cavity in the temporomandibular joint: A comparison between the oblique-lateral and the tomographic image. Medica Mundi 1970;15:27.
53. Rosenzweig D: Three-dimensional tomographic study of the temporomandibular articulation. J Periodontol 1975;46:348.
54. Tréheux A, Martin G: La tomographic sélective dans l'étude de l'articulation temporomandibulaire. J Radiol Electrol Med Nucl 1975;56:691.
55. Katzberg RW, Keith DA, Guralnick WC, et al: Internal derangements and arthritis of the temporomandibular joint. Radiology 1983;146:107–112.
56. Westesson P-L: Structural hard-tissue changes in temporomandibular joints with internal derangement. Oral Surg Oral Med Oral Pathol 1985;59:220–224.
57. Lindvall A-M, Helkimo E, Hollender L, Carlsson GE: Radiographic examination of the temporomandibular joint: A comparison between radiographic findings and gross and microscopic morphologic observations. Dentomaxillofac Radiol 1976;5:24–32.
58. Rohlin M, Åkerman S, Kopp S: Tomography as an aid to detect macroscopic changes of the temporomandibular joint. An autopsy study of the aged. Acta Odontol Scand 1986;44:131–140.
59. Brooks SL, Westesson P-L, Eriksson L, et al: Prevalence of osseous changes in the temporomandibular joint of asymptomatic persons without internal derangement. Oral Surg Oral Med Oral Pathol 1992;73:122–126.
60. Larheim TA, Storhaug K, Tveito L: Temporomandibular joint involvement and dental occlusion in a group of adults with rheumatoid arthritis. Acta Odontol Scand 1983;41:301–309.
61. Könönen M: Radiographic changes in the condyle of the temporomandibular joint in psoriatic arthritis. Acta Radiol Diagn 1987;28:185–188.
62. Wenneberg B, Hollender L, Kopp S: Radiographic changes in the temporomandibular joint in ankylosing spondylitis. Dentomaxillofac Radiol 1983;12:25–30.

CHAPTER FOUR

Temporomandibular Joint Arthrography

Section I · Single-Contrast Arthrography

HISTORY AND DEVELOPMENT OF TEMPOROMANDIBULAR JOINT ARTHROGRAPHY

Arthrography of the temporomandibular joint (TMJ) was first described by the Swiss radiologist Zimmer,[1] but the Danish professor of radiology, Flemming Nørgaard (Fig. 4–1), was the first to describe a standardized technique and to demonstrate its potential value in the diagnosis of soft tissue derangement of the joint.[2, 3] However, Nørgaard had few advocates, and the technique of arthrography of the TMJ had only limited clinical use for many years. Reasons for the skeptical attitude toward this examination can be attributed to at least three disadvantages: (1) puncture of the joint compartment may be technically difficult; (2) the examination may be painful for the patient; and (3) information gained from the examination at this early stage in development was usually of only limited value for treatment planning and evaluation of prognosis.[4, 5]

By the end of the 1970s the importance of arthrography gained increasing recognition, and this examination is now employed frequently at many institutions.[6] The change in attitude was probably the result of three factors: (1) application of the image intensifier to facilitate puncture of the joint[7, 8] and to observe and record joint dynamics;[9] (2) identification of anterior disk displacement as a common cause of TMJ pain and dysfunction;[7, 8, 10–15] and finally, but probably most importantly, (3) the introduction of new concepts in conservative and surgical methods to treat disk displacement that required an accurate assessment of the status and function of the joint.[16–22]

The improved quality of the images readily achieved by a combination of arthrography and tomography probably also favorably influenced the use of arthrography.[7, 8, 14, 15, 23, 24]

A technique for double-contrast arthrotomography of the TMJ was introduced by Arnaudow and colleagues in the late 1960s.[25, 26] This technique was further refined and introduced in routine clinical work during the early 1980s and is discussed in greater detail in Section II of this chapter.[27–30]

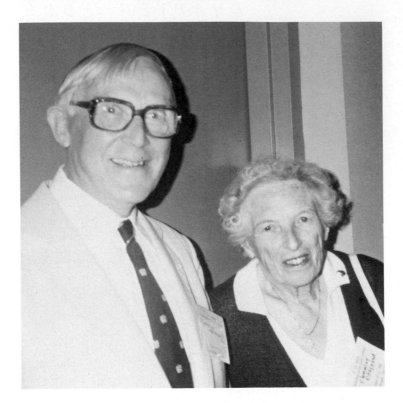

Figure 4–1
Dr. and Mrs. Flemming Nørgaard. Dr. Nørgaard is a pioneer in the development of arthrography of the TMJ. He published a thesis on the topic in 1947 while in Denmark.

INDICATIONS AND OBJECTIVES OF ARTHROGRAPHY

Temporomandibular joint arthrography is indicated to evaluate the soft tissue components, especially disk position, function, and morphology in those patients presenting with a suspected internal derangement of the TMJ (Table 4–1). The most common presenting complaints in these patients are TMJ pain, muscle tenderness, headaches, clicking, and limitation of jaw movement (locking) (Table 4–2). The ability to assess the soft tissue components of the TMJ allows arthrography to go beyond the simple delineation of osseous structures as in transcranial or tomographic radiographs (Fig. 4–2A to C).

Two major components to the clinical presentation are related to internal derangement and indicate the need for a definitive diagnosis of the TMJ: (1) the mechanical dysfunction of the joint, an objective component, manifested

Table 4–1
INDICATIONS FOR ARTHROGRAPHY

Common
- Assess position, function, and configuration of the disk
- Differential diagnosis in patients with diffuse facial and head pain
- Establish jaw position for protrusive splint therapy

Uncommon
- Diagnosis of loose bodies in the joint spaces
- Evaluation after trauma
- Aspiration of joint fluid
- Intra-articular injections

Table 4–2
COMMON PRESENTING COMPLAINTS OF INTERNAL DERANGEMENT

- Pain localized to the temporomandibular joint region
- Muscle tenderness around the temporomandibular joint region
- Clicking in the joint
- Limitation of jaw movement, often with asymmetric deviation on opening

by clicking or limitation of mouth opening or, more unusual, both; and (2) the subjective component manifested by pain and tenderness in and around the joint.[31] It is uncommon in our experience for patients to have an internal derangement of the TMJ when there is no current or previous evidence for range of motion abnormalities or joint noise. These clinical aspects of the physical findings and history should be clearly identified and communicated to the radiologist by the referring clinician prior to performance of the imaging procedure. The arthrogram can be used not only for the diagnosis of a specific

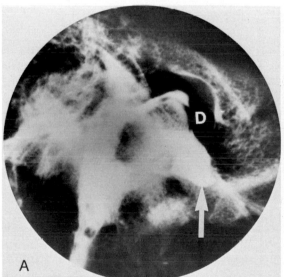
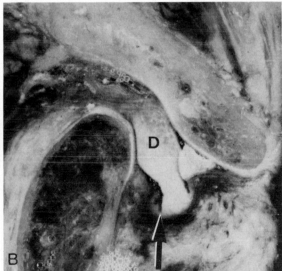

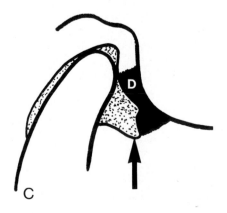

Figure 4–2
A, Transcranial arthrogram of specimen with anteriorly displaced disk. The anterior space (arrow) is larger than normal and the disk (D) is anteriorly displaced. B, The corresponding cryosection confirms the arthrographic observations of displaced disk (D, arrow) C, Schematic drawing with contrast medium injected into lower joint space (arrow) and demonstrating displaced disk (D).

Table 4–3
RELATIVE CONTRAINDICATIONS TO TEMPOROMANDIBULAR JOINT ARTHROGRAPHY

• Prior severe reaction to contrast material	• Infections in the preauricular area
• Excessive patient apprehension	• Bleeding disorder or anticoagulant medication

type of internal derangement but also to assist in the initial stages of protrusive splint therapy.

We strongly believe that TMJ imaging, whether arthrography or magnetic resonance (MR), is an integral component of the patient evaluation prior to the initiation of treatment, since the treatment can be more rigorously tailored to the specific type of disk abnormality. On the other hand, imaging of the soft tissue component of the TMJ is also valuable in those patients who have persistent complaints or vague symptomatology that does not respond to symptomatic therapy (Table 4–1).Uncommon indications for arthrography are for the delineation of loose bodies within the inferior and superior joint spaces, postoperative evaluation, recent injury, and diagnostic aspiration of joint fluid.

RELATIVE CONTRAINDICATIONS TO ARTHROGRAPHY

Arthrography in general is a safe procedure, and idiosyncratic reactions to intra-articular contrast media are rare. A review of 126,000 arthrographic examinations of many joints, not just the TMJ, revealed no deaths, 3 cases of infection, and 61 cases of hives.[6] Only a single case of idiosyncratic reaction to non-ionic contrast media injected into the TMJ has been reported.[32] Other acute but extremely uncommon reactions that have been reported for arthrography as a whole include hypotension, seizures, air embolism, and laryngeal edema. Minor complications were sterile chemical synovitis, pain after the procedure, and vasovagal responses.

However, arthrography is performed with caution and only after premedication with corticosteroids in patients who have a history of a prior severe reaction to iodinated contrast media (Table 4–3). With the advent of new imaging modalities such as computed tomography (CT) and magnetic resonance imaging (MRI), it is usually not necessary to obtain arthrograms on patients who have had previous severe reactions. However, after premedication with corticosteroids (Table 4–4), we have successfully obtained arthrograms on such patients without untoward reactions; and, indeed, serious and life-threatening reactions are extremely rare with arthrography as a whole. The utilization of air only as the contrast is another technique for evaluating the TMJ without the injection of iodinated material. With the introduction of the new non-ionic and dimeric contrast media, the risk of complication from arthrography is even less.[33]

Table 4–4
PREMEDICATION OF PATIENTS WITH PREVIOUS HISTORY OF REACTIONS TO CONTRAST MEDIUM

• 50 mg of prednisone orally every 4 hour three times prior to the procedure—the last dose one hour prior to the procedure
• 25–50 mg of diphenhydramine (Benadryl) orally prior to the procedure

Excessive patient apprehension can lead to a vagal response during the arthrographic procedure, and thus every attempt should be made to allay the patient's fears. If a vagal response should occur, the patient is aroused with ammonia and managed supportively; if the reaction is persistent and severe, 0.8 to 1 mg of atropine is administered intravenously.

Bleeding disorders and anticoagulation medication are relative contraindications to arthrography. Anticoagulants can be discontinued in advance of the procedure. Arthrography should be performed with caution in the presence of local skin infections to minimize the risk of introducing an infection into the joint space.

EQUIPMENT AND TECHNIQUE FOR SINGLE-CONTRAST ARTHROGRAPHY

The procedure is explained in full before beginning since patient cooperation is essential. The objective of the arthrogram, to assess the position, function, and integrity of the disk, is briefly discussed with the patient. The patient is instructed about the need to maintain a steady head position during the procedure, necessary for the rapid, successful completion of the intra-articular injection.

The sterile tray (Fig. 4–3) is prepared and the patient is then placed on the fluoroscopic table top in a laterally recumbent position (Fig. 4–4) with the

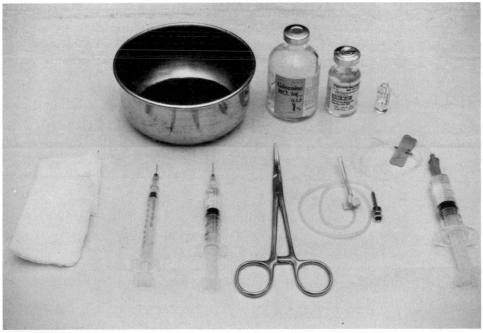

Figure 4–3
Sterile tray used in obtaining TMJ arthrograms. From left to right is a 1-ml tuberculin syringe for drawing up 0.03 ml of 1:1000 epinephrine to be mixed with the contrast material; a 3-ml syringe and 25-gauge needle to draw up 1 per cent lidocaine; a metal hemostat that can be used to mark the skin, similar to the device shown in Figure 4–5A; a 1.25-inch, 23-gauge needle for very deep joint spaces; and a 5-ml syringe with a 23-gauge scalp vein needle, which is the most commonly used method for injection of contrast material into the joint spaces. Three milliliters of contrast material has been drawn up in the 5-ml syringe for contrast medium administration, although only about 0.5 ml is usually necessary for the lower joint space. The basin contains povidone-iodine (Betadine.)

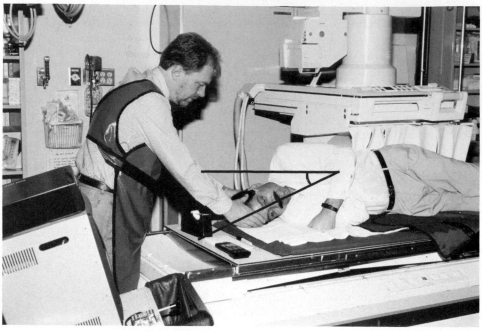

Figure 4–4
A patient on the fluoroscopic table. The head has been tilted as indicated by the lines drawn on the illustration. The tilt projects the left TMJ to be free of the base of the skull. Head positioning is adjusted under fluoroscopic observation to optimize the image of the joint.

head tilted. This allows the joint to project over the base of the skull and above the facial bones as in a transcranial radiograph. The side of the face to be examined is uppermost and accessible for skin preparation and draping. Allowing the patient to open and close the jaw several times during fluoroscopic visualization and recording allows rapid identification of the condylar head. Due to the small dimensions of the TMJ it is helpful to magnify the image electronically about two to three times.

Joint Puncture

Under fluoroscopic guidance, the posterosuperior quadrant of the mandibular condyle is identified (Fig. 4–5). This area is then marked with an indelible felt-tip marker (Fig. 4–6A and B) for guidance of local anesthesia and joint puncture. Using a 25-gauge needle, a local anesthetic, 1 or 2 per cent lidocaine, is infiltrated superficially into the skin and into the region of joint puncture (Fig. 4–7). A ¾-inch scalp vein needle infusion set with attached tubing is filled with contrast material (Omnipaque, 300 mg iodine per milliliter), with care taken to eliminate air bubbles. Air bubbles injected into the joint space may simulate loose bodies. The 23-gauge needle is introduced in a direction perpendicular to the skin surface and parallel to the x-ray beam, into the predetermined region of the condyle with the jaw in the fully closed position (Fig. 4–8A and B). After advancement of the needle, fluoroscopic observation ensures proper positioning. When the condyle is encountered by the needle tip, the needle is advanced in minute steps toward the back surface of the condylar head (Fig. 4–9). The needle is then guided by feel off the posterior

Text continued on page 111

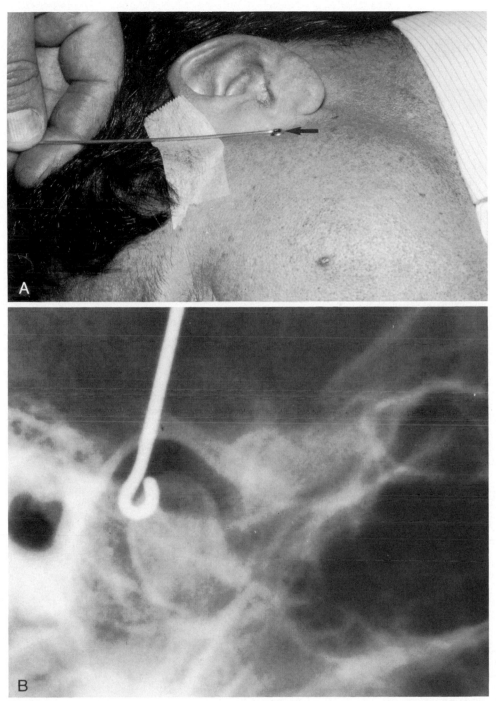

Figure 4–5
A, *A metal marker (arrow) is placed on the skin. B, Using fluoroscopy, the optimal position on the posterior aspect of the condyle is identified for joint puncture. A metal hemostat as shown in Figure 4–3 is also useful to mark the external skin surface.*

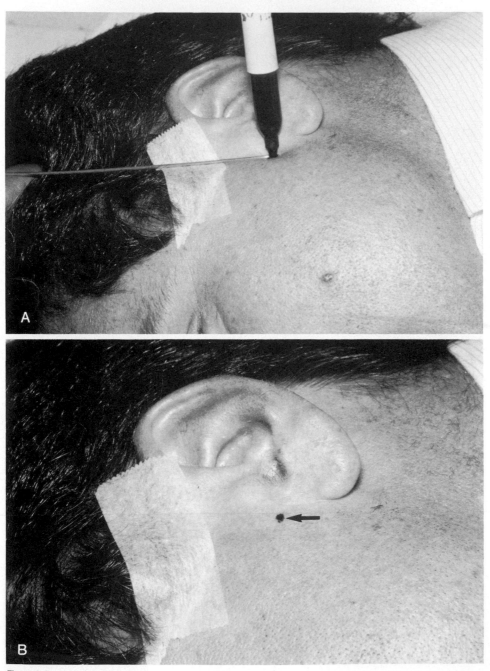

Figure 4–6
A, *The area of the joint puncture is marked with an indelible pen, as seen in B.*

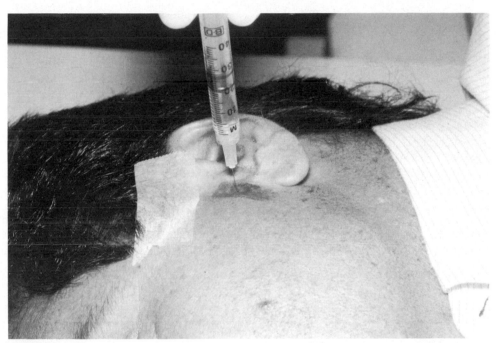

Figure 4–7
Injection of local anesthetic using a 3-ml syringe and 30-gauge needle.

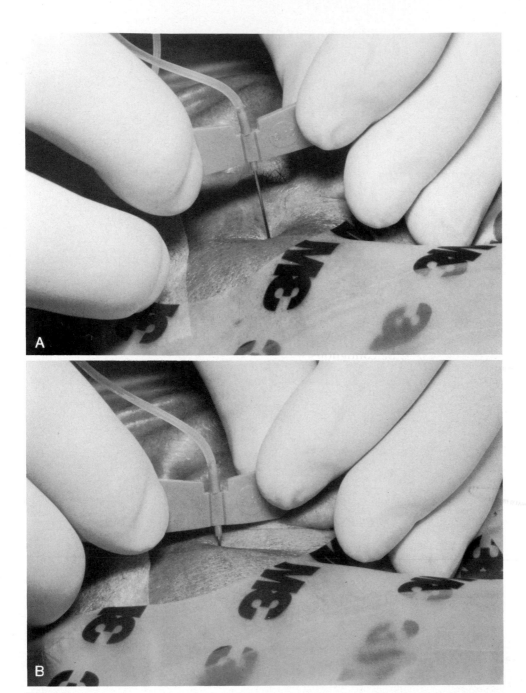

Figure 4–8
A, Joint puncture for contrast injection, using a 23-gauge butterfly needle. B, The needle has been advanced into the joint space. The direction of the needle is guided by the fluoroscopic impression of the location of the osseous anatomy versus the needle direction. The needle is actually advanced into the joint space by feel rather than by direct observation.

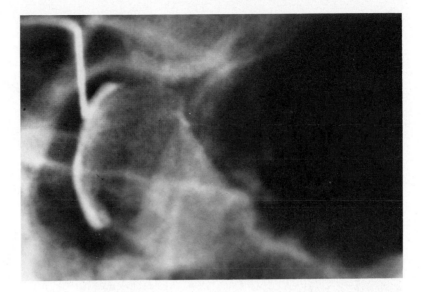

Figure 4–9
Fluoroscopic visualization of the needle in good position for injection of the lower joint space.

slope of the bony condylar margin. The needle will advance off the back surface of the condylar head without resistance if the examination is properly performed. The sensation of the needle rubbing (grazing) off the back surface of the condyle ensures correct needle handling. By fluoroscopic observation the needle will then appear to be contiguous with the posterior condylar edge (Fig. 4–9). The jaw is maintained in a stable, closed position, since condylar motion may displace the needle tip.

Contrast Injection into the Lower Joint Space

Approximately 0.2 to 0.4 ml of contrast material is then injected into the lower joint compartment under fluoroscopic observation. If desired, epinephrine can be mixed into the contrast medium to prolong the contrast density for arthrotomography. We add 0.03 ml of 1:1000 epinephrine to 3 ml of contrast medium. If the contrast material is successfully injected into the lower joint space, the opaque medium will be noted to flow freely anterior to the condyle into the anterior recess of the lower joint compartment (Fig. 4–10A and B). The contrast also will look perfectly contiguous to the posterior surface of the condylar head if the injection is intra-articular. A diffuse appearance of the injected contrast media appearing in the soft tissue outside the joint (Fig. 4–11) indicates extra-articular injection and the needle should be replaced. It is important to replace a needle before extensive contrast medium is injected, because extravasated contrast medium obscures major landmarks. Joint structures will be difficult to identify, and interpretation of the resulting arthrograms will be more difficult.

If there is simultaneous filling of the upper joint compartment with instillation of contrast material into the lower joint compartment, another 0.3 to 0.5 ml of contrast material may be needed for optimal visualization. It is imperative that fluoroscopic observation be used to determine whether the injection is successful and to monitor the appropriate amount of contrast material to be injected.

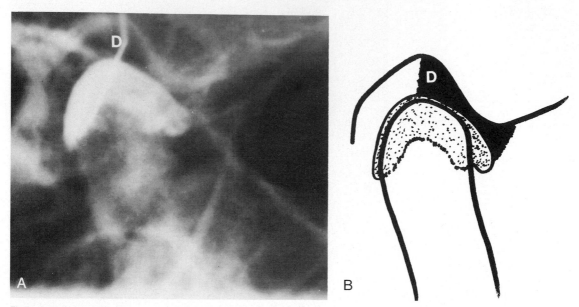

Figure 4–10
A, *Free flow of contrast medium into the lower joint space as seen on the fluoroscopic image and on the corresponding diagrammatic depiction (B). The disk (D) is located in a superior (normal) position.*

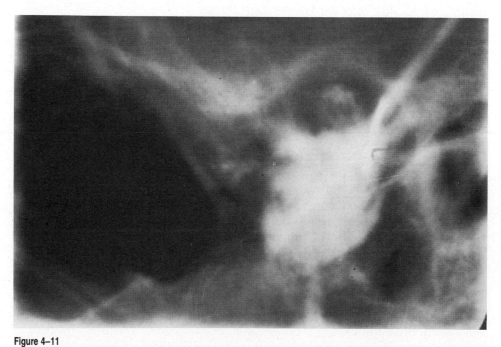

Figure 4–11
Diffuse extravasation of contrast material around the joint space due to faulty needle positioning. At this point it is usually best to terminate the examination since the anatomy is now very poorly visualized.

Once the contrast material is injected into the joint space, the needle is withdrawn approximately 1 cm but still remains in the skin. Fluoroscopic-dynamic-videotape images are recorded during opening and closing maneuvers of the jaw. Our average fluoroscopic time for observation and recording is 2 minutes. The examiner should ensure that the patient's degree of jaw opening is equal to that noted prior to the injection of the contrast material. Tightly collimated spot radiographs are obtained during the fluoroscopic procedure for subsequent analysis and for patient records. If multidirectional tomograms are needed for a more complete evaluation, the patient is moved with as little delay as possible to the multidirectional tomographic unit for arthrotomography since the contrast material dissipates rapidly.

Contrast Medium Injection into the Upper Joint Space

If a diagnosis on the lower space arthrogram is questionable or if the arthrographic findings do not correspond to the clinical findings, the next step is to inject contrast medium also into the upper joint space. With the patient's mouth open, the butterfly needle that is already inserted through the skin is redirected up into the glenoid fossa. The needle is advanced superiorly, anteriorly, and medially until there is bone contact in the anterior aspect of the glenoid fossa or against the posterior aspect of the articular eminence (Fig. 4–12). During needle advancement and contrast injection, the patient should maintain an open mouth. Once the needle is in contact with the bone and the bevel of the needle has been turned against the articular surface, approximately 0.3 to 0.5 ml of the contrast medium is injected under fluoroscopic observation. There should be an immediate free flow of the contrast medium in the upper joint space, and the resistance to the injection is minimal. No free flow of contrast medium in the joint spaces is a strong indication that the joint puncture was not successful and that the needle position has to be readjusted. After injection of contrast medium, the needle is withdrawn and left in the superficial skin. Transcranial closed- and open-mouth images are obtained. Joint function is also studied in fluoroscopy. A joint with injected lower and upper joint spaces is shown in Figure 4–13A through D.

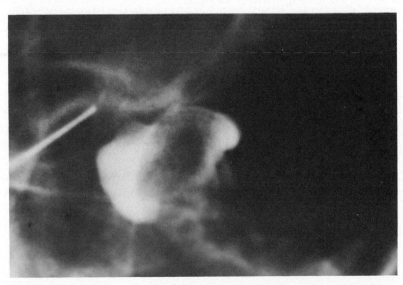

Figure 4–12
The needle is in good position for injection into the upper joint space.

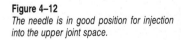

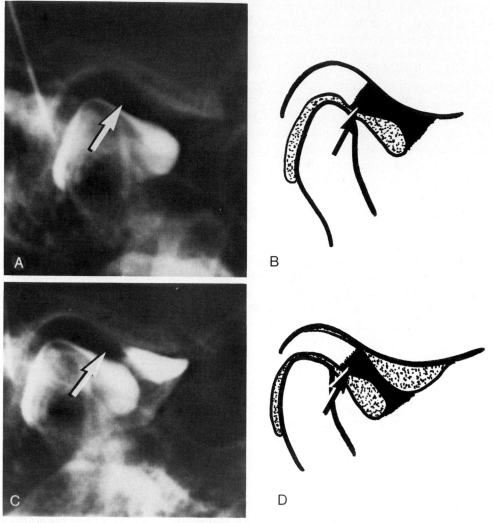

Figure 4–13
Injection into lower and upper joint spaces. A, Single-contrast arthrogram after injection of contrast medium into the lower joint space. B, Corresponding schematic drawing showing elongation of the anterior recess of the lower joint space. The disk is anteriorly displaced. Its posterior band (arrow) is located on the anterior-superior aspect of the condyle. C and D, Contrast medium into the upper joint space confirms the diagnosis of anterior disk displacement. The upper joint space further delineates the configuration of the disk. The posterior band of the disk is indicated by arrows.

Arthrotomography

For the arthrotomographic phase of the examination, the patient lies prone on the radiographic table top with the face oriented in a lateral position or in a position so that the flat surface of the ramus of the mandible is against the table top (Fig. 4–14). Multidirectional tomography is performed optimally with a hypocycloidal motion. Images are obtained in the closed- and open-jaw positions. If hypocycloidal tomographic movement is used, the images should be approximately 3 mm in thickness.[34] With linear tomography, the images are more likely to have streak artifacts. Images should be obtained throughout the medial lateral dimension of the joint, at least at the closed-mouth position. Since the most lateral and most medial parts of the joint usually cannot be clearly visualized on a tomographic image, four to six images will cover the

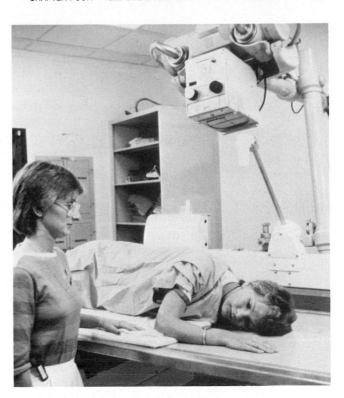

Figure 4–14
Patient positioning on the tomographic table following the injection of contrast material into the joint space. The side injected is against the table top, closest to the film.

medial lateral dimension of the joint, using a hypocycloidal motion pattern. Images should be obtained at closed-mouth and open-mouth positions.

Objectives of Arthrography

The objective of the dynamic-fluoroscopic phase of the examination is to evaluate disk function during opening and closing maneuvers of the jaw. These maneuvers are recorded on videotape for future analysis.[9] If the disk is displaced and reduces on jaw opening, these dynamic events are more clearly depicted with the fluoroscopic analysis, obviating the need for arthrotomography. The smooth to-and-fro flow of contrast material from the anterior recess in the closed-jaw position to the posterior recess in the open-jaw position indicates normal function. A continual collection of contrast material in the anterior recess of the lower joint compartment and progressive deformity of the anterior recess with jaw opening help confirm the diagnosis of disk displacement without reduction. The reciprocal incoordination between the disk and condyle, signifying disk displacement with reduction, is usually most obvious in the dynamic mode of the assessment. The arthrographer's impression during the initial phase of the examination is vital for a complete and accurate diagnosis.

The objective of the arthrotomogram is to survey the joint completely over its medial, central, and lateral aspects. This is important since many disk displacements are only partial. Frequently the lateral part of the disk is anteriorly displaced, whereas the central and medial parts are located in a normal superior position.[35–37] In other patients, the disk is not in a purely anterior direction but in an anteromedial or anterolateral displaced direction.

This means a medial or lateral component to the displacement, in addition to the anterior displacement. Thus, part of the joint space configuration might look normal and other parts clearly abnormal. For the arthrogram to be confidently normal, the joint space should appear normal in the lateral, central, and medial regions by arthrotomography. The fluoroscopic phase of the examination identifies only the lateral third of the joint space in clear profile, thus displacements might be missed without tomography. The patient's head should be turned during arthrography to optimize the demonstration of an abnormality. Thus, when the head is turned with the nose down, the lateral portion of the joint is visualized in profile. When the head is turned nose up, the medial portion of the joint is visualized in greater profile in the transcranial projection.

In unusual circumstances, if one elects to obtain arthrotomograms in patients with clicking of the jaw, images are made in three jaw positions: closed, just before the click, and at maximal jaw opening. If the jaw does not click, images are simply acquired with the jaw closed and at maximal opening only. Patients with painful locking of the TMJ and fluoroscopic diagnosis of anterior disk displacement with reduction also may be evaluated solely by fluoroscopy and videotape recording if the findings are certain. When both lower and upper joint spaces have been opacified, arthrotomography is usually a valuable addition to the diagnosis (Fig. 4–15*A* to *C*).

Potential Errors in Technique

Some errors during the learning phase of lower joint space TMJ arthrography will be encountered. The most common mistake is a joint puncture that results in extravasation of contrast material (Figs. 4–16*A* and *B*, 4–17). Most commonly, the contrast medium is extravasated over the lateral pole of the condyle or into the loose connective tissues posterior to the condyle. The latter may occur when the needle is placed too deeply behind the back surface of the condyle. The desired tactile sensation is a rubbing or "grazing" feeling as the needle slides off the posterior bony surface of the condylar head. After this, the needle is advanced only about 1 to 2 mm, followed by the injection of a small test dose of contrast material monitored with fluoroscopy. The bevel of the needle should be against the articular surface and not against the internal capsule. In this way, injected contrast medium will flow into the joint space instead of into the soft tissue.

Another common error is positioning the needle too superficially into the lateral capsular tissues of the TMJ, resulting in extravasation of contrast material over the lateral pole of the condyle and the lateral condylar neck (Fig. 4–16). This may cause additional patient discomfort. Using the hard, bony surface of the posterior aspect of the condyle as a guide to needle depth is invaluable to minimize this error. Injection of large amounts of contrast material into the capsule can lead to an arthrographic failure, since extravasated contrast material may obscure the anatomic landmarks that must be visualized for successful interpretation of the arthrogram. Using contrast media without sodium or administration of non-ionic contrast media can minimize the amount of patient discomfort when contrast medium is injected outside the joint.

Placement of the needle too caudally along the condylar surface makes the injection inferior to the posterior recess of the lower joint compartment. Contrast material will be noted to extravasate far down along the posterior neck of the condyle (Fig. 4–17).

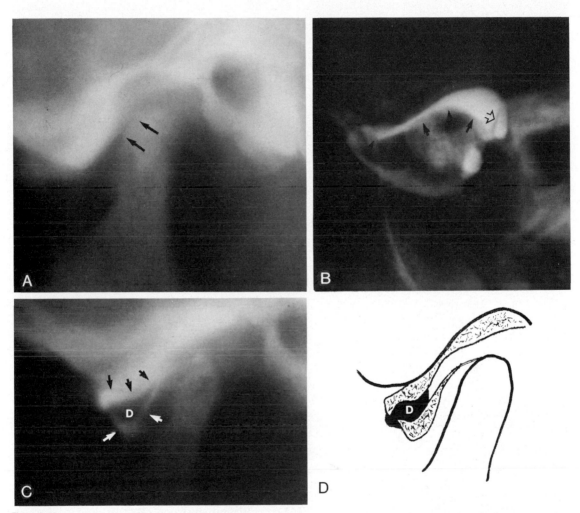

Figure 4–15
Value of arthrotomography. A, *Plain, multidirectional tomogram of the jaw in the closed position shows flattening of the condylar head (arrows) and sclerosis. B, Contrast material has been injected into the lower joint space and there is flooding of contrast material into the upper joint space (arrows) due to a perforation. Incidental note is made of a fibrous adhesion in the posterior aspect of the upper joint space (open arrow). C, Multidirectional tomography following the injection of contrast material is invaluable in sorting out the details of the position of the disk. An arthrotomogram of the same patient shows a clear distinction between the lower joint space (white arrows) and the upper joint space (black arrows). The disk (D) is anteriorly displaced. D, Diagrammatic depiction of the arthrotomogram, showing the disk (D) being displaced relative to the condyle.*

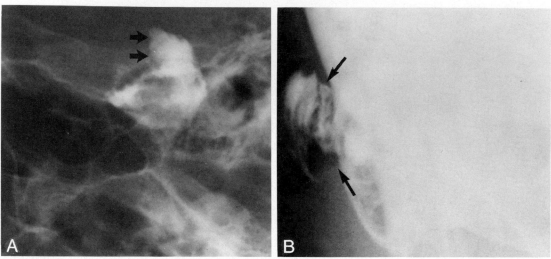

Figure 4–16
Lateral extravasation of contrast material. A, Transcranial radiograph with contrast material injected into the lower joint space shows a moderate amount of extravasation (arrows) along the lateral pole of the condyle in a patient with psoriatic arthritis. B, Anteroposterior spot radiograph of the same joint following the injection of contrast material, showing extensive extravasation of contrast material (arrows) from the lateral capsule of the joint space.

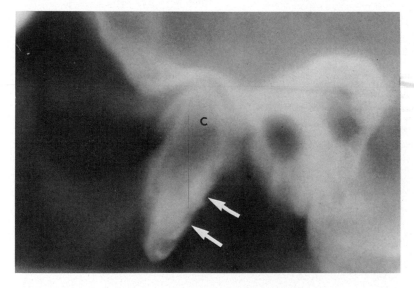

Figure 4–17
A common occurrence is placement of the needle too far posterior relative to the condylar head, with consequent posterior extravasation of contrast material (arrows). C, Condyle.

Finally, another error occurs when the injection of contrast material is solely into the upper joint compartment (Fig. 4–18). It is usually not possible to make a clear assessment of the disk with contrast material only in the upper joint compartment. This can be avoided by placing the needle firmly over the lateral pole of the condyle and using this bony landmark as the guide. The needle tip is then moved posteriorly and medially along the surface of the condyle into a position for successful injection of contrast medium into the lower joint space.

RADIOGRAPHIC INTERPRETATION: SINGLE-CONTRAST ARTHROGRAM

Normal Arthrogram

Jaw opening requires a coordinated movement of the condyle, muscles of mastication, and the disk. The disk and condyle move anteriorly in a smooth, synchronized fashion, with the biconcave disk being interposed between the convex condylar surface inferiorly and the convex margins of the temporal bone superiorly. During jaw closing, the disk also maintains its interposed position and moves in a coordinated fashion with the condyle. Mechanical dysfunction results when the disk is no longer correctly positioned, leading to a mechanical incoordination and internal derangement. An important, but often unappreciated, aspect of jaw mechanics is the necessity for a coordinated action by both TMJs that are functionally unified by the bony yoke formed by the mandible itself. This explains the high prevalence of bilateral abnormalities in contradistinction to other joints of the body such as the knee, ankle, shoulders, elbow, and so on.

The normal disk and posterior disk attachment allow no communication of contrast material between the upper and lower joint spaces (Fig. 4–19A through D). The position and integrity of the disk are interpreted indirectly by the configurations of the joint spaces. In the normal case, the posterior band of the disk can be estimated to be located in the superior or 12 o'clock position relative to the condylar head. Another helpful anatomic landmark to determine

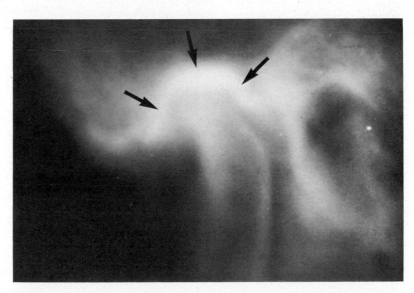

Figure 4–18
Upper joint space injection (arrows) of contrast material following multiple attempts to inject into the lower joint space. Diagnosis of the position of the disk cannot be made on this radiograph. The study is of a 29-year-old professional boxer with multiple past hemarthroses following repeated mandibular trauma.

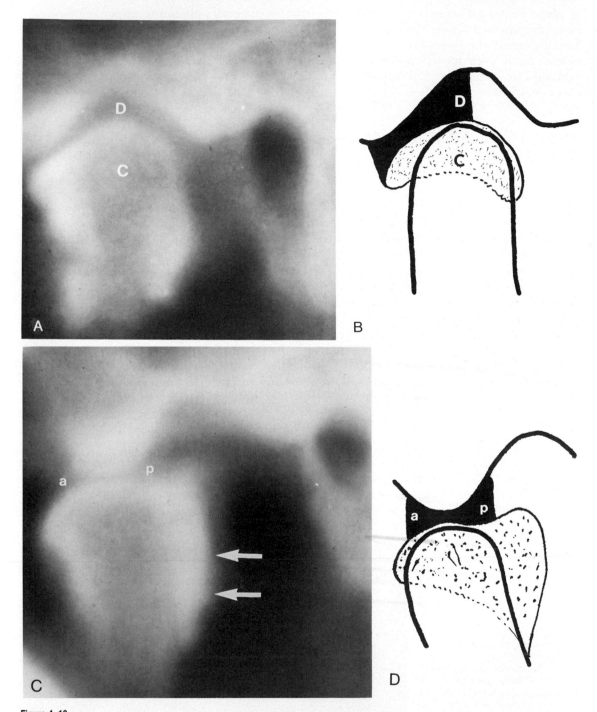

Figure 4–19
Normal arthrotomogram. A, Single-contrast arthrotomogram after injection of contrast material into the lower joint space. B, Corresponding schematic drawing showing normal position of the disk (D) relative to the condyle (C). In A and B, the jaw is in the closed position. C, Open jaw position, with contrast material in the lower joint space. D, The corresponding diagram shows the anterior (a) and posterior (p) bands of the disk to be in a normal relationship to the condyle. The bulk of the contrast material is now in the posterior recess (arrows) of the lower joint space.

disk position is to relate the central thin zone of the disk to the anterior prominence of the condyle. In a normal joint, the anterior prominence of the condyle should articulate directly against the inferior concavity of the central thin zone of the disk. Any separation of these two articulating surfaces indicates that the condyle-disk relationship is not normal. The posterior margin of the normal lower joint space has a very thin, curvilinear configuration hugging the posterior aspect of the condyle. The lower joint space is wider anteriorly, with a smooth, teardrop configuration directed obliquely downward. The superior margin of the teardrop delineates the anterior extent of the disk. The slight convex configuration of the upper margin of the anterior recess delineates the thin zone of the disk. By extrapolation, the posterior margin of the disk is at the apex of the condyle.

The anterior band of the disk may create a slight concave impression on the anterior recess of the joint space in some cases. This is to be distinguished from disk displacement with reduction. Dynamic videofluoroscopy usually confirms that the joint is normal. Magnetic resonance imaging (MRI) also may be useful (Fig. 4–20A through D).

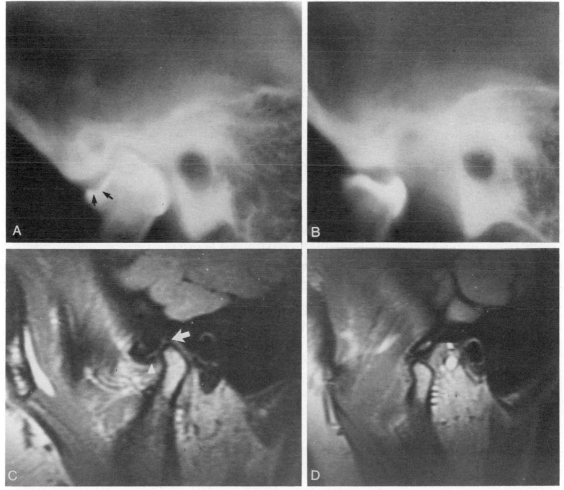

Figure 4–20
This arthrotomogram shows a prominent indentation (arrows in A) of the anterior band on the anterior recess of the lower joint space, which is a normal variant. This is not to be mistaken for an anteriorly displaced disk. A shows the jaw in the closed position, and B shows the jaw in the open position. By videofluoroscopy, there was no incoordination. C, The MR scan shows the disk to be in a normal position (posterior band of the disk, large arrow, and anterior band of the disk, arrowhead) in the closed jaw position and in the open jaw position (D).

Table 4-5
INTRA-ARTICULAR CHANGES ASSOCIATED WITH TEMPOROMANDIBULAR JOINT CLICKING

Common	Uncommon
• Disk displacement with reduction	• Disk displacement without reduction
• Jaw subluxation, eminence impediment	• Adhesions
• Deviation in the form of the articulating surfaces	• Loose joint bodies
	• Vacuum phenomenon

Disk Displacement with Reduction

Temporomandibular joint sounds are the most frequent finding in patients with TMJ disorders and represent a salient component for any imaging assessment. According to epidemiologic studies, clicking has been recognized to occur in between 14 and 44 per cent of the general population.[38–42] Clicking sounds have been ascribed to a variety of mechanisms, including disk displacement, condylar subluxation, deviations in the form or shape of any of the articulating surfaces, loose bodies, and fibrous bands or adhesions within the joint spaces (Table 4–5). Arthrographic observations and direct inspections in patients and cadaver material support the concept that clicking is frequently associated with disk displacement with reduction. However, there are also joints with clicking that have disk displacement without reduction. In a study by Miller and associates, 15 per cent of patients with clicking actually had disk displacement without reduction.[43] In these joints, the clicking was due to something other than the recapturing of the disk. At the other end of the spectrum, there are joints with disk displacement with reduction but not clicking.[44, 45]

Various characteristics of the TMJ clicking sound are listed in Table 4–6; these have been derived mainly from detailed analyses by means of high-speed cinematography of the movement of the disk and condyle in cadaver TMJ with clicking.[41, 42] The opening click is associated with an event that occurs in the range of 12 to 36 milliseconds, and the closing click in the range of 6 to 8 milliseconds. The opening click is produced when the condyle and recaptured disk have an impact on the temporal bone. The condyle eminence incoordination associated with jaw subluxation, on the other hand, is usually a jolting type of sound, rather than the snapping sound that occurs with disk displacements.[46] Macroscopically detectable alterations in the shape of the articular surfaces of the TMJ were reported in as many as 45 per cent of autopsy specimens.[47] These deviations in form are local thickenings of the articular tissue layers, usually focal in nature and usually occurring in the lateral regions of the joint surfaces.

The absence of joint sounds, it is stressed, is not an indication of a normal joint.[48–50] We have noted disk displacement with reduction by arthrographic analysis in some patients who have no signs of clicking at all. The presence of

Table 4-6
ASPECTS OF CLICKING DUE TO DISK DISPLACEMENT WITH REDUCTION

• Usually reciprocal	• Clicks occur in 6 to 36 msec
• Deflection in condylar path associated with both the opening and closing clicks	• Eminence "click" is a jolting sound
• Change in velocity of condylar movement associated with the opening and closing clicks	• Deviation of jaw from midline greater with eminence than with disk clicks

disk displacement with reduction in silent joints has been documented in autopsy material.[51] Also, advanced degenerative changes have been seen in joints that are silent.[48]

Clinically and radiographically, disk displacement with reduction, associated with clicking sounds, is often associated with joint, muscular, and facial pain. Disk displacement with reduction is both an anatomic and a functional disorder that is cyclic in nature (Fig. 4–21). This has been termed "reciprocal clicking."[12]

In the clicking joint, a major advantage of arthrography over other imaging modalities is that it allows a detailed assessment of the dynamic aspects of joint function and dysfunction. An appreciation of these dynamic aspects can be effectively used to initiate treatment with protrusive jaw splints. The precise position of the displacement of the disk during jaw closing and the tooth position can be determined at the time of the arthrogram.[52, 53] The relationships of the upper and lower teeth can thus be documented in conjunction with the arthrographic diagnosis. Re-establishment of normal disk/condyle anatomic relationships can also be confirmed. This subject is discussed later.

Disk displacement with reduction is generally considered an early phase of the entire spectrum of internal derangement. In this situation the posterior band of the disk is anterior to the 12 o'clock position of the condyle, and the posterior band creates a concave impression on the anterior recess of the joint space (Figs. 4–13, and 4–22A and B). The anterior recess tends to be more elongated and larger in volume than in the normal condition, and the impression created by the anteriorly displaced posterior band of the disk on the lower joint space is usually prominent. In the earliest of displacements, however, the configuration of the anterior recess must be distinguished from variations in normal in which a slightly prominent anterior band of the disk (Fig. 4–20A through D) may create a similar joint space configuration.[45, 54] Again, these

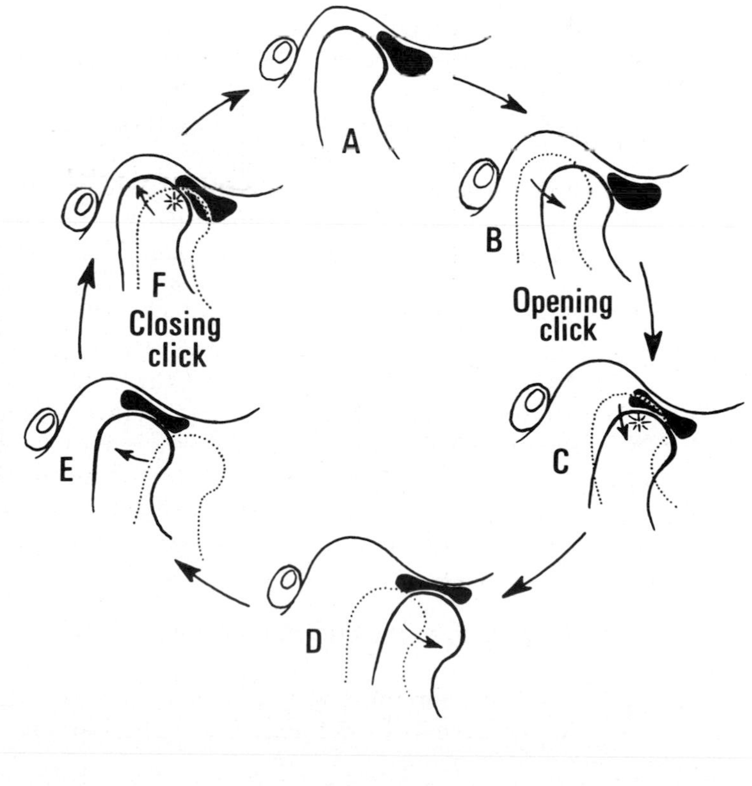

Figure 4–21
Disk displacement with reduction and the association of an opening click (between B and C) and the closing click (E and F). This is a modification of the diagrammatic depiction of reciprocal clicking first described by William Farrar, DDS. If a protrusive splint is to be fashioned for recapture of the disk, position E is optimal rather than position C. This is because the condylar head is closer to the fossa and in a more physiologic position than in position C. (Modified from Farrar WB, McCarty WL Jr: The TMJ dilemma. J Alabama Dent Assoc 63:19–26, 1979.)

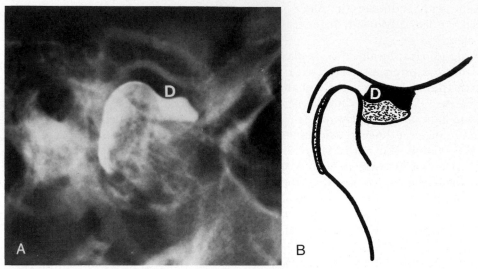

Figure 4–22
Characteristic example of anterior disk displacement. The disk (D) is seen anterior to the condyle. The anterior recess of the lower joint space is elongated, as seen both in the arthrogram (A) and in the schematic drawing (B).

conditions can be distinguished by noting whether the patient has a clicking sound with opening and closing maneuvers of the jaw and by demonstrating incoordination between the disk and condyle during repeated opening and closing maneuvers observed during dynamic video fluoroscopy. Upper space injection or MR imaging is also valuable when the diagnosis is not obvious on the lower space arthrogram.

After reduction of disk displacement, the arthrographic pattern is then as noted for the normal patient. Thus, the contrast material clears from the anterior recess of the joint space and flows into the posterior recess. Since the disk has recaptured at this jaw position, it is usually indistinguishable from any normal open jaw arthrogram. However, since the anterior recess is usually more elongated in disk displacement with reduction than with normal disk position, a pocket of contrast material is frequently demonstrated anterior to the condylar head even following disk recapture (Fig. 4–23A through D). In disk displacement with reduction, anteromedial or anterolateral displacements are common. These are difficult to depict with arthrography and are better demonstrated using the multiplanar capabilities of MRI. An arthrographic report has described an "edge-sign" of the medial or lateral recess of the lower joint compartment as an indication of the sideways component of disk displacement.[35] We have not been able to rely on this observation consistently.[37] Further study is needed to define better the criteria of lower joint space arthrography for rotational and sideways displacements. Rotating the patient's head during the arthrographic examination sometimes will be helpful in identifying oblique types of displacement. Thus, if the displacement is more prominent in one part of the joint, the anterior recess of the lower joint space will be accentuated if the head is turned so that this part of the joint is imaged in profile.

Staging the Opening Recapture

We stage the position of recapture as early, mid, or late (Fig. 4–24). Early recapture may be defined as the repositioning of the disk related to the condyle

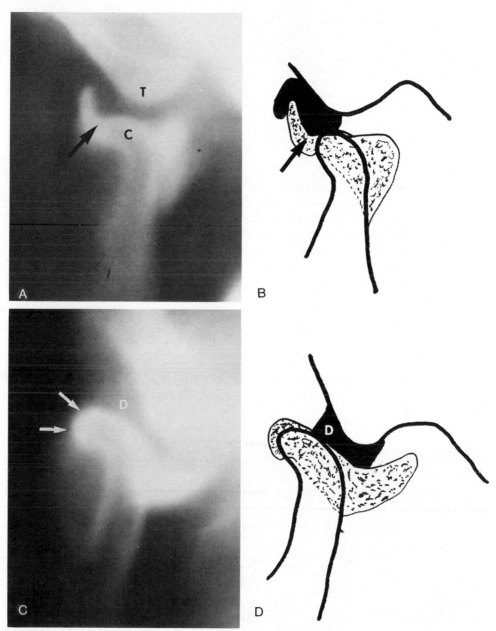

Figure 4–23

This arthrotomogram demonstrates anterior disk displacement with late opening reduction. A, Single-contrast lower joint space arthrotomogram showing the posterior band of the disk (arrows in A and B) to be displaced even though the condyle (C) is at the apex of the tubercle (T). C and D, With continued jaw opening, the disk (D) recaptures into a normal relationship relative to the condyle. The arrows in C delineate a small amount of contrast material remaining in the anterior recess.

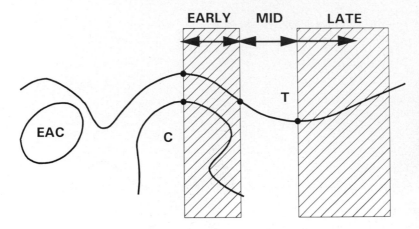

Figure 4–24
Staging of disk displacement with reduction: disk reduction in the early translation of the condyle, midpoint of anterior translation of the condyle or far anterior position of the condyle. C, Condyle; T, tubercle; EAC, external auditory canal.

when the condyle has moved along the posterior half of the slope of the articular eminence. A midopening recapture is noted when the disk assumes a normal relationship to the condylar head when the condyle is at the position between the midpoint of the slope of the articular eminence to the apex of the articular eminence. A late opening click is noted when the disk assumes a normal relationship with the condyle at or beyond the apex of the articular eminence.

Disk Deformation

Deformation of the disk is also sometimes demonstrable by lower joint space arthrography in patients with clicking (Figs. 4–25*A* and *B* and 4–26*A* and *B*), although double-space arthrography and MRI are more accurate in

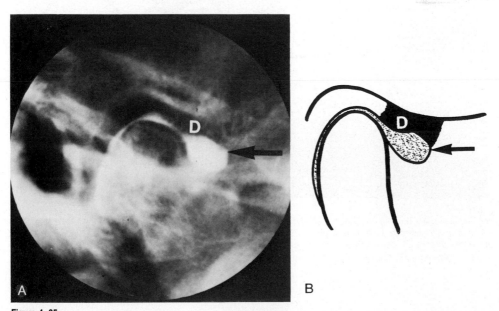

Figure 4–25
A, *Single-contrast lower space arthrogram and* B, *schematic drawing showing anterior disk displacement. The disk (D) is not significantly deformed.*

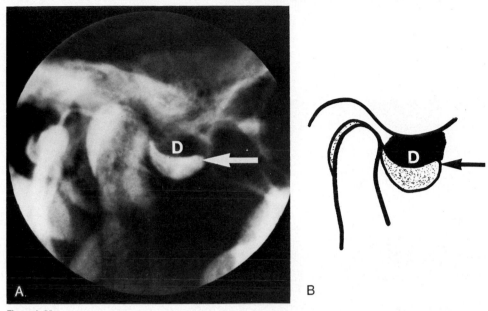

Figure 4–26
A, Single-contrast lower space transcranial arthrogram and B, schematic drawing showing anterior disk displacement with deformation. The disk (D) is deformed. The anterior recess of the lower joint space (arrow) is elongated.

the assessment of deformations of the displaced disk. The deformation of the disk sometimes can be appreciated with the single-contrast lower compartment arthrogram as shown in Figures 4–25 and 4–26. Deformation of the disk is probably important to determine the prognosis. If the deformation of the disk with thickening of the posterior band is more pronounced, as shown in Figure 4–26, there is a greater tendency to progress from clicking to locking than if the disk is less deformed, as shown in Figure 4–25. Deformation with thickening of the posterior band can thus be used to predict which patients with disk displacement with reduction are more likely to progress to locking.

Arthrographically Assisted Recapture of the Disk

In patients with disk displacement with reduction shown by arthrography, we are able to assess an optimal disk-condyle relationship during the fluoroscopic observation. We are also able to document a mandibular position in which the condyle-disk relationship is normal using fast-setting material injected between the teeth (Figs. 4–27A through D and 4–28A through C). This material sets in 2 to 3 minutes and allows us to document the optimal mandibular position with the disk in a recaptured position. This jaw registration position is then sent to the referring clinician to reproduce it for the construction of a protrusive splint. The additional time to accomplish this procedure is usually about 5 minutes.

It is important to recognize that the recapture position of the disk and condyle optimal for the protrusive splint is determined during jaw closing and just before the closing displacement (Figs. 4–21E and 4–27B). A position for recapturing the disk can also be documented clinically. However, studies have shown a relatively low success rate with this technique.[52, 53] The reason is probably that the disk starts to displace anteriorly before the closing click is

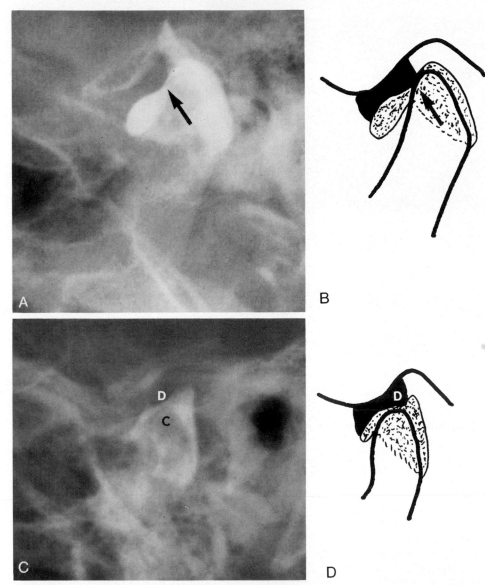

Figure 4–27
These lower space arthrograms (A through D) demonstrate disk displacement with reduction and show an optimal position of the condyle relative to the disk (C and D) for splinting the jaw using the fast-setting material Ramitech. A, Lower joint space arthrogram showing an anteriorly displaced disk (arrows in A and B). C, Position of the condyle (C) relative to the lower joint space and disk with recapture and in an optimal position for initiating splint therapy. D, Diagrammatic depiction of the recaptured position of the disk (D) relative to the condyle, in preparation for the splinting phase of the procedure (Figure 4–28).

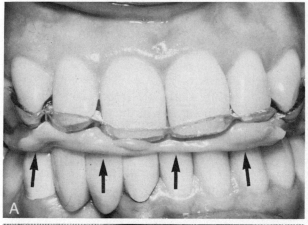

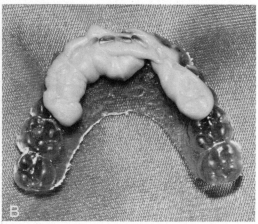

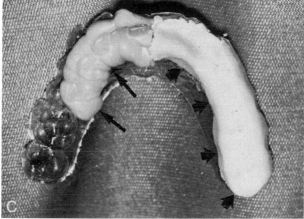

Figure 4–28

A, Fast-setting putty-like material (long arrows) between the teeth in concert with the appropriate position of the condyle (see Figure 4–27C and D) determined by the arthrogram. B, This material hardens in approximately 2 to 3 minutes and serves as an impression that can be utilized by the referring dental clinician to fashion a splint (C). In C, the putty-like material is noted (long arrows) and the permanent splint (short arrows) is partially completed. The putty-like material that forms an impression of the lower jaw relative to the upper incisors establishes a reproducible jaw position that was determined by the arthrogram to give the optimal recaptured disk position.

heard. That means if a position is documented that is close to the closing click, the disk already will be partially anteriorly displaced. To maintain a stable condyle-disk relationship, the condyle has to be right under the posterior band of the disk, and this is not possible if the disk has already started to displace anteriorly. Splinting the patient just following the opening click (recapture) is not possible, as the degree of jaw protrusion or jaw opening would be excessive and would necessitate placing the mandible in a very anterior position with undue stretch on the posterior ligament.

Several studies have suggested that recapturing a displaced disk and stabilizing the mandible in the therapeutic position effectively reduce pain and dysfunction associated with disk displacement and internal derangement.[21, 55] The long-term results of this treatment also have been encouraging.[55] The therapeutic position must be maintained for a long time and possibly permanently in order to avoid redisplacement of the disk[56] and can be maintained by orthodontic treatment or prosthetic reconstruction. This is a disadvantage compared with other methods because it requires more extensive dental treatment. The extent of the dental treatment necessary should be considered relative to the severity of the patient's initial symptoms.

Disk Displacement Without Reduction

Disk displacement with reduction is often a precursor to complete anterior displacement of the disk that does not reduce (locking). Our experience is that disk displacement with reduction is only very rarely associated with perforation or tears of the posterior attachment, whereas this is quite commonly encountered in disk displacement without reduction.[15, 29, 31, 44] Displacement is usually easily demonstrable by lower joint space video-dynamic arthrography; arthrotomography or upper joint space opacification is usually not necessary to make the diagnosis of disk displacement without reduction.

Disk displacement without reduction (Fig. 4–29) is a progression of internal derangement compared with disk displacement with reduction. This stage of internal derangement also represents the most significant type of mechanical dysfunction of the disk and condyle. It is manifest clinically as acute unilateral limitation of anterior condylar translation, resulting in restriction of mouth opening and deviation to the affected side upon opening. If preceded by disk displacement with reduction, the patient will relate that the clicking disappeared when the jaw restriction began. The displaced disk, per se, is probably a significant cause of the physical limitation of condylar translation, and this situation has been termed the "closed lock."[7, 8] Damage to the disk attachments, both posteriorly and laterally, is probably also a component of the pathophysiologic mechanism. The squeezing force of the condyle upon the well-innervated posterior disk attachment up against the superior surface of the temporal bone may well be a cause of pain. Other sources of TMJ pain are trauma from the disk impinging on the inner aspect of the anterior capsule and inflammatory changes in the joint and joint capsule secondary to disk displacement.

The disk is often more abnormal in shape in disk displacement without reduction than in the earlier stages of internal derangement. The thin zone of the disk is nearly obliterated by progressive thickening of the posterior band of the disk, leaving only a small groove on the undersurface (Fig. 4–30*A* and *B*). This is sometimes a useful anatomic landmark demarcating the thickened posterior band from the smaller anterior band.

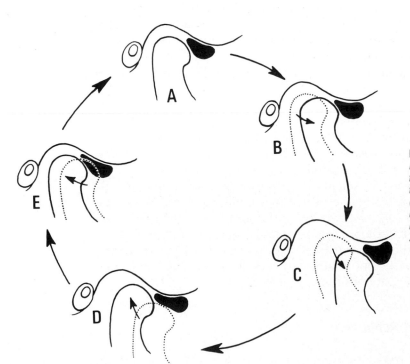

Figure 4–29
Disk displacement without reduction, modified from Dr. William Farrar's conceptual presentation. Note that at all jaw positions the disk (black structure) remains displaced. There is usually no clicking sound. (Modified from Farrar WB, McCarty WL Jr: The TMJ dilemma. J Alabama Dent Assoc 63:19–26, 1979.)

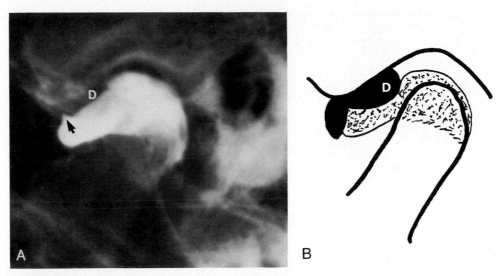

Figure 4–30
A, *The lower joint space single-contrast arthrogram shows disk displacement without reduction. The anterior recess of the lower joint space has a "beak" in its upper margin (arrow) that demonstrates the location of the deformed, thin, or central zone of the disk (D).* B, *Diagrammatic depiction of displaced disk (D).*

The arthrographic findings of anterior disk displacement without reduction are usually characteristic (Fig. 4–31A and B). In all jaw positions the entire disk remains anterior to the condylar head and is often deformed (Figs. 4–30 and 4–32). The anterior recess of the lower joint space is more elongated than in the normal condition and has a characteristic, cup-shaped configuration (Fig. 4–31). The more elongated and deeper the cup of the anterior recess, the more deformed is the posterior band of the disk. The deformation of the anterior recess can be accentuated by instructing the patient to open the mouth maximally. Furthermore, this characteristic configuration is usually more apparent in the lateral third of the articulation than in the medial third, since most disk displacements frequently are more pronounced in the lateral than in the medial part of the joint. Most often the findings of disk displacement without reduction are clearly demonstrated during the fluoroscopic procedure;

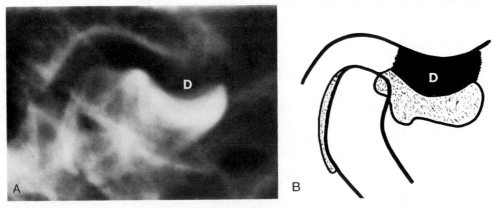

Figure 4–31
A, *Transcranial arthrogram with contrast injection into the lower joint space.* B, *Schematic drawing showing anterior disk displacement with significant deformation of the disk (D). The anterior recess of the lower joint space is cup-shaped, and the posterior recess of the lower joint space is thin.*

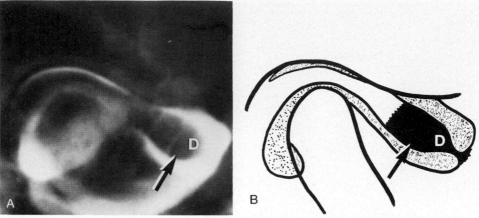

Figure 4–32
Anterior disk displacement, deformation of the disk, and perforation. A, Single-contrast arthrogram with contrast medium in the lower and upper joint spaces. B, Schematic drawing showing the deformed disk (D). The approximate position of the posterior band of the disk is indicated by an arrow. Contrast medium was injected into the lower joint space and resulted in immediate filling of both the upper and lower spaces, indicating a perforation.

however, arthrotomography may help clarify these findings and should be readily available if there is any doubt. Again injection of contrast medium into the upper space is a possibility to enhance the diagnostic information from arthrography.

The arthrographic findings of disk displacement without reduction are often very similar to those of disk displacement with reduction when the closed-jaw position only is compared. Thus, it is imperative that the patient open maximally at the time of the examination and the arthrographic findings be recorded to assess whether or not recapture of the disk has occurred.

Greater detail with regard to the configuration of the disk is possible with dual space double-contrast arthrotomography, which is discussed in detail later.

Disk Displacement with Perforation

In our experience with a relatively young adult patient population, the great majority of patients with perforation of the tissues within the TMJ have disk displacement without reduction. This clinical experience is consistent with the pathophysiology and progression of the disorder, as discussed in Chapter 2. Indeed, these patients have a history of chronic symptomatology of internal derangement related to disk dysfunction. A high percentage of these patients will also show osseous abnormalities compatible with degenerative arthritis. In one series, it was noted that approximately two thirds of patients with disk displacement and perforation had plain film findings of degenerative joint disease.[15, 51] Flattening of the condyle with osteophytosis in association with flattening of the articular eminence is almost pathognomonic. In these chronic stages of the disorder, the condylar translation is usually normal. These patients relate a history of chronic limitation of jaw opening that slowly resolved and preceded the current signs and symptoms by a reasonably long period of time.

Arthrographic detection of perforation is demonstrated by simultaneous opacification of the upper joint space when contrast material is introduced into the lower joint compartment (Fig. 4–33A through D). Anterior disk displace-

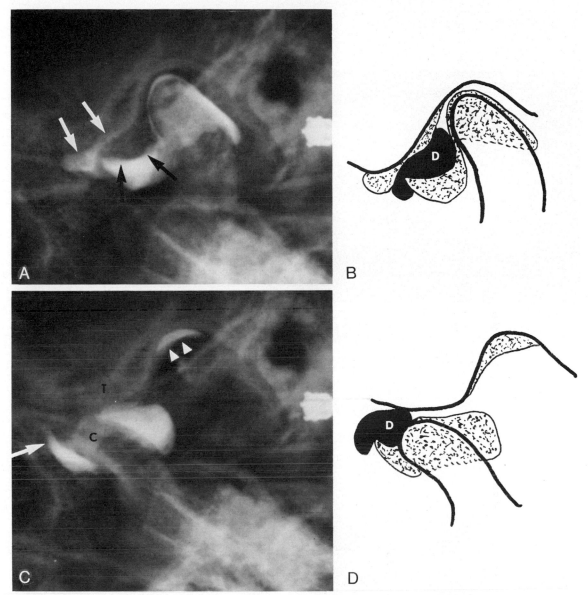

Figure 4–33

Transcranial demonstration of disk displacement without reduction and an associated perforation. A, The closed jaw position with contrast medium in the lower joint space (black arrows), with some contrast in the upper joint space (white arrows). B, The disk (D) is shown diagrammatically. C and D, Maximal jaw opening that shows persistent displacement of the disk (D). Note the high peaked shape of the anterior recess (arrow). Contrast medium is noted in the upper joint space (arrowheads). C, Condyle; T, tubercle.

ment without reduction will usually be demonstrated as well. When filling of the upper and lower compartments is noted at fluoroscopy, arthrotomography is sometimes necessary for a complete evaluation, since the upper joint compartment superimposes over the lower joint compartment. If a complete, solid column of contrast material is noted posterior to the displaced disk, then a diagnosis of complete disk detachment is likely (Fig. 4–34A and B). Normally the perforation cannot be demonstrated directly. Occasionally, however, we obtain images that actually show the perforation between the lower and upper joint spaces (Figs. 4–35A and B and 4–36A and B). The literature has reported

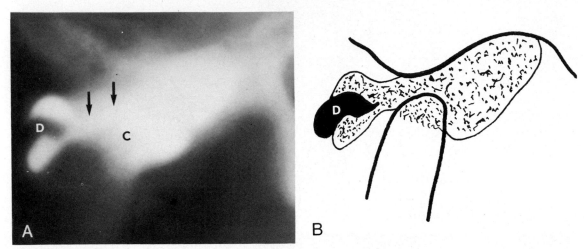

Figure 4–34
Arthrotomogram following injection of contrast material into the lower joint space, and with flooding of contrast into the upper joint space as well. This indicates a perforation or detachment of the disk. A, With maximal jaw opening, the disk (D) is noted to be displaced anterior to the condyle (C). In addition, there is a solid collection of contrast material posterior to the disk (arrows) indicating complete detachment and destruction of the posterior disk ligament. This is diagrammatically depicted in B.

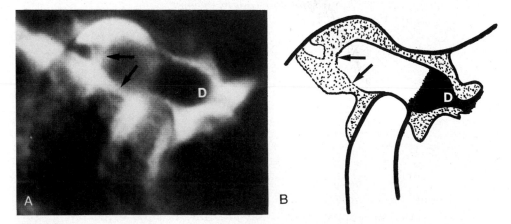

Figure 4–35
A, Single-contrast transcranial arthrogram and B, schematic drawing showing contrast filling of both upper and lower joint spaces. The disk (D) is anteriorly displaced and deformed. Contrast medium is seen to connect the posterior recess of the lower joint space and posterior recess of the upper joint space, indicating the position of the perforation (arrows).

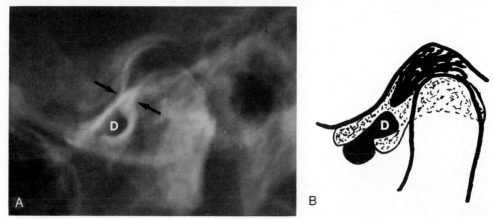

Figure 4–36
A, *Transcranial arthrogram and* B, *diagrammatic depiction showing disk (D) displacement and perforation. The exact site of the perforation (arrows) is demonstrated in this example. It is unusual for the exact site of the perforation to be directly visualized.*

and we also have occasionally encountered surgical follow-up of false-positive arthrographic diagnosis of perforation. These artificial perforations are probably due to a straddling of the needle between the upper and lower joint spaces during joint puncture, resulting in simultaneous opacification during injection of the contrast material. An experienced examiner could suspect this at the time of the procedure. It is fortuitous, however, that virtually all the perforation cases are associated with anterior disk displacement without reduction. Therefore, the primary diagnosis is disk displacement without reduction and perforation is a secondary diagnosis. The findings of perforation stage the disorder as long-standing and chronic.

Disk Displacement Without Reduction That Is Associated with Clicking Sounds

Some patients have clicking sounds emanating from the joint and yet will be diagnosed by arthrography to have disk displacement without reduction (Fig. 4–37A through D). This condition also represents chronic displacement of the disk but is associated with adhesions or advanced degenerative changes of the condyle, disk, and temporal bone. These multiple irregular surfaces provide frictional restrictions that can cause clicking sounds. This is an important clinical pitfall to avoid, since these patients are often indistinguishable from those with the earlier stage of disk displacement, disk displacement with reduction. The association of crepitus or degenerative joint disease or both should increase the level of suspicion.

Eminence Click

Loud popping sounds of the TMJ that occur in patients with large degrees of vertical jaw opening may be associated with bony incoordination between the condyle and articular eminence (Fig. 4–38A through C). The patients may also present with a history of jaw dislocation or subluxation. Typically they do

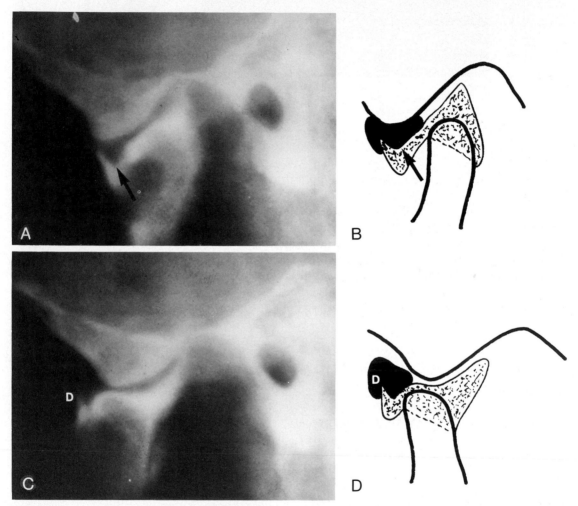

Figure 4–37

*An example of disk displacement **without reduction** that is associated with a clicking sound. This uncommon presentation can lead to clinical understaging of the severity of the internal derangements. A and B are images with the jaw closed, showing disk displacement (arrows). C and D show the arthrotomogram and diagrammatic depiction of the arthrotomogram with the jaw maximally opened and beyond the opening click. The disk (D) is still displaced.*

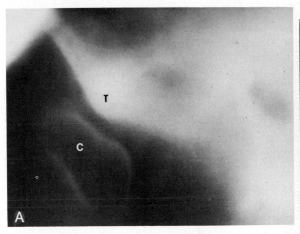

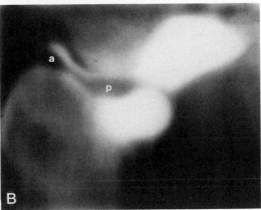

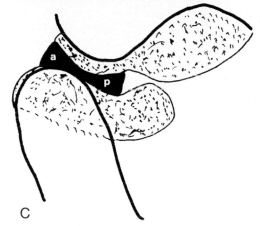

Figure 4–38
Loud popping sounds of the TMJ that occur in patients with large degrees of vertical jaw opening may be associated with bony incoordination between the condyle and bony tubercle. A, Extreme anterior translation of the condyle (C) beyond the tubercle (T). This is associated with a loud popping or clicking sound. B and C are the arthrotomogram and diagrammatic depiction of the position of the disk relative to the condyle and tubercle with jaw opening. The disk (a, anterior band; p, posterior band) is in a normal relationship to the condyle and temporal bone at all jaw positions. Thus, the popping or clicking sounds emanating from the joint are due to a mechanical incoordination between the condyle, disk complex, and tubercle.

not have pain, and their clicks occur at the same locations of jaw opening and closing. Frequently, the patients will have normal disk function and position. Clinically, however, this is difficult to differentiate from a true internal derangement.

Displacement of the Condyle Anterior to the Anterior Band of the Disk

On rare occasions we have demonstrated the condyle to translate anterior to the anterior band of the disk (Fig. 4–39*A* and *B*). This is a form of posterior displacement of the disk in which the condyle articulates against the anterior capsule wall anterior to the anterior band of the disk. This has been seen to occur late during opening under or anterior to the articular eminence. This has been associated with clicking and sometimes also with locking on closing. In rare instances the disk has been folded behind the condyle on closing (see Chapter 10).

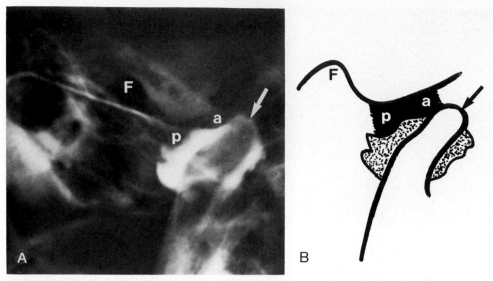

Figure 4–39
A, *Transcranial arthrogram with a contrast injection into the lower joint space and B, schematic drawing showing the condylar head (arrow) translating beyond the anterior band of the disk at maximal jaw opening. The anterior (a) and posterior (b) bands of the disk are indicated. The glenoid fossa (F) is also indicated for orientation.*

ARTHROGRAPHY OF MISCELLANEOUS CONDITIONS

Trauma

No systematic evaluation of internal derangement by arthrography related to trauma severe enough to result in fractures of the condyle or condylar neck has been reported. Our limited experience with these types of patients suggest that internal derangements may occur. However, ankylosis of the TMJ is much more common, and this makes the arthrographic technique extremely difficult to perform (Fig. 4–40A and B). It is our feeling that magnetic resonance

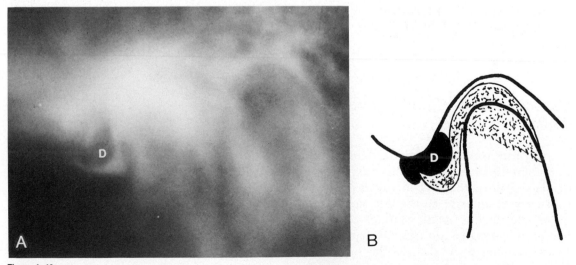

Figure 4–40
Lower joint space ankylosis. A, Arthrotomogram and B, diagrammatic depiction of a lower joint space ankylosis. The contrast material was injected into the lower joint space with great difficulty. The lower joint space is very small in volume and the disk (D) is noted to be displaced anteriorly. With attempted maximal jaw opening the condyle does not translate but simply rotates within the glenoid fossa. With suspected ankylosis, magnetic resonance is clearly the modality of choice for this evaluation.

imaging is a more effective modality for evaluating patients who have sustained severe mandibular trauma. MR imaging will allow an examination of these patients during the acute phase of the injury and permit an earlier assessment of the extent of hard and soft tissue damage.

Loose Bodies

Patients presenting with symptomatology suggesting internal derangement may on rare occasions be diagnosed as having loose bodies ("joint mice").[57] These loose bodies may or may not be calcified, and the diagnosis may be appreciated on the plain radiographs alone. Arthrography ensures a correct preoperative diagnosis (Fig. 4–41A through C). The cause of loose bodies is unknown, but they have been noted to occur in association with degenerative arthritis.

Arthrographic Imaging of Sideways Disk Displacement

It is difficult to evaluate the mediolateral position of the disk using arthrography in the transcranial projection. Attempts have been made to use anteroposterior arthrography and arthrotomography; by these techniques it is

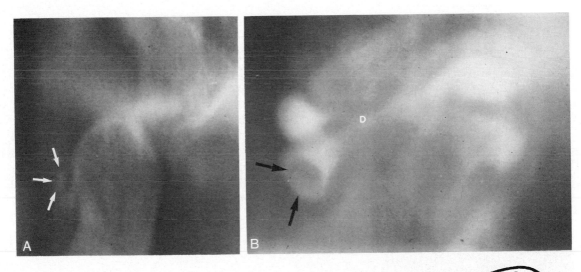

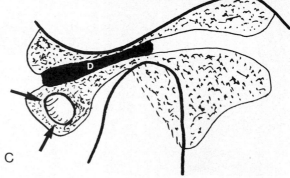

Figure 4–41
A, Multidirectional tomogram, B, arthrotomogram, and C, diagrammatic depiction of a large, partially calcified loose body (arrows) located within the lower joint space in a patient with degenerative arthritis of the TMJ. The disk (D), though apparently elongated, is only slightly displaced. (Courtesy of Dr. Quentin Anderson.)

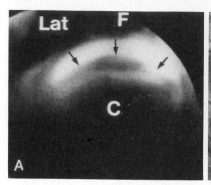

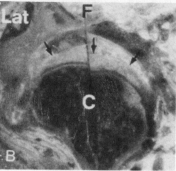

Figure 4–42
A, Anterior/posterior dual-space arthrotomogram and B, corresponding cryosection
showing the disk (arrows) in a normal superior position over the condyle (C). The
glenoid fossa (F) is indicated for orientation.
Lat, lateral.

difficult to determine whether a disk is medially or laterally displaced (Figs. 4–
42A and B and 4–43A and B).[58, 59]

The edge-sign is regarded as a contrast medium margin passing over the
lower part of the condyle at the closed- or open-mouth position. The edge-sign
was described by Khoury and Dolan and may be an indication of sideways
displacement of a disk.[35] Our experience is that the edge-sign is reliable if it is
clearly depicted, as in Figure 4–44A through D. In this joint the displacement
in a sideways fashion was accentuated on opening, which facilitated the diagnosis
of an anterior and sideways disk displacement without reduction. However, in
our experience, the absence of an edge-sign does not rule out a sideways disk
displacement.

Rupture of the Posterior Disk Attachment

Perforations between the lower and upper joint usually occur in the
posterior disk attachment and less often in the disk itself. Before a perforation
occurs there are small ruptures of the posterior disk attachment. Usually these
are seen on the inferior surface and can be described as partial perforations or
ruptures (Fig. 4–45A and B). If contrast medium is injected into the lower joint
space, sometimes filling of these defects can be seen in the posterior disk
attachment (Fig. 4–45A and B). These ruptures are a sign of a more advanced
stage and should be considered as the beginning of a perforation.

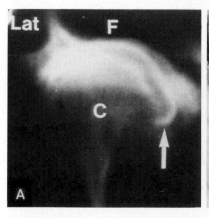

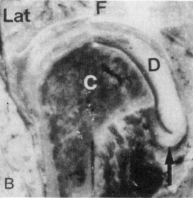

Figure 4–43
A, Dual-space anterior/posterior arthrotomogram and B, corresponding cryosection,
showing medial disk (D) displacement (arrow). The condyle (C) and glenoid fossa (F)
are indicated for orientation. Lat, lateral.

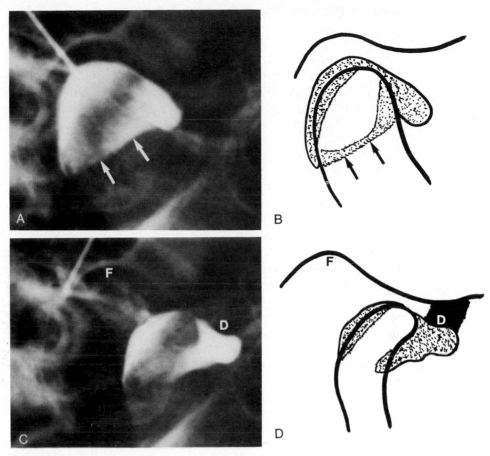

Figure 4–44

A, *Transcranial arthrogram with injection of contrast medium into the lower joint space and B, schematic drawing showing a contrast medium margin (arrows) passing over the lower part of the condyle. C and D, On opening, this contrast medium margin is accentuated and the disk (D) remains anterior to the condyle. The arthrographic diagnosis was anterior and medial disk displacement without reduction. The glenoid fossa (F) is indicated for orientation.*

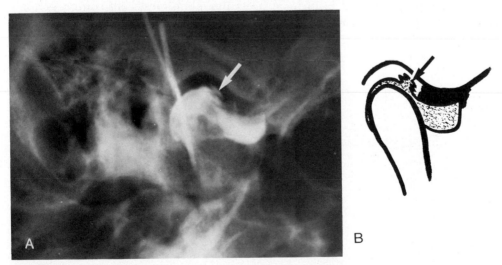

Figure 4–45

A, *Transcranial arthrogram with contrast medium injected into the lower joint space and B, schematic drawing showing anterior disk displacement and deformation. In addition, there is a partial perforation or rupture (arrow) on the undersurface of the posterior disk attachment. See also Figure 4–36A and B.*

Inflammatory Arthritis

A diagnosis of inflammatory arthritis of the TMJ can be established on clinical parameters. In rheumatoid arthritis the patients generally have multiple joint involvement, an elevation of the sedimentation rate, and an elevated rheumatoid factor. Other forms of inflammatory arthritis occur in association with skin lesions (psoriasis) or other stigmata such as inflammatory bowel disease. These conditions are discussed in greater detail in Chapter 10.

COMPLICATIONS

Serious complications following TMJ arthrography are extremely uncommon. The TMJ is quite resistant to infection; we have experienced no cases of infection, nor have any cases been reported in the literature.

One of the most frequent complications of TMJ arthrography is contrast medium extravasation into the joint capsule and soft tissues around the joint causing pain. Non-ionic contrast media are the agents of choice to minimize this discomfort.

A case of parotiditis has been reported following arthrography with larger needles and cannulas. A cannula tip can be lost in the region of the joint with this technique.[7]

Some patients show a great deal of anxiety during the arthrographic procedure, and these patients will infrequently experience a vagal reaction (fainting episode). Such a response will be associated with hypotension and bradycardia. In rare instances one must be prepared to administer 0.8 to 1 mg of atropine intravenously.

Transient facial nerve palsy may result from too vigorous infiltration of the local anesthetic. We do not recommend a nerve block during the arthrographic procedure, and therefore some patients may experience pain as the needle is placed on the periosteum of the condyle and as the joint is distended with the contrast injection. The discomfort is transient in the great majority of cases. The use of non-ionic contrast medium will help minimize this problem. If persistent joint pain occurs following the procedure, we recommend an oral anti-inflammatory agent (aspirin or acetaminophen) and cold compress application to the affected side.

HISTORY

The introduction of double-contrast arthrography as an alternative to single-contrast arthrography was an attempt to improve and refine the accuracy of this examination. Double contrast is a variant of arthrography in which the injection of iodinated contrast medium is combined with a gas contrast medium. The iodinated contrast medium is dense while the gas is lucent. The joint space and disk margins are thus outlined more clearly when compared with an iodinated medium alone.

Double-contrast arthrography has been used extensively for examination of the knee and was first described by Bircher in 1931[60] and more extensively by the same author in 1934.[61] Double-contrast arthrography is performed with the injection of a small amount of iodinated contrast medium followed by the injection of a larger amount of gas. The most commonly used gas for double-contrast arthrography today is unsterilized room air. In the past different gases have been used, such as carbon dioxide, but postarthrographic symptoms have been found to be lowest with regular room air.[62] The purpose of injecting air is distention of the joint space so that the articular surfaces, coated with iodinated contrast, stand out and can be more clearly evaluated.

Although double contrast mainly has been used for examination of the knee,[63–66] it also has been employed in examination of the ankle,[67] the elbow,[68–73] the shoulder,[65, 72–76] and the TMJ.[25–30, 77]

DOUBLE-CONTRAST ARTHROGRAPHY OF THE TMJ

The first description of double-contrast arthrography of the TMJ came from a German research group in the late 1960s.[25, 26] These investigators presented a single patient case and concluded that double-contrast arthrography was valuable for detection of early cartilage defects. More recently, double-contrast arthrography has been refined and systematically evaluated in a series of clinical and experimental studies.[27–30, 77–79]

Double-contrast arthrography, or more specifically dual-space double-contrast arthrography, is technically more difficult to perform and usually takes longer than a single-contrast examination. The resulting images, however, depict with greater detail the articular surfaces, the extent of the joint spaces, and the configuration of the disk. Examples of single-space, single-contrast and dual-space, double-contrast arthrography of a normal (Fig. 4–46) and an abnormal TMJ (Fig. 4–47) with correlation to cryosectional morphology clearly show the different characters of the two examinations. A patient case with dual space arthrotomography and dual-space double-contrast arthrotomography is shown in Figure 4–48.

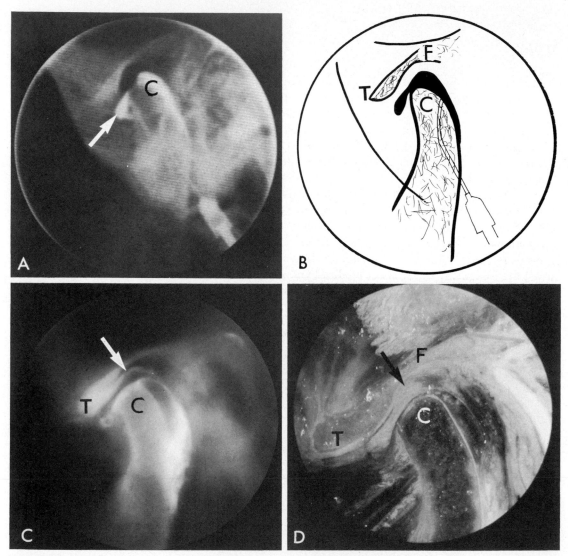

Figure 4–46
Comparison of single- and double-contrast arthrography in normal joint. A, Lower space, single-contrast arthrogram, B, corresponding schematic drawing, C, dual space double-contrast arthrotomogram, and D, corresponding cryosection. The configuration of the lower joint space (arrow in A) suggests normal superior disk position. This is confirmed in the dual space double-contrast arthrotomogram (C) and in the cryosection (D). The posterior band of the disk (arrows in C and D), the condyle (C), the tubercle (T), and the fossa (F) are indicated for orientation.

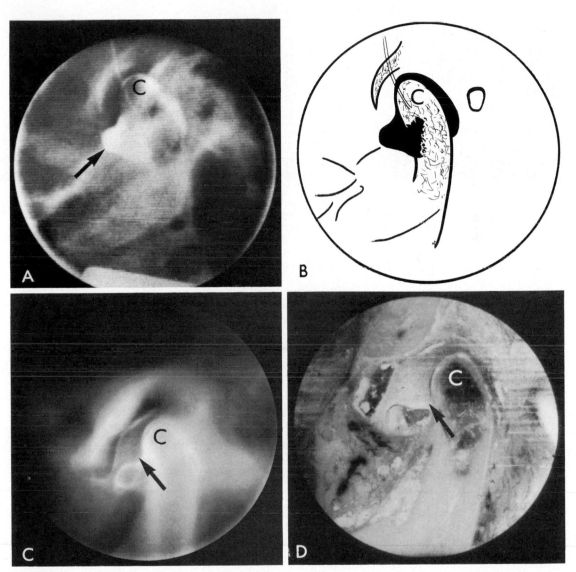

Figure 4–47
Comparison of single and double contrast in abnormal joint. A, Lower space, single-contrast arthrogram, B, corresponding schematic drawing, C, dual-space double-contrast arthrotomogram, and D, corresponding cryosection of a joint with anterior disk displacement. The configuration of the lower joint space (arrow in A) suggests anterior disk displacement. This is confirmed in the dual-space double-contrast arthrotomogram (C) and in the cryosection (D). The posterior band of the disk (arrows in C and D) and the condyle are indicated for orientation.

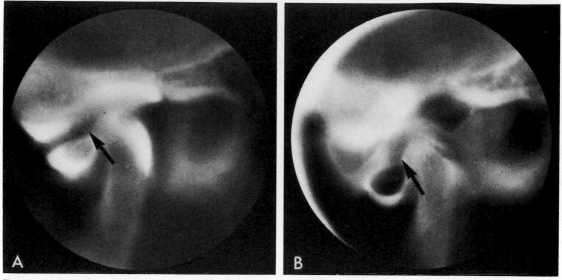

Figure 4–48
Comparison of single- and double-contrast arthrotomography in a patient. A, Dual-space, single-contrast arthrotomogram, and B, dual-space double-contrast arthrotomogram of a patient, showing anterior disk (arrow) displacement. The posterior band of a disk is located anterior to the condyle. The outline of the joint compartments and the form and configuration of the disk are better visualized with the double-contrast technique.

Technique

As with the single-contrast arthrogram, the arthrographic procedure and possible complications are explained to the patient before starting the study. Usually open- and closed-mouth lateral transcranial films or corresponding tomograms are obtained before arthrography. The purpose of these initial views is to document the range of motion and to obtain an impression of the condition of the osseous components of the joint.

A fluoroscopic table or a C-arm (Fig. 4–49) with an x-ray tube and image intensifier is adequate equipment for the first part of the examination. The image intensifier has to have high resolution and a magnification capacity up to about three times, since the joint is small and the condyle measures only about 10 mm anteroposteriorly.

The patient should lie on the side with the head oriented so that the site to be injected is located superiorly. If a fluoroscopic table is used, the head should be tilted, with the top of the head downward as illustrated for single-contrast examination (see Figure 4–4). This head tilt will project the joint to be examined free of the base of the skull. If a C-arm (Fig. 4–49) is used, it should be tilted caudally instead to obtain the same effect. Joint visualization is optimized by slightly adjusting the amount of head tilt and turning the head left to right until an optimal image of the joint is obtained.

Opening and closing movements are studied and recorded on videotape. The area of joint puncture is localized and marked on the skin with a permanent marker, as described for single-contrast examination (see Figure 4–6). Local anesthetic is injected in the preauricular region specifically where the joint is going to be punctured; between 0.75 and 1 ml of 2 per cent solution is usually administered for a double-contrast examination, which is slightly more than for a single-contrast examination.

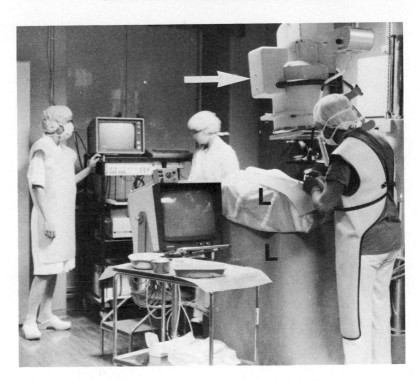

Figure 4–49
Clinical setup for joint puncture, using a C-arm with an image intensifier (arrow) located above the patient. The patient is covered with lead shields (L) and is not seen.

Joint Puncture

The lower and upper joint spaces are punctured in the same area as for the single-contrast examination. Thus, the lower joint space is punctured in its posterior recess along the posterior margin of the condyle, and the upper joint space is punctured in the glenoid fossa or along the posterior surface of the articular eminence.

For double-contrast examination, it is preferable to use catheters (Fig. 4–50) instead of needles. This is because two contrast media are injected; since there is a need for aspiration, it is necessary to leave the catheters in the joint space during the examination. We advocate using angiographic catheters (The Desert Company, Sandy, Utah). The 21- or 20-gauge sizes are adequate for the TMJ and have a length of 1 to 1.25 inches. These are 0.25 to 0.5 inch longer than the butterfly needle used for the single-contrast arthrogram. These longer catheters are desirable because during jaw movement the tip of the catheter should remain in the joint space and not slip out at the maximal open-mouth views. The standard catheter that can be used in most patients is 21-gauge and 1-inch. For a large patient, a 1.25-inch catheter could be recommended in the lower joint space. In the upper joint space the 1-inch catheter is useful for most patients. The longer catheter is needed in the lower joint space because movement is greater than in the upper joint space.

After the catheters have been correctly inserted into the joint space, the outer parts should be affixed to the skin with tape (Fig. 4–51). At this point attempts can be made to aspirate possible joint effusion. This is only rarely successful, probably because joint effusion is located medially in the joint space with the patient lying on the side. If joint effusion can be aspirated or spontaneously flows out of the joint space, this is clearly abnormal.

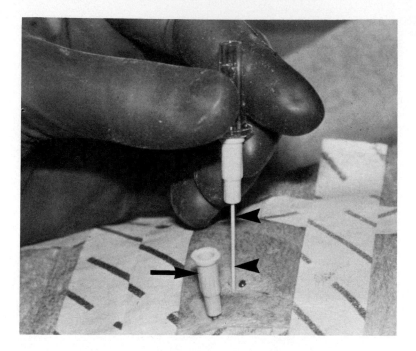

Figure 4–50
Cannulation of the upper and lower joint spaces using catheters. A catheter has been placed into the lower joint space (arrow). A second catheter (arrowheads) is inserted into the upper joint space.

Contrast Injection

After aspiration, a few drops of contrast medium are dropped into the hubs of the catheters to avoid injecting air with the iodinated contrast medium into the joint space. Air bubbles should be avoided since they may be confused with loose bodies. The extension tubes filled with contrast medium and connected to syringes are connected to the catheters. Contrast medium is injected into the lower joint space first, as described for single-contrast arthrography. Between 0.2 and 0.5 ml is usually optimal for visualization of the lower joint space. Joint movements are studied during fluoroscopy, as in single-

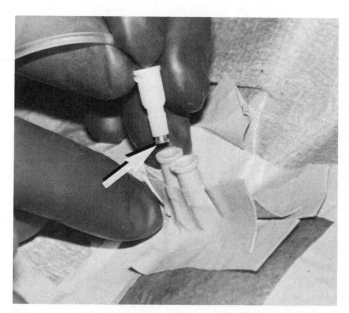

Figure 4–51
Catheters in the joint space have been affixed to the skin with tape. An extension set (arrow) and tubing where contrast is injected into catheters is shown.

contrast arthrography, and spot films are obtained at the closed- and open-mouth positions. Additional spot films may be obtained at positions between closed- and open-mouth positions, where abnormalities are optimally visualized.

Contrast medium is then also injected into the upper joint space. Approximately 0.3 to 0.5 ml is used. Again, joint movement is studied during fluoroscopy, and spot films are again obtained at the closed- and open-mouth positions. Additional spot films should be obtained at positions where abnormalities are optimally visualized. Up to this point this examination is not different from a dual-space single-contrast examination, with the exception of the use of two catheters instead of the one scalp vein needle.

Double-Contrast

The actual double-contrast technique begins with aspiration of the contrast medium from both joint spaces. As much of the contrast medium as possible should be aspirated. This is best done while the patient is sitting up and opens and closes the mouth slowly. Because the catheters move slightly in the joint space, it is possible to aspirate more contrast medium than if they stayed in the same place.

After the contrast medium has been aspirated, the extension tubes are removed and the patient is transported from the fluoroscopic table to the tomographic unit. We have been using a Philips Polytome U (Massiot, Paris, France). With this radiographic unit it is possible to use both upright sitting and supine patient positions. The sitting position is advantageous for double-contrast arthrotomography of the TMJ because more accurate joint localization is possible, and this posture provides a more natural position for the mandible relative to the maxilla.

Air Injection and Double-Contrast Arthrotomography

Once the patient has been positioned in the tomographic unit and the head has been oriented and fixed to a predetermined position by the aid of the head holder (Fig. 4–52), new extension tubes are connected to the catheters. These are necessary because otherwise small amounts of iodinated contrast medium will be reinjected into the joint spaces and reduce the quality of the double-contrast arthrotomograms. Glass syringes of about 2 to 3 ml are connected to the extension tubes. We have tried both plastic disposable and glass syringes. The glass syringes are preferable over regular disposable plastic syringes because of lower friction, which makes it easier to feel how much air should be injected.

The patient is asked to open the mouth slightly, corresponding to a rest position, and about 0.5 to 1 ml of air is injected simultaneously into both upper and lower joint spaces (Fig. 4–52). Both joint spaces should be injected at the same time, otherwise the disk has a tendency to move toward the noninjected joint space and lie close to the articular surface. This makes it more difficult to outline the configuration of the disk. The amount of air to be injected is determined by the resistance to the injection; approximately 0.5 to 1 ml of air in each joint space is usually optimal. More air usually can be injected at maximal mouth opening. If more air has been injected for the open-mouth images, this should be aspirated before the mouth is closed. If the mouth is

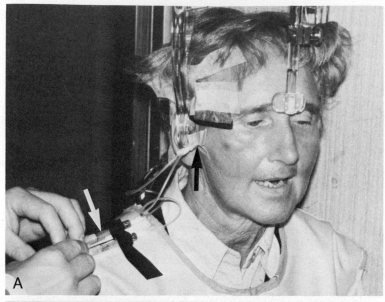

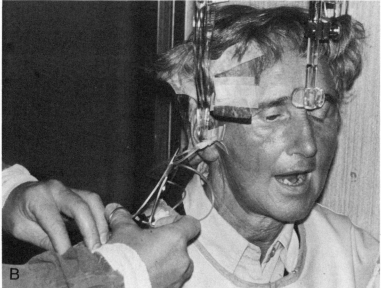

Figure 4–52
Injection of air for double contrast. The patient has been positioned in the tomographic unit and extension sets have been connected to the catheters (black arrow). A, Air is injected with a glass syringe (white arrow) simultaneously into both upper and lower joint spaces. B, After injection, a clamp is put on the extension sets to prevent the air from flowing out of the joint space.

closed without aspiration of extensive air in the joint space, emphysema in the soft tissues around the joint could result. After the appropriate amount of air has been injected, a clamp is placed on the extension tubes to prevent air from escaping from the joint spaces (Fig. 4–52*B*). It is desirable to have tested the tomographic layers and patient positioning before arthrography so that once contrast and air have been injected, successful arthrotomography can be accomplished in the first attempt.

Many different film-target movements are available, such as hypocycloidal, linear, and spiral movements. We prefer the hypocycloidal or spiral movements, since these provide the clearest images. The arthrotomographic images with these movements should be acquired with a tissue thickness of approximately 3 mm.[34] Linear tomography also can be used, but there is incomplete blurring of structures outside the joint, creating artifacts that degrade the image quality.

Multifilm Cassette

The arthrotomographic images can be obtained on single films or multiple film cassettes. We have been using two multifilm cassettes with five or seven films. These provide five or seven arthrotomographic images in one exposure. The use of a multifilm cassette is valuable because it saves time, which is essential in arthrography. The first images are the sharpest; the contrast medium will diffuse into the surrounding soft tissue within 10 to 15 minutes. The multifilm cassette also reduces the radiation dose compared with the same number of single-film images. Finally, the fact that all the images were obtained in the same mandibular position is valuable knowledge when the images are interpreted. We recommend the use of a multifilm cassette both for tomography and arthrotomography of the TMJ.

Mandibular Positions for Double-Contrast Arthrotomography

Double-contrast arthrotomography is performed at the rest position and at maximal mouth opening. In patients with clicking, arthrotomograms also could be obtained before and after clicking; if there are positions in between when abnormalities are better visualized, additional images should be obtained. Patients with symptoms of open lock also should be imaged in the open lock position in order to determine whether the disk or the anterior aspect of the articular eminence is the etiology of the open lock.

DOUBLE-CONTRAST ARTHROTOMOGRAPHIC FINDINGS

Arthrographic findings are classified like other imaging modalities, mainly into normal superior disk positioning, disk displacement with reduction, disk displacement without reduction, and perforation. Perforations are usually associated with disk displacement without reduction and are rarely seen in joints with disk displacement with reduction or in joints with normal superior disk position.

Normal Joint

The normal joint is characterized by a biconcave disk located superior to the condyle, with the posterior band of the disk riding on top of the condyle and the thin central part of the disk located between the anterior prominence of the condyle and the posterior prominence of the articular tubercle (Fig. 4–53). With normal superior disk position the lower joint space is relatively small. Studies of normal volunteers without symptoms have indicated that there is a substantial variation in the sizes of the anterior recesses of lower joint spaces in individuals with normal superior disk position.[45] Double-contrast arthrotomography is specifically valuable for studying joints when a single-contrast arthrogram in the transcranial projection is not conclusive.

On opening, the disk translates along the articular eminence in the upper joint space and the condyle rotates against the inferior surface of the disk. The central thin zone of the disk consistently lies between the prominence of the

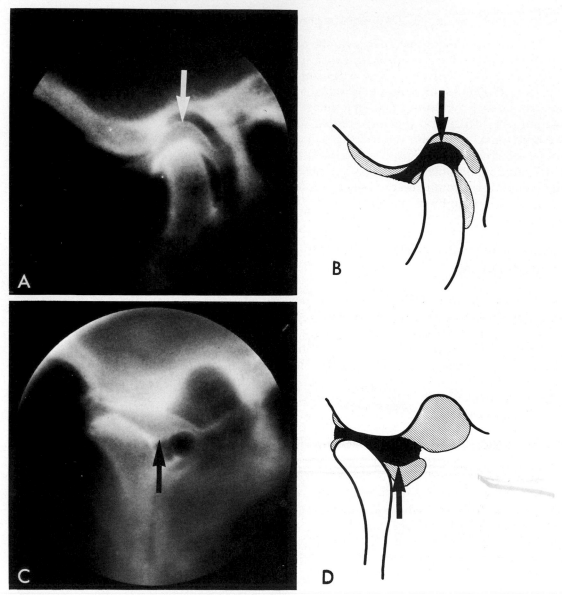

Figure 4–53
Normal temporomandibular joint. Dual-space double-contrast arthrotomograms at the closed (A) and maximal mouth opening (C). B and D, Corresponding schematic drawings. The disk is located with its posterior band (arrows) superior to the condyle in the closed mouth image and posterior to the condyle in the maximal open mouth images (C).

condyle and the prominence of the articular tubercle during joint function (Fig. 4–54). Normally the disk is biconcave, and it merges with even thickness into the posterior disk attachment.

False-Negative Diagnosis with Arthrography

During arthrography, especially double-contrast arthrotomography, the joint spaces are expanded. Expansion of the joint spaces is necessary for a clear delineation of the articular surfaces. It is our experience that expansion of the

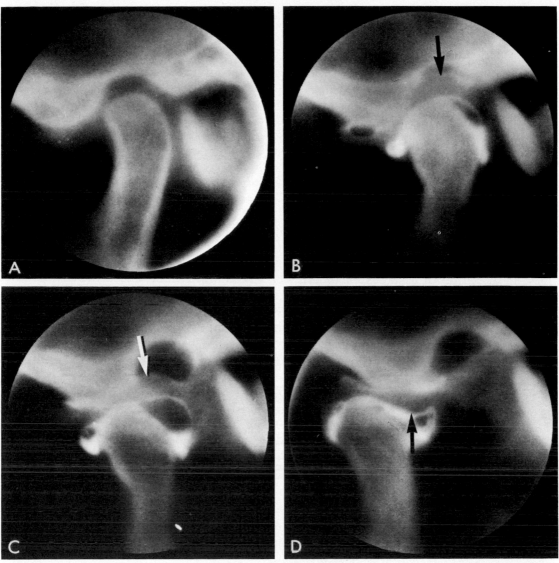

Figure 4–54
Normal joint function. A, Prearthrographic tomogram showing normal osseous structures. B, Closed mouth dual-space double-contrast arthrotomogram, showing the posterior band of the disk (arrow) in normal superior position in this asymptomatic volunteer. C, At half-open mouth position, the disk is located between the condyle and temporal component. D, At maximal mouth opening, the biconcave disk is located between the articular eminence and the posterior surface of the condyle.

joint spaces does not result in displacement of the disk (false-positive diagnosis). However, if displacement of a disk is minimal and reduction occurs early, there might be the risk of a false-negative diagnosis, since images may be obtained after the position of the disk has normalized, yet the disk would be slightly anteriorly displaced when the patient closes the mouth firmly on the back teeth without any material injected into the joint spaces. It is our experience that the risk of false-negative diagnosis of disk displacement is greater than the risk of false-positive diagnosis of disk displacement using arthrography. To overcome this minimal risk, single-contrast arthrography is done before double-contrast examination. In the single-contrast examination, only a small amount of contrast medium is injected to begin with. It is important to ensure that the patient closes the mouth all the way to the intercuspal position to show an early reduction of disk displacement.

Another small risk of false-negative diagnosis occurs if the disk is only partially anteriorly displaced, and the displacement is confined to the most lateral part of the joint. Then a normal disk position will be seen in the rest of the joint and the diagnosis is dependent on the depiction of the most lateral part of the joint. Here, the transcranial projection may sometimes be better than tomographic images.

We have attempted anteroposterior or coronal arthrography in patients but with only limited success. It seems that there are too many dense osseous structures anteroposterior to the joint that obscure the image. Good and clear anteroposterior arthrograms or arthrotomograms have not been routinely obtained in clinical work. An example from our autopsy studies of an antero-posterior dual-space double-contrast arthrotomogram is shown in Figure 4–55. This clearly shows the relationship between the upper and lower joint spaces, the disk, and the medial and lateral recesses. The same high-quality images have not been possible to obtain routinely in patients.

Anterior Disk Displacement with Reduction

The two most common findings in patients suffering from TMJ pain, clicking, and limitation of opening are different forms of disk displacement and degenerative joint disease. The different forms of disk displacement are listed in Chapter 2. The most common displacement is in an anterior direction, but there are medial and lateral components to the displacement in up to one fourth to one third of patients.[36] Anteroposterior or coronal arthrograms have been attempted both in patients and in cadaver material[58, 59] (see Figs. 4–42 and 4–43). However, results have not been consistent since too many overlapping structures and too little distention result in inferior image quality. An example of double-contrast arthrography from our cadaver studies is shown in Figure 4–55.

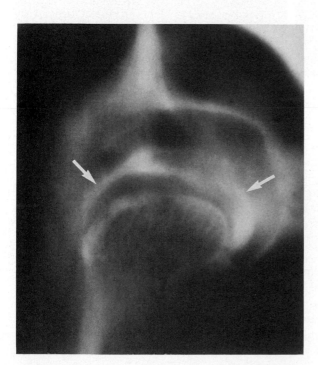

Figure 4–55
Anterior-posterior dual-space double-contrast arthrotomogram from a cadaver joint showing the disk (arrows) in a normal superior position over the condyle. The upper and lower joint spaces are distended by the injected air. The disk is flattened in its lateral aspect.

Anterior disk displacement with reduction (Fig. 4–56) implies that the disk is anteriorly displaced at the closed-mouth position and on opening the disk position is normalized.

Partial Anterior Disk Displacement

It has been seen in both patients and cadaver material that the disk is frequently rotated around its medial attachment to the condyle. This means that the disk is anteriorly displaced in the lateral part of the joint and remains in a normal superior position in the medial part of the joint (Fig. 4–57). This

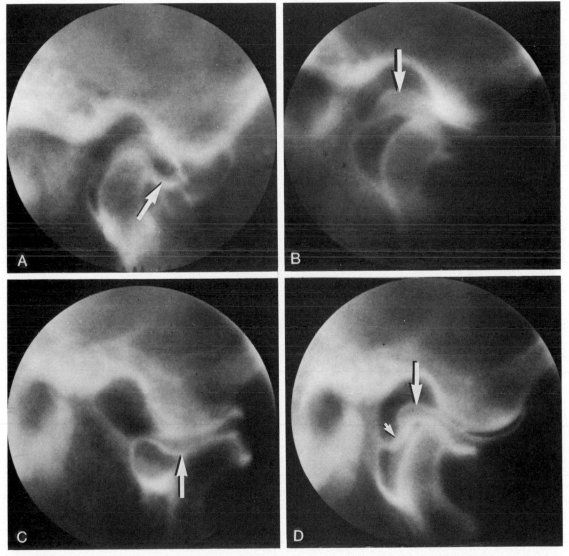

Figure 4–56
Anterior disk displacement with reduction. A, Dual-space double-contrast arthrotomogram at the rest position, showing the disk (arrow) anterior to the condyle. B, After the opening click, the disk is in a normal relationship to the condyle. C, At maximal mouth opening, the disk is located between the articular tubercle and the posterior surface of the condyle. D, This image was obtained during closing, just before the closing click and displacement of the disk. The disk (arrow) is located superior to the condyle. The posterior disk attachment is elongated and hanging down (small arrow). C and D are from a different joint than A and B.

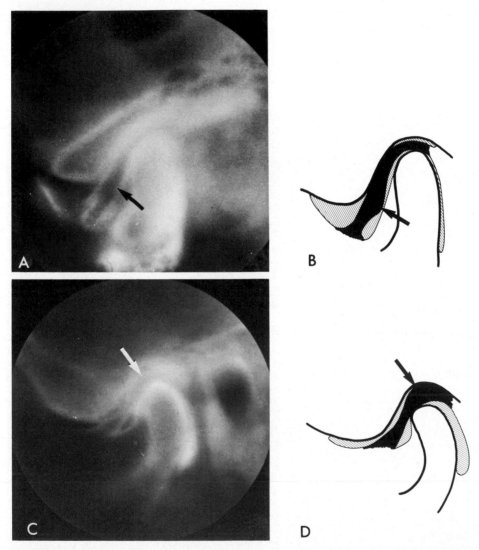

Figure 4–57
Partial anterior disk displacement. Dual-space double-contrast arthrotomograms from lateral (A) and medial parts (C) of a joint with partial anterior disk displacement. Diagrammatic depictions are seen in B and D. In the lateral part of the joint (A and B), the disk is anteriorly displaced. The posterior band of the disk is indicated by an arrow. In the central part of the joint (C and D), the disk is in a normal position. The images in A and C were obtained in the same exposure using the multifilm cassette. The information combined suggested partial anterior disk displacement.

has been termed partial anterior disk displacement,[29, 30, 80] and it is clearly seen on double-contrast arthrotomograms (Fig. 4–57) when multiple sagittal sections of the different mediolateral parts of the joint are compared. Most commonly the disk is anteriorly displaced in the lateral part of the joint and normal in the central and medial parts. However, the opposite occurs when the disk is anteriorly displaced in the medial part and remains in a normal superior position in the lateral part of the joint. In order to detect and clearly describe a partial anterior disk displacement, it is important to obtain arthrotomographic images all the way from the lateral to the medial part of the joint.

Disk Deformation

Advanced disk deformation is probably a result of displacement. Once the disk is anteriorly displaced and functions in the abnormal position, it becomes deformed as a result of the abnormal function. Thickening occurs on the inferior surface of the disk under the posterior band (Fig. 4–58). If disk deformation continues, the disk will get thicker, and eventually it will be a biconvex disk (Fig. 4–59). Extensive deformation with total loss of morphology of the disk may occur in late-stage internal derangement and degenerative joint disease (Fig. 4–60). Most commonly, disk deformation occurs with more advanced stages of internal derangement, but in some patients there might be extensive deformation although the position of the disk normalizes on opening. The longer the disk has been functioning in an anterior position, the more extensive could be the deformation. Deformation of the disk is probably more precisely assessed with double-contrast arthrotomography than with single-contrast lower-space arthrography.[81]

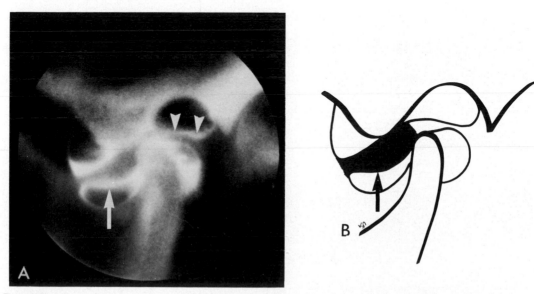

Figure 4–58
Deformation of disk. Dual-space double-contrast arthrotomogram (A) and schematic drawing (B) showing deformation of a disk (arrow). The anteriorly displaced disk shows a marked thickening of the posterior band. The posterior disk attachment (arrowheads) is elongated.

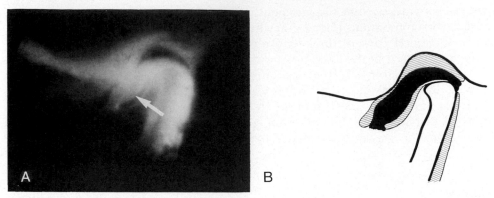

Figure 4–59
Deformation of disk. Dual-space double-contrast arthrotomogram (A) and schematic drawing (B) showing deformation of disk (arrow).
The anteriorly displaced disk shows a marked thickening of the posterior band and elongation of the posterior disk attachment.

Anterior Disk Displacement Without Reduction

This is characterized by the disk being anterior to the condyle on all mandibular movements (Fig. 4–61). This means that the position of the posterior band will not be normal relative to the condyle at any mandibular position. This condition is usually associated with disk deformation. Disk displacement without reduction is frequently associated with deformation of the disk ranging from thickening of the posterior band (see Figs. 4–58 and 4–59) to a totally biconvex disk (Fig. 4–60).

Perforation

Perforation is frequently associated with late-stage internal derangement. Perforation is rarely seen in a joint with normal superior disk position. Only a

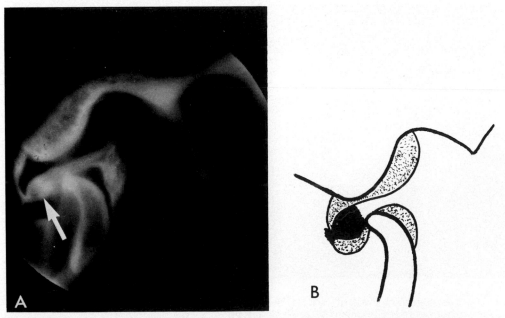

Figure 4–60
Biconvex disk. Dual-space double-contrast arthrotomogram (A) and schematic drawing (B) showing significant deformation of the disk
(arrow). The posterior band of the disk is biconvex. The central thin zone and the anterior third of a disk are almost nonexistent.

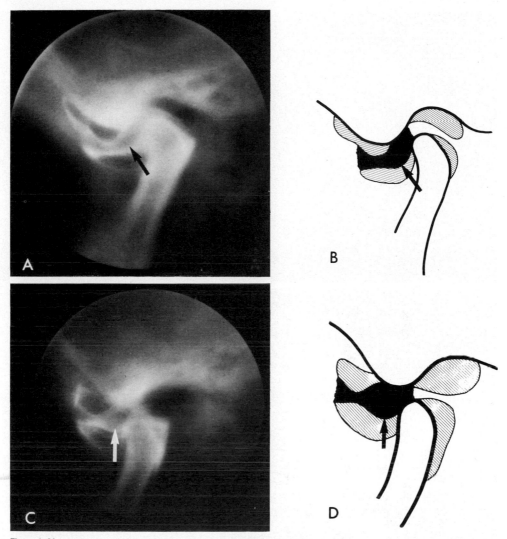

Figure 4–61

A, *Dual-space double-contrast arthrotomogram at rest position; C, at maximal mouth opening; and B and D, schematic drawings show anterior disk displacement without reduction. The posterior band of the disk (arrows) remains anterior to the condyle at maximal mouth opening. There is some deformation of the disk, with thickening of the posterior band.*

few joints with disk displacement with reduction show perforation. Perforations are usually located in the posterior disk attachment and not in the disk itself.[44] In a series of autopsy material, about 90 per cent of the perforations were located in the posterior disk attachment and only about 10 per cent in the disk per se.[44] Similar observations have been made in multiple patient studies.[28–30] A posterior disk attachment perforation in a cadaver specimen is seen in Figure 4–62. A perforation in the central thin zone of the disk in a patient is shown for comparison in Figure 4–63.

Adhesions

Adhesions are usually diagnosed with arthroscopy but can occasionally be seen with the use of double-contrast arthrotomography (Fig. 4–64). An example

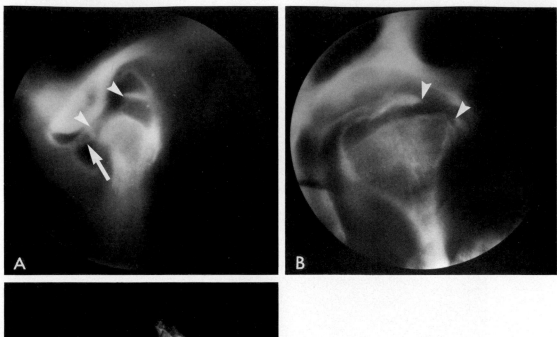

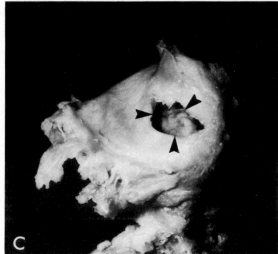

Figure 4–62
Perforation. Dual-space double-contrast arthrotomograms in sagittal (A) and coronal (B) planes, showing anterior displacement of the disk (arrow) and perforation of the posterior lateral third of the posterior disk attachment (arrowheads). C, Corresponding cadaver specimen showing perforation (arrowheads).

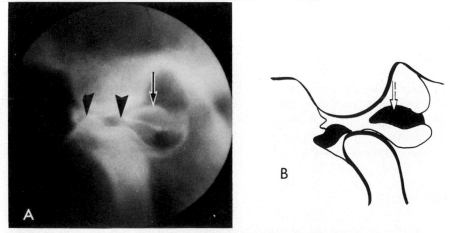

Figure 4–63
Perforation. Dual-space double-contrast arthrotomogram (A) and corresponding schematic drawing (B) showing perforation (arrowheads) in the central thin zone of the disk. The posterior band of the disk (arrow) remains in a normal position.

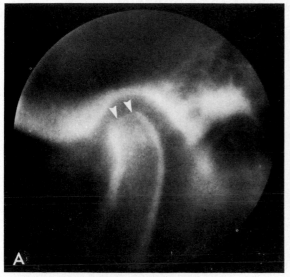
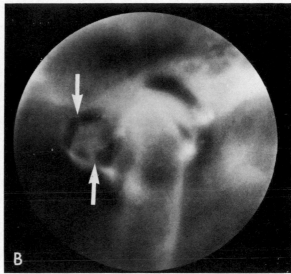

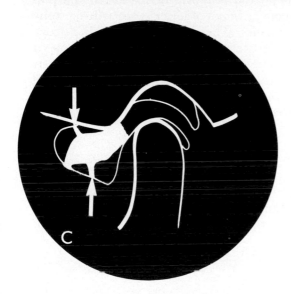

Figure 4–64
Adhesions. A, Sagittal tomogram, B, dual-space double-contrast arthrotomogram, and C, schematic drawing of a joint with anterior disk displacement without reduction and with adhesions. A shows a minimal flattening of the superior surface of the condyle (arrowheads). In B, the disk is anteriorly displaced and deformed. Adhesions exist between the upper and lower surfaces of the disk and the capsule (arrows).

of a joint with adhesions in a patient who suffered facial trauma is seen in Figure 4–64. Another relatively rare finding that can be diagnosed with double-contrast arthrotomography is synovial chondromatosis with loose bodies. A more extensive discussion of tumors of the TMJ is given in Chapter 10.

Imaging After Treatment

Imaging after surgical disk repositioning can be done with double-contrast arthrotomography, but this is usually technically difficult because peripheral intra-articular adhesions make joint puncture technically difficult. Today MR imaging is the preferred technique for imaging evaluation after surgical disk repositioning as well as after disk removal. The purpose of imaging evaluation is to assess the position of the disk and delineate intra-articular adhesions.

Imaging after diskectomy has also been done with double-contrast arthrotomography[82] and is extensively discussed in Chapter 7.

COMPLICATIONS OF DOUBLE-CONTRAST ARTHROGRAPHY

Complications after double-contrast arthrotomography are essentially the same as those of single-contrast arthrography and are extremely rare. Transient pain and discomfort are commonly encountered and treated symptomatically.[83] The use of air in the joint spaces includes the potential risk of causing emphysema in the soft tissues surrounding the joint. In our experience, a small emphysema in the soft tissue around the TMJ has occurred only in a few patients during early development of the technique. These cases resolved without treatment.

COMPARISON BETWEEN DOUBLE- AND SINGLE-CONTRAST ARTHROGRAPHY

A systematic study comparing double- and single-contrast arthrography in the same joint has been performed using fresh autopsy specimens.[79] Examples of these are shown in Figures 4–46, 4–47, and 4–48. A side-by-side comparison has shown that the single-space lower compartment of lower-space arthrography is better for demonstrating joint dynamics. The double-contrast dual-space arthrotomographic technique is better for demonstrating anatomic features of the joint, such as shape of the joint spaces and configuration of the disk in its different mediolateral sections. Perforation between the lower and upper joint spaces is best diagnosed with single-contrast arthrography as an overflow of contrast from the lower to the upper joint space.

CONCLUSION

Double-contrast arthrotomography is a refined technique that provides exquisite detail of the intra-articular anatomy of the joint. The technique is recommended when this information is clinically desirable and when a radiologist's skill in the technique is available.

References

1. Zimmer EA: Die Röntgenologie des Kiefergelenkes. Schweiz Monatsschr Zahnheilkd 1941;51:12–24.
2. Nørgaard F: Artrografi af kaebeleddet. Preliminary report. Acta Radiol 1944;25:679–685.
3. Nørgaard F: Temporomandibular arthrography. Thesis, Munksgaard, Copenhagen, 1947.
4. Campbell W: Clinical radiological investigations of the mandibular joints. Br J Radiol 1965;38:401–421.
5. Toller PA: Opaque arthrography of the temporomandibular joint. Int J Oral Surg 1974;3:17–28.
6. Neuberg AH, Munn CS, Robbins AH: Complications of arthrography. Radiology 1985;155:605–606.
7. Wilkes CH: Arthrography of the temporomandibular joint in patients with the TMJ pain-dysfunction syndrome. Minn Med 1978;61:645–652.
8. Wilkes CH: Structural and functional alterations of the temporomandibular joint. Northwest Dent 1978;57:287–294.
9. Bell KA, Walters PJ: Videofluoroscopy during arthrography of the temporomandibular joint. Radiology 1983;147:879.
10. Farrar WB: Diagnosis and treatment of anterior dislocation of the articular disk. NY J Dent 1971;41:348–351.

11. Farrar WB: Differentiation of temporomandibular joint dysfunction to simplify treatment. J Prosthet Dent 1972;*28*:629–636.
12. Farrar WB: Characteristics of the condylar path in internal derangement of the TMJ. J Prosthet Dent 1978;*39*:319–323.
13. Farrar WB, McCarty WL Jr: Inferior joint space arthrography and characteristics of condylar paths in internal derangements of the TMJ. J Prosthet Dent 1979;*41*:548–555.
14. Katzberg RW, Dolwick MF, Bales DJ, Helms CA: Arthrotomography of the temporomandibular joint: New technique and preliminary observations. AJR 1979;*132*:949–955.
15. Katzberg RW, Dolwick MF, Helms CA, et al: Arthrotomography of the temporomandibular joint. AJR 1980;*134*:995–1003.
16. McCarty WL Jr, Farrar WB: Surgery for internal derangements of the temporomandibular joint. J Prosthet Dent 1979;*42*:191–196.
17. Farrar WB, McCarty WL Jr: A Clinical Outline of Temporomandibular Joint Diagnosis and Treatment. 9th ed. Montgomery, Alabama, Normandie Publications, 1982, pp 165–167.
18. Bellavia WD: A functional jaw device to aid in treating anterior displaced disks. J Craniomandib Pract 1983;*1*:53–60.
19. Dugal GL: Closing a minor unilateral open bite on TMJ patients. J Craniomandib Pract 1983;*1*:39–41.
20. Dolwick MF, Riggs RR: Diagnosis and treatment of internal derangements of the temporomandibular joint. Dent Clin North Am 1983;27:561–572.
21. Lundh H, Westesson P-L, Kopp S, Tillström B: Anterior repositioning splint in the treatment of temporomandibular joints with reciprocal clicking. Comparison with a flat occlusal splint and an untreated control group. Oral Surg 1985;*60*:131–136.
22. Lundh H: Correction of temporomandibular joint disk displacement with occlusal therapy. Swed Dent J Suppl 1987;(51):1–38.
23. Frenkel G: Untersuchungen mit der Kombination Arthrographie und Tomographie zur Darstellung des Diskus articulares des Menschen. Dtsch Zahnaerztl Z 1965;*20*:1261–1274.
24. Blaschke DD, Solberg WK, Sanders B: Arthrography of the temporomandibular joint: Review of current status. J Am Dent Assoc 1980;*100*:388–395.
25. Arnaudow M, Haage H, Pflaum I: Die Doppelkontrast arthrographie des Kiefergelenkes. Dtsch Zahnarztl Z 1968;*23*:390–393.
26. Arnaudow M, Pflaum I: Neue Erkenntnisse in der Beurteilung bei der Kiefergelenktomographie. Dtsch Zahnarztl Z 1974;*29*:554–556.
27. Westesson P-L, Omnell K-Å, Rohlin M: Double-contrast tomography of the temporomandibular joint. A new technique based on autopsy specimen examinations. Acta Radiol (Diagn) (Stockh) 1980;*21*:777–784.
28. Westesson P-L: Double-contrast arthrography and internal derangement of the temporomandibular joint. Swed Dent J Suppl 1982;(13):1–57.
29. Westesson P-L: Double-contrast arthrotomography of the temporomandibular joint: Introduction of an arthrographic technique for visualization of the disk and articular surfaces. J Oral Maxillofac Surg 1983;*41*:163–172.
30. Westesson P-L: Arthrography of the temporomandibular joint. J Prosthet Dent 1984;*51*:535–543.
31. Katzberg RW: Temporomandibular joint imaging. Radiology 1989;*170*:297–307.
32. Westesson P-L, Manzione JV: Contrast media reaction during TMJ arthrography. AJR 1990;*154*:344.
33. Katzberg RW, Miller TL, Hayakawa K, et al: Temporomandibular joint arthrography: Comparison of morbidity with ionic and low osmolality contrast media. Radiology 1985;*155*:245–246.
34. Eckerdal O: Tomography of the temporomandibular joint. Correlation between tomographic image and histologic sections in a three-dimensional system. Acta Radiol (Diagn) (Suppl 329) (Stockh) 1973:196–197.
35. Khoury MB, Dolan E: Sideways dislocation of the temporomandibular joint meniscus: The edge sign. AJNR 1986;*7*:869–872.
36. Katzberg RW, Westesson P-L, Tallents RH, et al: Temporomandibular joint: MR assessment of rotational and sideways disk displacements. Radiology 1988;*169*:741–748.
37. Liedberg J, Westesson P-L, Kurita K: Sideways and rotational displacement of the temporomandibular joint disk: Diagnosis by arthrography and correlation to cryosectional morphology. Oral Surg Oral Med Oral Pathol 1990;*67*:757–763.
38. Helkimo M: Studies on function and dysfunction of the masticatory system. Thesis, University of Gothenburg, Sweden, 1974.
39. Hansson T, Nilner M: A study of the occurrence of symptoms of diseases of the temporomandibular joint masticatory musculature and related structures. J Oral Rehabil 1975;*2*:313–324.
40. Solberg WK, Woo MW, Houston JB: Prevalent mandibular dysfunction in young adults. J Am Dent Assoc 1979;*98*:25–34.
41. Isberg-Holm AM, Westesson P-L: Movement of disk and condyle in temporomandibular joints with clicking. An arthrographic and cineradiographic study on autopsy specimens. Acta Odontol Scand 1982;*40*:153–166.

42. Isberg-Holm AM, Westesson P-L: Movement of disk and condyle in temporomandibular joints without clicking: a high-speed cinematographic dissection study in autopsy specimens. Acta Odontol Scand 1982;*40*:167–179.
43. Miller TL, Katzberg RW, Tallents RH, et al: Temporomandibular joint clicking with nonreducing anterior displacement of the meniscus. Radiology 1985;*154*:121–124.
44. Westesson P-L, Bronstein SL, Leidberg J: Internal derangement of the temporomandibular joint: Morphologic description with correlation to function. Oral Surg Oral Med Oral Pathol 1985;*59*:323–331.
45. Westesson P-L, Eriksson L, Kurita K: Temporomandibular joint: Variation of normal arthrographic anatomy. Oral Surg Oral Med Oral Pathol 1990;*69*:514–519.
46. Ireland VE: The problem of "the clicking jaw." Proc R Soc Med 1951;*44*:363–372.
47. Hansson T, Oberg T: Arthrosis and deviation in form of the temporomandibular joint: A macroscopic study on human autopsy material. Acta Odontol Scand 1976;*35*:167–174.
48. Eriksson L, Westesson P-L, Rohlin M: Temporomandibular joint sounds in patients with disk displacement. Int J Oral Surg 1985;*14*:229–237.
49. Eriksson L, Rohlin M, Westesson P-L: The correlation of temporomandibular joint sounds with joint morphology in fifty-five autopsy specimens. J Oral Maxillofac Surg 1985;*43*:194–200.
50. Widmalm S-E, Westesson P-L, Brooks SL, et al: Temporomandibular joint sounds: Correlation to joint structure in fresh autopsy specimens. Am J Orthod Dentofac Orthop 1992;*101*:60–69.
51. Westesson P-L: Structural hard tissue changes in temporomandibular joints with internal derangement. Oral Surg Oral Med Oral Pathol 1985;*59*:220–224.
52. Manzione JV, Tallents R, Katzberg RW, et al: Arthrographically guided splint therapy for recapturing the temporomandibular joint meniscus. Oral Surg 1984;*57*:235–240.
53. Tallents RH, Katzberg RW, Miller TL, et al: Arthrographically assisted splint therapy. J Prosthet Dent 1985;*53*:235–238.
54. Kaplan PA, Tu KH, Sleder PR, et al: Inferior joint space arthrography of normal temporomandibular joints: Reassessment of diagnostic criteria. Radiology 1986;*159*:585–589.
55. Lundh H, Westesson P-L, Kopp S: A three-year follow-up of patients with reciprocal temporomandibular joint clicking. Oral Surg Oral Med Oral Pathol 1987;*63*:530–533.
56. Lundh H, Westesson P-L: Long-term follow-up after occlusal treatment to correct an abnormal temporomandibular joint disk position. Oral Surg Oral Med Oral Pathol 1989;*67*:2–10.
57. Anderson QN, Katzberg RW: Loose bodies of the temporomandibular joint: Arthrographic diagnosis. Skeletal Radiol 1984;*11*:42–46.
58. Kurita K, Westesson P-L, Tasaki M, Liedberg J: Temporomandibular joint: Diagnosis of medial and lateral disk displacement with anteroposterior arthrography. Correlation with cryosections. Oral Surg Oral Med Oral Pathol 1992;*73*:364–368.
59. Kurita K, Westesson P-L, Tasaki M: Diagnosis of medial disk displacement with dual space anteroposterior arthrotomography: Correlation with cryosectional morphology. J Oral Maxillofac Surg 1992;*50*:618–620.
60. Bircher E: Pneumoradiographie des Knies und der anderen Gelenke. Schweiz Med Wochenschr 1931;*50*:1210–1211.
61. Bircher E, Oberholzer J: Die Kniegelenkkapsel im Pneumoradiographie-Bilde. Acta Radiol Diagn (Stockh) 1934;*15*:452–466.
62. Hall FM, Goldberg RP, Wyshak G, Kilcoyne RF: Shoulder arthrography: Comparison of morbidity after use of various contrast media. Radiology 1985;*154*:339–341.
63. Freiberger RH, Kaye JJ: Arthrography. New York, Appleton-Century-Crofts, 1979.
64. Thijn CJP: Arthrography of the Knee Joint. Berlin, Springer-Verlag, 1979.
65. Dalinka MK: Comprehensive Manuals in Radiology: Arthrography. New York, Springer-Verlag, 1980.
66. Horns JW: Arthrography of the knee. *In* Arndt R-D, Horns JW, Gold RH, eds: Clinical Arthrography. Baltimore, Williams & Wilkins, 1981, pp 1–53.
67. Olsen RW: Ankle arthrography. Radiol Clin North Am 1981;*19*:255–268.
68. delBuono MS: Die Doppelkontrastarthrographie des Ellbogens. Schweiz Med Wochenschr 1961;*91*:1466–1470.
69. delBuono MS, Solarino GB: Arthrography of the elbow with double contrast media. Ital LA Clin Orthop 1962;*14*:223–228.
70. Eto RT, Anderson PW, Harley JD: Elbow arthrography with the application of tomography. Radiology 1975;*115*:283–288.
71. Pavlov H, Ghelman B, Warren RF: Double-contrast arthrography of the elbow. Radiology 1979;*130*:87–95.
72. Horns JW: Arthrography of the elbow. *In* Arndt R-D, Horns JW, Gold RH, eds: Clinical Arthrography. Baltimore, Williams & Wilkins, 1981, pp 119–140.
73. Hudson TM: Elbow arthrography. Radiol Clin North Am 1981;*19*:227–241.
74. Ghelman B, Goldman AB: The double-contrast shoulder arthrogram: Evaluation of rotator cuff tears. Radiology 1977;*124*:251–254.
75. Goldman AB, Ghelman B. The double-contrast shoulder arthrogram. A review of 158 studies. Radiology 1978;*127*:655–663.
76. Resnick D: Shoulder arthrography. Radiol Clin North Am 1981;*19*:243–253.

77. Westesson P-L, Rohlin M: Diagnostic accuracy of double-contrast arthrotomography of the temporomandibular joint: Correlation with postmortem morphology. AJNR 1984;5:463–468, and AJR 1984;143:655–660.
78. Westesson P-L, Bronstein SL, Liedberg J: Temporomandibular joint: Correlation between single-contrast videoarthrography and postmortem morphology. Radiology 1986;160:767–771.
79. Westesson P-L, Bronstein SL: Temporomandibular joint: Comparison of single- and double-contrast arthrography. Radiology 1987;164:65–70.
80. Eriksson L, Westesson P-L: Clinical and radiological study of patients with anterior disc displacement of the temporomandibular joint. Swed Dent J 1983;7:55–64.
81. Westesson P-L, Bronstein SL, Liedberg JL: Internal derangement of the temporomandibular joint: Morphologic description with correlation to joint junction. Oral Surg Oral Med Oral Pathol 1985;59:323–331.
82. Westesson P-L, Eriksson L: Diskectomy of the temporomandibular joint: A double-contrast arthrotomographic follow-up study. Oral Surg Oral Med Oral Pathol 1985;59:435–440.
83. Westesson P-L, Eriksson L: Morbidity after temporomandibular joint arthrography is lower than after removal of lower third molars. Oral Surg Oral Med Oral Pathol 1990;70:72–74.

CHAPTER FIVE

Magnetic Resonance Imaging

DEVELOPMENT

Magnetic resonance (MR) imaging became a realistic possibility for the diagnosis of temporomandibular joint (TMJ) internal derangement in the clinical setting in 1984 following the development of surface coil technology.[1–3] MR imaging is now a proven method in the assessment of soft tissue and osseous structures of the TMJ, as well as other joints of the body. In recent publications MR imaging has been recommended as the first choice for imaging of most disorders of the TMJ.[4–6] In general it has become a dominant imaging modality in neurologic and musculoskeletal imaging.[7]

The technology of nuclear magnetic resonance emerged from the laboratory and into the clinical setting as an imaging modality of potential importance in the early 1980s.[8, 9] The major events in the development of this technology for imaging occurred in the early 1970s when Damadian introduced the concept of deliberately modulating the external magnetic field so that only a small volume element of the sample was in resonance with the radiofrequency field.[9] At about the same time Lauterbur developed a method of utilizing back projection technology to create an image in a manner similar to that which had been developed for computed tomography (CT).[10] These investigators were able to scale the size of their magnets up to the point at which the small specimen became the whole human body, and thus MR imaging became a clinical reality.

MR imaging produces cross-sectional images similar to those of CT but does not rely on ionizing radiation and involves an apparently safe interaction between radio waves and certain atomic nuclei in the body when they are in the presence of a strong magnetic field. At this time there are no known harmful biologic side effects of MR imaging.

The MR image, like CT, is composed of picture elements (pixels) and is generated by computer technology. However, the numerical value of each pixel in MR imaging reflects the intensity of the MR signal that is emitted by the tissue in this specific location following the phenomenon of resonance rather than representing a numerical value reflecting x-ray attenuation, as in CT, or reflection of an external beam, as in ultrasound. The relative brightness of a dot that appears on the final MR image is directly proportional to MR signal strength recorded from the volume element (voxel) of tissue represented by the dot.

PHYSICAL PRINCIPLES

The physical and chemical characteristics of a tissue being imaged determine the brightness of the signal that the tissue emits when stimulated into

Table 5–1
SIGNAL INTENSITY DETERMINANTS OF TISSUE

Concentration of hydrogen protons in the tissue (predominantly water and fat)
Velocity at which these protons are moving
T1 relaxation effects
T2 relaxation effects

magnetic resonance. The four most significant properties are listed in Table 5–1; probably the most significant for TMJ imaging is the concentration of hydrogen protons in the tissue because the difference between the water content in the disk and the water content in the surrounding disk attachment and joint capsule is the basis for imaging the disk. The T1 and T2 relaxation times for the TMJ tissues have not been determined, and the significance of

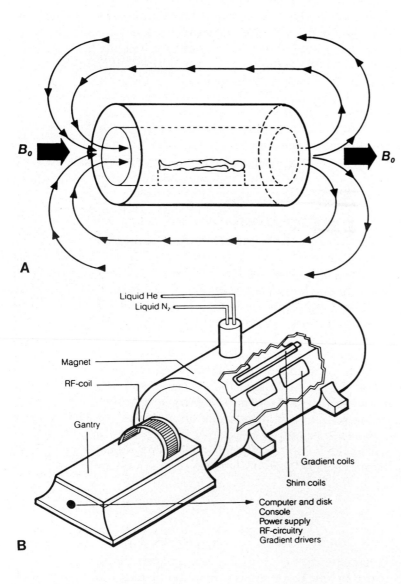

Figure 5–1
Schematic drawing of a magnetic resonance (MR) scanner. A, The static magnetic field (B_0) for a superconductive MR scanner. B, The major components of a superconductive scanner. (Reproduced with permission from Elster AD: Magnetic Resonance Imaging. A Reference Guide and Atlas. Philadelphia, Lippincott, 1986.)

possible alterations in T1 and T2 relaxation times is not known. Initially, during the early era of MR imaging, there was a great deal of enthusiasm and hope that the T1 and T2 relaxation times would be valuable for characterization of tumors. Further experience has not substantiated the initial high expectations.

The first process of MR imaging takes place when the patient is placed within the bore of a large magnet. The magnet produces a tremendously powerful static field, denoted by a B_o (Fig. 5–1A and B). The most commonly utilized magnetic field strength in the United States is 1.5 tesla (Fig. 5–2), which represents a static magnetic field with a strength 30,000 times that of the earth's magnetic field. Scanners work at 1.0, 0.5, and down to around 0.02 tesla. There is a relationship between the magnetic field strength, image quality, and imaging time.[11] One study compared the quality of MR images of the TMJ obtained at 0.3 and 1.5 tesla and showed that the image quality at equal scanning times is significantly better and the diagnostic accuracy significantly higher using the 1.5-tesla scanner.[11] This study also showed that it takes approximately four times longer on the 0.3-tesla scanner to acquire similar image quality and diagnostic accuracy as with the 1.5-tesla scanner (Fig. 5–3). The static magnetic field (B_o in Fig. 5–1A) in the scanner remains constant throughout the imaging process.

The second magnetic component that MR refers to is the hydrogen proton itself. Each proton may be thought of as a tiny spinning magnet because of its

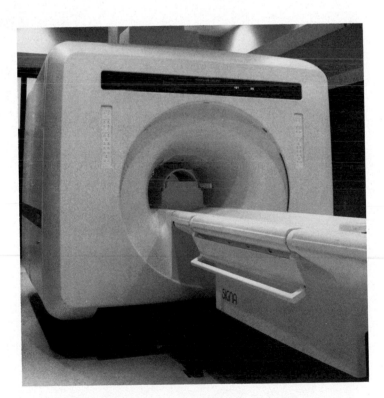

Figure 5–2
General Electric 1.5-tesla MR scanner with head coil.

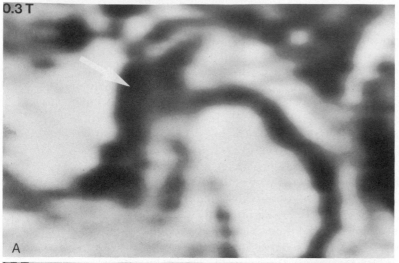

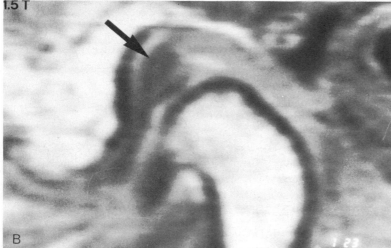

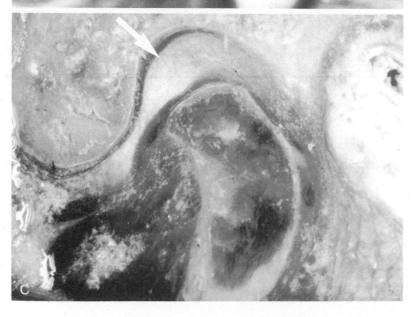

Figure 5–3
Comparison between 0.3- and 1.5-tesla MR images in sagittal MR scans obtained at 0.3 tesla (A) and at 1.5 tesla (B) and the corresponding cryosection (C). The posterior band of the disk is indicated with arrows in A, B, and C. The imaging time for the 0.3- and the 1.5-tesla images was 2.5 minutes in these T1-weighted images.

electrical charge. When a body is placed in the strong magnetic field present in the bore of the magnet, many of these small protons align with the external magnetic field. These many tiny magnetic poles add together and produce a small magnetic field of their own within the body tissue, parallel to the main static field of the MR scanner (B_o in Fig. 5–1*A*), although it is millions of times smaller. When the magnetized objects, which are the protons in the human body, are exposed to short bursts of radio-frequency energy (radio waves) at exactly the same frequency as that of the precessing nuclei, the nuclei start precessing in phase and emit a coherent signal similar to the coherent light of a laser. This radio-frequency signal is detectable by the nearby head, body, or surface coil and is then converted into an image by the powerful computer of the MR scanner.

The process by which these stimulated protons release their energy to return to their original alignment is known as relaxation. Release of energy in the form of radio waves is the fundamental basis for MR imaging. The MR imaging signal from each small volume of tissue is a little different, because it has been coded to have a slightly different frequency in phase by the gradient magnetic fields built into the MR scanner. The location of each signal from within the human tissue is computed by the mathematical process known as the Fourier transformation. This signal is then represented as a bright dot on the video display, with stronger signals producing brighter dots.

CHARACTERISTICS OF THE MAGNETIC RESONANCE IMAGE

The fundamental characteristics of the MR images are listed in Table 5–2 and include (1) the anatomic plane of the image; (2) slice thickness of each anatomic plane; (3) the matrix (pixel) size; (4) the number of signal averages; (5) the pulse sequence; and (6) pulse-time intervals.

The imaging plane refers to the angle of anatomic sectioning and typically includes the sagittal and coronal planes for the TMJ. Recent computer technology for MR also provides the capability for an infinite array of imaging

Table 5–2
PARAMETERS THAT MUST BE SPECIFIED TO PERFORM AN MR SCAN

Parameters	Typical Options	Comments
Imaging plane	Axial	Axial plane is used for localizing the condyle and programming the imaging angles for the sagittal and coronal scans
	Sagittal	Sagittal is the standard plane of imaging, and images are obtained at closed- and open-mouth positions. Oblique images perpendicular to the horizontal long axis of the condyle are preferable to straight sagittal images
	Coronal	Coronal images should be parallel to the horizontal long axis of the condyle. Coronal images are important for studying medial and lateral disk displacement. Coronal images are usually obtained only at the closed-mouth position
Slice thickness	3 mm	Slices as thin as possible are desirable, because these provide better anatomic detail. The disadvantage of thin slices is a lower signal-to-noise ratio
Matrix size	192 × 256	The finer the matrix the better the resolution, but the longer imaging time
Number of averages (NEX)	0.5, 0.75, 1.0, 2.0	More averages improve image quality but require longer scanning time and increase risk for motion artifacts. Between 0.5 and 1 is usually employed for the TMJ
Pulse sequence	Spin-echo	Spin-echo is most frequently used for TMJ imaging
		Inversion recovery
		Partial saturation
Pulse-time intervals (in msec)		See Table 5–7 for TMJ imaging
		TR = 600–2000
		TE = 10–200

planes. Studies have shown that the image quality of the TMJ can be improved by using oblique scanning planes compared with regular coronal and sagittal planes.[12] Examples of images obtained in the regular sagittal and in the corrected oblique sagittal plane of the same patient are shown in Figure 5–4. Examples of coronal images that were obtained in the true coronal and oblique coronal plane of the same patient are shown in Figure 5–5.

Slice thickness used in imaging of the head and body usually varies from 3 to 10 mm. Slice thicknesses down to 0.7 mm are possible with three-dimensional acccquisition technique, but the amount of chemical shift artifact is greater than with regular spin-echo technique and the technology has not gained wide acceptance for TMJ imaging. In MR imaging, there is a tradeoff between slice thickness, signal-to-noise ratio, and scanning time. Thinner slices improve visualization of anatomic detail but require longer scanning times to maintain an equivalent signal-to-noise ratio. Three-millimeter slice thicknesses of the TMJ appear adequate for routine use. There is evidence, however, that thinner slices may improve quality, especially in the coronal plane.[13] The reason for the improved image quality by the thinner sections is probably reduced volume averaging of rounded structures. Since the anteroposterior dimension

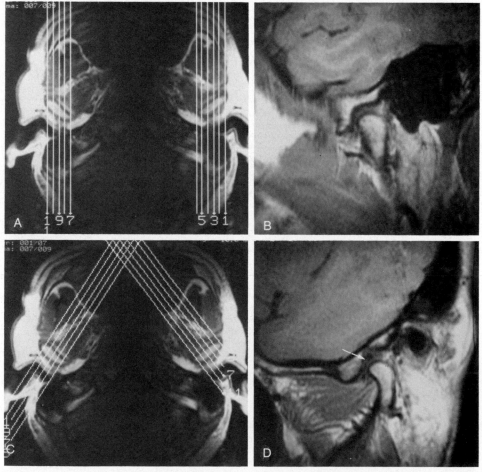

Figure 5–4
Improvement of imaging quality by oblique scanning planes, sagittal. A and B, Sagittal MR scans obtained with the straight and C and D, the oblique technique. The disk is better delineated in the oblique sagittal scan (D) than in the straight sagittal scan (B). The posterior band of the disk is indicated by an arrow in D.

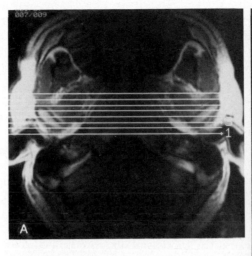

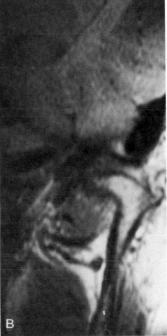

Figure 5–5

Improvement of image quality by oblique scanning planes, coronal. A and B, Coronal MR scans obtained with the straight and C and D, the oblique technique. There is improvement of image quality with the oblique scanning plane. The lateral displacement of the disk (arrow in D) on the left side is seen only in the oblique image.

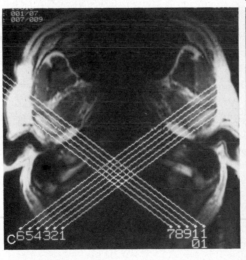

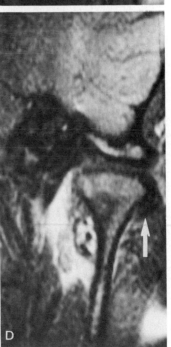

of the condyle is smaller than its mediolateral dimension, the improvement of image quality appears more obvious in the coronal plane than in the sagittal plane (Fig. 5–6).

Matrix sizes vary from 128 × 128 to 512 × 512 and relate to the in-plane resolution or fineness of anatomic detail. The out-of-plane resolution is perpendicular to the plane of imaging and is equal to the slice thickness. Again, tradeoffs similar to those noted with slice thickness also exist with the selection of finer matrices. Thus, one must expend twice the imaging time to obtain a 256 × 256 matrix versus a 128 × 256 matrix. A 192 × 256 matrix seems adequate for imaging of the TMJ. For the open-mouth images, we use a 128 × 256 matrix in order to reduce the imaging time.

Signal averaging is the technique of repeating the image acquisition sequence in order to gain a better signal-to-noise ratio to improve image quality. Imaging time is increased in direct proportion to the number of signal averages, or excitations. Image quality is better with more excitations, but again there is a tradeoff because of the risk of patient motion with longer imaging times. An example of images obtained with one versus four excitations on a midfield 0.3-tesla scanner is shown in Figure 5–7. The increased anatomic detail is obvious. The improvement is usually not as prominent in patients as in these cadaver specimens, because the increased imaging time also increases the risk of patient motion that deteriorates the image quality in longer scans.

An unlimited number of combinations of pulse sequences (radio-frequency pulses) may be utilized to generate an MR signal. The most commonly used pulse sequence is the spin-echo, which is a train of alternating 90-degree and 180-degree RF pulses. The time delay between the original 90-degree pulse and the echo signal is known as the echo time (TE). The entire pulse sequence can be repeated at a certain operator-prescribable interval called the repetition time (TR). If the TR and TE are short, then a "T1-weighting" effect in the signal occurs that highlights fat (Table 5–3). If one sets the imaging parameters for a long TR and a long TE, then a "T2-weighting" effect occurs that highlights water-containing structures (Fig. 5–8). A "proton-weighted" or balanced-pulse sequence employs the effects of these variables on imaging characteristics of the TMJ, as shown in Tables 5–3 and 5–4. For the TMJ, there is not a great difference between a T1 and a proton density image as long as the TE is no longer than 20 msec. The fat in the bone marrow of the condyle and in the parotid gland will be brighter on the T1-weighted images, making them appear more contrasty than with the proton density image.

CONTRAINDICATIONS TO MAGNETIC RESONANCE IMAGING

At present, there are only two absolute contraindications to MR imaging (Table 5–5). One includes ferromagnetic cerebral aneurysm clips, since the rapidly changing magnetic fields might induce motion in such a clip, shearing the vessel or causing injury to adjacent tissue. The second absolute contraindication to MR imaging involves cardiac pacemakers. The rapidly changing magnetic fields can induce dysfunction of the pacemaker and lead to arrhythmias that could be fatal. Relative contraindications are also listed in Table 5–5. There is no harm from dental apparatuses as long as they are nonferromagnetic or secured tightly. However, the signal in and around these materials may be completely lost (Figure 5–9), and thus an image cannot be obtained in the

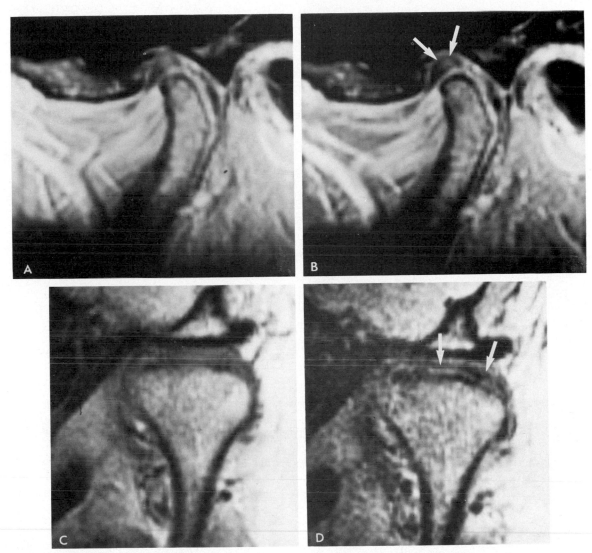

Figure 5–6
Improved image quality by thinner sections—MR images obtained with 3.0- (A and C) and 1.5-mm slice thickness (B and D) in the sagittal and coronal planes. Significant improvement of the delineation of the disk is seen with the thin-slice technique. The disk is indicated by arrows in the 1.5-mm images (B and D).

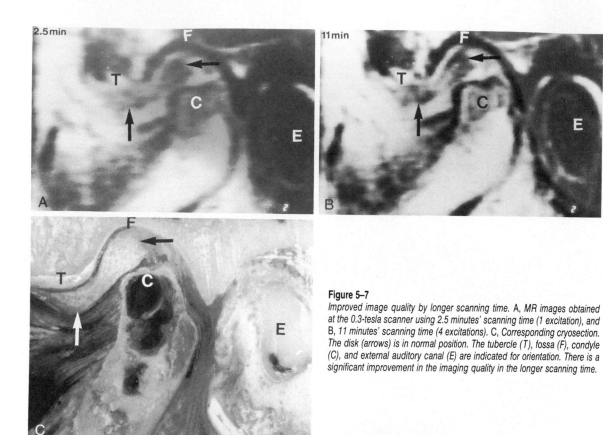

Figure 5–7
Improved image quality by longer scanning time. A, MR images obtained at the 0.3-tesla scanner using 2.5 minutes' scanning time (1 excitation), and B, 11 minutes' scanning time (4 excitations). C, Corresponding cryosection. The disk (arrows) is in normal position. The tubercle (T), fossa (F), condyle (C), and external auditory canal (E) are indicated for orientation. There is a significant improvement in the imaging quality in the longer scanning time.

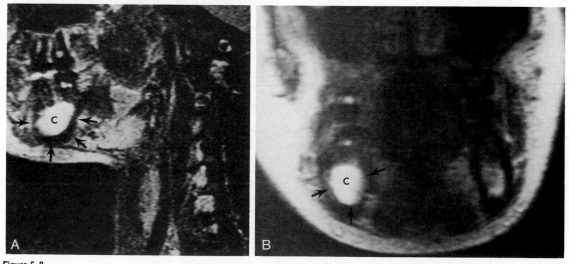

Figure 5–8
These T2-weighted MR scans of the mandible demonstrate a fluid-filled cyst (C, arrows) that is of a bright signal intensity but was not visible on T1-weighted images. A, Sagittal MR scan. B, Coronal MR scan.

Table 5–3
TMJ ANATOMY AND MR PARAMETERS

TR	TE	Effect	Terminology	Results
Short	Short	Highlights Fat	T1-weighting	Lateral pterygoid fat pad accentuated Posterior disk ligament accentuated Disk signal low Marrow signal of condyle accentuated Excellent anatomic detail
Long	Short	Highlights Fat	Proton density	Similar effects as T1-weighting
Long	Long	Highlights Water	T2-weighting	Joint effusion accentuated Bone marrow edema accentuated Signal of fat pad, posterior ligament, and marrow decreased Poor anatomic detail

Table 5–4
RELATIVE BRIGHTNESS OF BODY TISSUES SEEN ON A T1- OR PROTON-WEIGHTED SPIN-ECHO SEQUENCE*

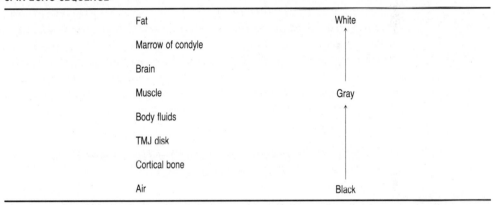

*For example: TE = 11 msec, TR = 500 msec.
Modified from Elster AD: Magnetic Resonance Imaging: A Reference Guide and Atlas. Philadelphia, JB Lippincott, 1986, pp 1–56.

Table 5–5
CONTRAINDICATIONS TO MR SCANNING

Absolute
Cerebral aneurysm clips
Cardiac pacemakers

Relative
Claustrophobic or uncooperative patients
Pregnancy
Metallic prosthetic heart valves
Ferromagnetic foreign bodies in critical locations (e.g., eye)
Implanted stimulator wires for pain control

No Contraindications
Orthodontic braces, dental material
Surgical clips outside the brain
Metallic prostheses

Modified from Elster AD: Magnetic Resonance Imaging: A Reference Guide and Atlas. Philadelphia, JB Lippincott, 1986, pp 1–56.

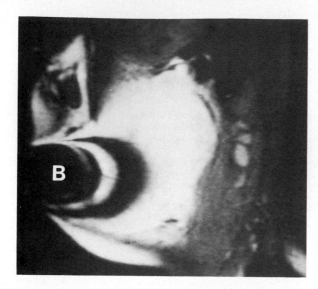

Figure 5–9
Signal intensity loss and artifact from braces (B) on the teeth.

immediate vicinity of these metallic devices. Metallic plates or screws in the jaws are not a contraindication to MR imaging of the TMJ. Again, no image can be created in the area around the metallic device. Usually the metallic device is somewhat away from the joint region, and an adequate image can be obtained of the joint itself, even if there are artifacts in the mandible. We have attempted to image a patient with a total TMJ prosthesis that has an entire metallic condyle, but the metallic artifacts were so extensive that these MR images were not diagnostic (see Chapter 7 on post-treatment imaging).

COMPARISON OF MAGNETIC RESONANCE, COMPUTED TOMOGRAPHY, AND ARTHROGRAPHY

MR imaging with surface coils is now a proven method for the assessment of internal derangement of the TMJ and is rapidly surpassing arthrography and CT as the prime imaging modality. The major advantages of MR imaging in comparison with arthrography are (1) MR is noninvasive; (2) it requires no ionizing radiation for image acquisition; (3) multiplanar imaging is readily obtained in an infinite array of anatomic sections; (4) it permits a direct visualization of soft tissue components, including disk and joint structures; (5) it allows easy bilateral assessment; (6) it permits an assessment of joint effusion and inflammation; and (7) structures outside the joint, such as the joint capsule and the muscles of mastication, can be easily assessed. The disadvantages are (1) high cost; (2) it does not permit a true dynamic assessment of joint function; (3) perforations of the posterior attachment or of the disk are not usually visible; and (4) one cannot easily assess the accurate jaw position for the initiation or adjustment of protrusive splint therapy.

The relative advantages and disadvantages of MR imaging versus CT are listed in Table 5–6. Because of the multiplanar capabilities, the superior anatomic detail, and the lack of ionizing radiation for image acquisition using MR imaging, CT is no longer a competitive modality in the assessment of internal derangement. Comparative studies using cryosectional cadaver material in conjunction with multiplanar imaging have demonstrated the high accuracy of MR imaging.[14–16]

Table 5–6
MR ADVANTAGES AND DISADVANTAGES AS COMPARED WITH CT

Advantages
No ionizing radiation
Primary imaging in multiple planes without moving the patient
Superior image detail of articular soft tissue components
Fewer artifacts from metal clips and dense bone
Images bone marrow of condyle

Disadvantages
High initial cost of the scanner
Special site planning and shielding
Danger to patients with cerebral aneurysm clips, pacemakers
Claustrophobia in magnet
Inferior image of hard tissues

TECHNIQUES FOR TEMPOROMANDIBULAR JOINT IMAGING

Our suggested method acquires MR images from the left and right TMJs at the same time, using two 6.5-cm surface coil receivers (Fig. 5–10). The patient is positioned supine, and the surface coils are placed against both TMJ regions with the condyles in the center of the coil. A set of images is obtained in both the closed- and open-jaw positions. A basic imaging protocol that we have found useful is outlined in Table 5–7. This protocol includes closed- and

Table 5–7
SCANNING PARAMETERS FOR MR IMAGING USING BILATERAL SURFACE COILS

Image	Scanning Time
1. **Axial Localizer** TR – 400* TE = 16 NEX = 0.5 FOV = 18 Thickness = 3 mm Matrix = 256 × 128	52 sec
2. **Sagittal, Closed** TR – 2000 TE = 19 and 80 NEX = 0.5 FOV = 10 cm Thickness = 3 mm Matrix = 256 × 192	3 min, 52 sec
3. **Sagittal, Open** TR = 1500 TE = 19 and 80 NEX = 0.75 FOV = 10 cm Thickness = 3 mm Matrix = 256 × 192	2 min, 42 sec
4. **Coronal, Closed** TR = 2000 TE = 19 and 80 NEX = 0.5 FOV = 10 cm Thickness = 3 mm 256 × 192 matrix	3 min, 52 sec

*TR, TE values in msec.
If a splint is provided by the clinician, additional sagittal scans can be performed with the splint in place.
Total scanning time for a complete bilateral TMJ examination is about 12 minutes. Table time is approximately 30 minutes.

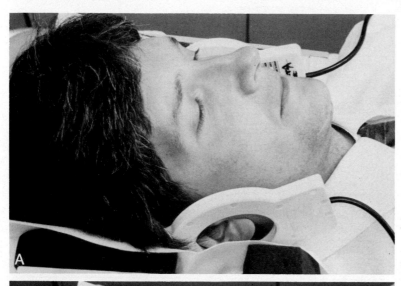

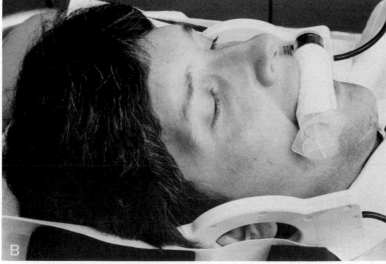

Figure 5–10
Dual coil technique. A, Placement of 6.5-cm surface coils for bilateral TMJ imaging with the jaw closed. B, Bilateral TMJ imaging with the jaw open; a syringe wrapped in saline-soaked gauze is used as a bite block.

open-mouth images in the sagittal plane and coronal images in the closed-mouth position. The closed-mouth position images are obtained using a long TR and both long and short TEs (proton density and T2-weighting imaging sequences). The scanning protocol has to be adjusted for the type of scanner and surface coil technology, as well as for the specific clinical needs. We interspace the scans by approximately 0.5 to 1.0 mm. We have not found it useful to interleave considering the extra time this would require. We routinely obtain T2-weighted images in both the sagittal and coronal plane in order to determine the presence of joint effusion (Fig. 5–11) or bone marrow edema (Fig. 5–12). We have found it valuable to identify the joint effusion in both sagittal and coronal planes, since the diagnostic confidence increases and, in some cases, the joint effusion is seen only in one plane. The closed-mouth images are obtained with the jaw in the closed, rest position. A clenched-tooth position would be painful for many patients to maintain over a 4-minute scanning period. We have found it useful to obtain T2-weighting also for the open-mouth images. This allows the joint effusion to relocate, which occasionally may be useful in the differentiation from synovial proliferation. The total table time for a study as described in Table 5–7 is about 30 minutes.

We attempted to obtain coronal open-mouth images but have discontinued them since they did not contribute significantly to the diagnosis. The condyle moves in an anterior direction on opening, and it is frequently difficult to identify anatomic landmarks upon which the disk could be related. For these reasons, we do not recommend coronal open-mouth images routinely.

We use 0.5 excitations for the closed-mouth position in the sagittal and coronal plane and 0.75 for the open-mouth images. This reduces the imaging time by 50 per cent and 25 per cent, respectively, without significant degradation of image quality compared with one full excitation. We have found the signal-to-noise ratio in these images to be sufficient. The shorter imaging time is valuable in reducing patient motion and thereby improves image quality.

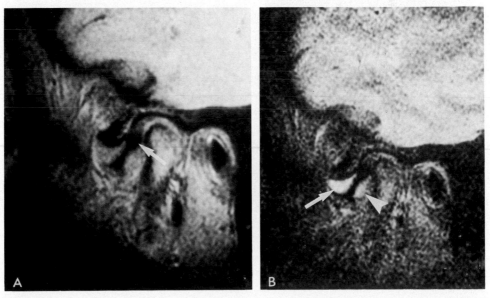

Figure 5–11
T2-weighted image showing joint effusion. A, Proton density and B, T2-weighted image of TMJ with disk displacement and joint effusion in the upper (arrow in B) and lower (arrowhead in B) joint spaces. The posterior band of the disk is indicated by an arrow in A.

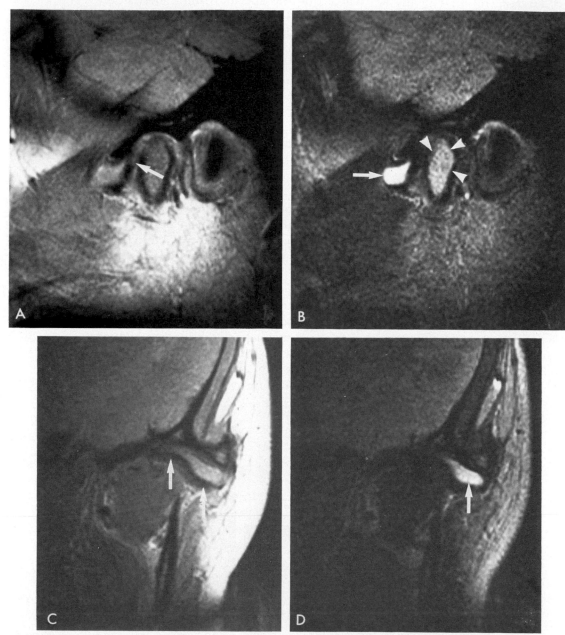

Figure 5–12

Joint effusion and bone marrow edema. A, Sagittal proton density; B, T2-weighted images; C, coronal proton density; and D, T2-weighted images, showing disk anterior (arrows in A and C). There is a significant amount of joint effusion in the anterior recess of the upper joint space (arrow in B and D). The bone marrow of the mandibular condyle shows increased signal in the T2-weighted image (arrowheads in B). The bone marrow is not depicted in the coronal image because these images represent a section anterior to the condylar head.

We have tested many different pulse sequences for TMJ MR imaging on our 1.5-tesla General Electric Signa scanner and have found that one of the most important principles is to ensure that the TE is as short as possible. When the TE is increased from 19 to 30 msec, for example, the differentiation between the disk and surrounding soft tissue is marginal. Scans acquired with a TE of 30 msec or longer are frequently nondiagnostic for disk position. We have also tested different TRs and have found that a TR of 1000 or 2000 msec provides excellent image quality, provided the signal-to-noise ratio is equivalent. Thus, more excitations are used for the TR 1000-msec image compared with the TR 2000-msec image. In our experience, there is a slight advantage of TR 2000 versus TR 1000 msec in producing optimal quality MR images. A TR shorter than 1000 can be used if only one side is imaged at a time. Four our imager we need a TR equal to 1000 msec or longer in order to acquire enough slices to cover both left and right joints in one sequence set. A lower signal-to-nose ratio is acceptable in the open-jaw position when the disk has been clearly depicted in the closed-jaw position, and consequently, imaging time can be decreased. It is necessary to minimize the imaging time during which the patient must keep the jaw open. This can be uncomfortable following acute trauma to the TMJ, especially when associated with condylar fractures and suspected intra-articular injuries.

It should be noted that the scanning protocol continually changes with increasing experience and advances in the technology.

Fast Scan

Short flip angle (gradient-recalled acquisition in the steady state, or GRASS) "fast-scanning" techniques may be employed for assessment of functional joint dynamics.[17] Some investigators recommend use of these techniques routinely to assess the joint at a series of different degrees of jaw opening and evaluate disk function relative to the condyle and temporal bone with simulated movement.[18, 19] These images, however, are not true dynamic depictions, since the imaging times are at a minimum several seconds long. They can be formatted in a "snapshot" manner to provide the illusion of a dynamic assessment. The value of a pseudodynamic study of the TMJ has not been established. It has been our clinical experience with the use of pseudodynamic TMJ MR that occasionally we are able to determine that the disk is not moving relative to either the condyle or temporal component. So far, these observations have not been confirmed surgically or arthroscopically, but they might indicate the presence of adhesions in either the upper or lower joint spaces. Short flip angle techniques also can be utilized to highlight different tissue elements in a manner similar to the spin-echo technique. By setting the imaging parameters to highlight fluid, a T2-weighted effect can be obtained (Table 5–8). The disad-

Table 5–8
CONTRAST CHARACTERISTICS IN FAST-SCAN GRADIENT-ECHO IMAGES

	T1-Weighted	Proton Density	T2-Weighted
TR (msec)	200–400	200–400	200–400
TE (msec)	12–15	12–15	30–60
θ (degrees)	45–50	5–20	5–20

Modified from Wehrli FW: Principles of magnetic resonance. *In* Stark DD, Bradley WG Jr, eds: Magnetic Resonance Imaging. St Louis, CV Mosby, 1988, pp 3–23.

vantages of the short flip angle techniques with short imaging times are the very poor signal-to-noise ratio and the accentuated motion artifacts from vascular pulsations.

Fat Suppression

We have used fat suppression (chemical shift imaging) in association with T2-weighted imaging of the TMJ. Fat suppression does not improve the depiction of anatomic details. Instead, fat suppression eliminates some of the contrast between the disk and the higher fat-containing tissues surrounding the joint capsule. Therefore, fat suppression images are not valuable for delineating the anatomy. However, we have found that a combination of T2 weighting and fat suppression sometimes can be helpful in identifying an increased signal from the bone marrow of the mandibular condyle that might indicate marrow edema (Fig. 5–13). It seems as though the bright signal in the bone marrow of the mandibular condyle sometimes stands out even more clearly on fat-suppressed T2-weighted images, compared with regular T2-

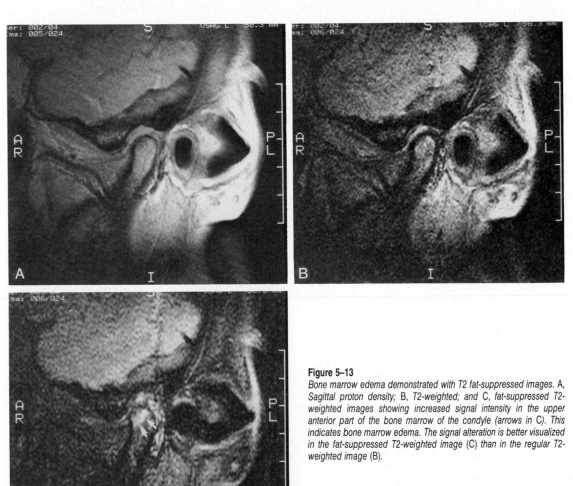

Figure 5–13
Bone marrow edema demonstrated with T2 fat-suppressed images. A, Sagittal proton density; B, T2-weighted; and C, fat-suppressed T2-weighted images showing increased signal intensity in the upper anterior part of the bone marrow of the condyle (arrows in C). This indicates bone marrow edema. The signal alteration is better visualized in the fat-suppressed T2-weighted image (C) than in the regular T2-weighted image (B).

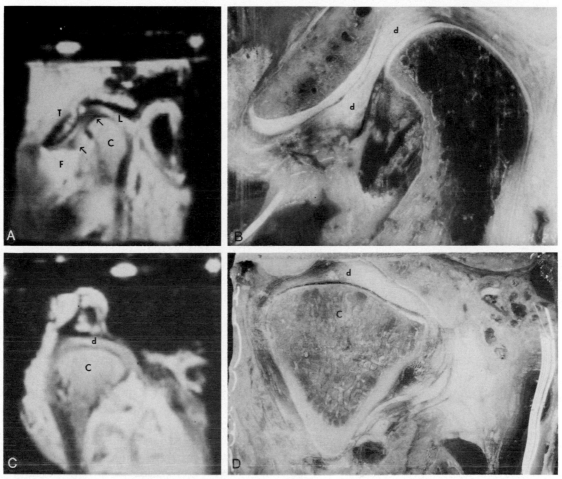

Figure 5–14
Normal disk comparing MR with anatomic specimen. A, Sagittal MR scan of a normal anatomic specimen showing the disk (arrows) in a normal relationship to the condyle (C) and temporal bone (T). The disk has a low signal intensity, whereas the signal intensity of the lateral pterygoid fat pad (F) and posterior disk ligament (L) have a bright signal. B, Corresponding sagittal anatomic specimen showing the biconcave disk (d) in a normal relationship to the condylar head. C, Coronal MR scan showing the relationship of the disk (d) and condyle (C). D, Corresponding coronal anatomic specimen.

weighted images (Fig. 5–13). Our experience with fat-suppressed T2-weighted images of the TMJ is limited at this time. We do not recommend a fat suppression technique for routine use until further experience has been gained. The technique has two disadvantages compared with regular MR images: a lower signal-to-noise ratio and a higher sensitivity to metallic artifacts, even from metal outside the joint area.

NORMAL MAGNETIC RESONANCE IMAGE ANATOMY OF THE TEMPOROMANDIBULAR JOINT

The normal TMJ demonstrated by MR imaging in the sagittal and coronal closed-jaw position is depicted in Figure 5–14*A* through *D* in a comparison with the corresponding cryosectional anatomy. The low signal intensity of the fibrous disk is clearly demonstrated because of the relatively bright signal intensity emanating from the surrounding soft tissues and the lateral pterygoid fat pad, as outlined in Table 5–3. The cortex of the condylar head has an absence of signal but is well depicted because of the relatively bright signal intensity of the contiguous fibrocartilage and synovial tissues superiorly and the bright signal of the fatty marrow inferiorly.

The MR imaging anatomy of an asymptomatic volunteer is shown in Figure 5–15A through D. The disk has a "bowtie"-like configuration with maximal jaw opening (Fig. 5–15B) and maintains its position interposed between the convexity of the condyle inferiorly and the convexity of the tubercle superiorly. The posterior disk attachment has a bright signal owing to the rich network of fatty tissue. This contrasts extremely well with the low signal intensity of the fibrous disk. In some instances, there is a small region of high signal intensity within the posterior band of the disk, as has been described for the meniscus of the knee (Fig. 5–16). This can be a normal anatomic landmark and probably represents mucin deposits in this region of disk tissue. This has been seen in both normal and abnormal joints. The insertion of the superior belly of the lateral pterygoid muscle is often demonstrated on MR imaging as a low intensity, threadlike structure attaching on the anteromedial aspect of the disk and condyle (Fig. 5–15). In the coronal plane, the disk has an arc-shaped configuration, with the medial margin of the disk attaching just inferior to the medial pole and to the neck of the condyle. The lateral margin is attached just underneath the lateral pole and to the lateral capsule wall (see Fig. 5–14).

The arthrographic correlation with MR imaging in the lateral and sagittal imaging projections, respectively, is excellent and is demonstrated in Figure 5–17. The arthrogram is an indirect asssessment of the position of the disk, whereas MR imaging is a direct image of the anatomic structures. Thus, not only can the disk be demonstrated directly, but also the other soft and hard tissue elements of the articulation and its vicinity can be clearly depicted.

It has not yet been demonstrated that the axial plane of imaging is valuable in depicting the anatomic location of the disk. However, this imaging plane is important in determining the long axis of the condyle for programming the sagittal and coronal set of MR images (see Fig. 5–4). Occasionally, the disk can be clearly identified also in the axial images (Fig. 5–18). The clinical significance of axial imaging is still unclear. There are many variations in both the length and configuration of the disk. A relatively elongated normal disk is shown in Figure 5–19.

A pitfall in interpretation could occur when the joint capsule is interposed between the condylar head and glenoid fossa with a medially displaced disk. Figure 5–20A through C compares an MR imaging scan with an anatomic specimen in conjunction with the coronal MR imaging plane, depicting a sideways, medial displacement. The sagittal plane of imaging demonstrates a low signal intensity structure interposed between the condyle and the glenoid fossa, which is, in reality, the low signal intensity of the fibrous capsule that has herniated into the joint space. This is an important pitfall to keep in mind and can be avoided by obtaining coronal images. A clinical example is demonstrated in Figure 5–21A and B.

MAGNETIC RESONANCE IMAGING CHARACTERISTICS OF DISK DISPLACEMENT

The same general clinical criteria that have been discussed as indications for arthrography also apply for MR imaging. Thus, imaging is recommended for those patients who are experiencing TMJ pain and who have a suspected

Text continued on page 191

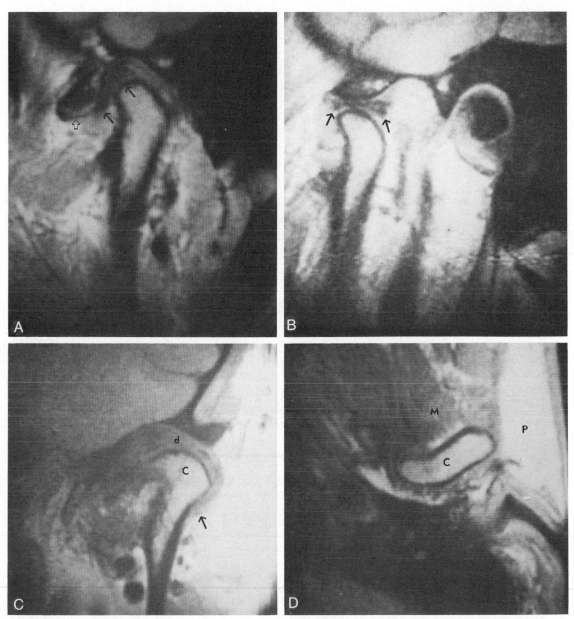

Figure 5–15

Images of a normal asymptomatic volunteer. A, Sagittal MR image with the jaw closed. The biconcave, low signal intensity disk (arrows) is situated in the proper relationship between the anterior convexity of the condyle inferiorly and the superior convexity of the temporal bone. Notice the fine pencil-thin insertion (open arrow) of the superior belly of the lateral pterygoid muscle to the anterior band of the disk. B, Sagittal MR image with the jaw maximally opened shows the biconcave lenslike configuration of the disk (arrows) in a correct anatomic position to the convex surface of the condyle inferiorly and the convex surface of the tubercle of the temporal bone superiorly. C, Coronal MR image of the left TMJ of the same subject with the jaw in the closed position. The disk (d) and condyle (C) are well-delineated, as is the lateral capsular insertion (arrow) to the lateral aspect of the neck of the condyle. D, Axial MR image, closed jaw. This image does not demonstrate the normally positioned disk but is valuable in determining the orientation of the condyle (C) for programming the corrected sagittal images. The inferior belly of the lateral pterygoid muscle (M) is noted anteromedial to the condyle and the parotid gland (P), and subcutaneous tissues are noted lateral to the articulation.

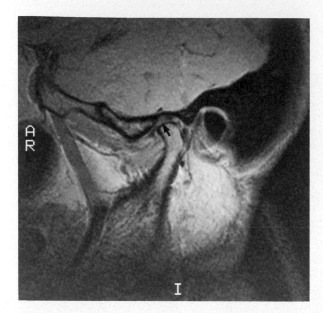

Figure 5–16
Bright signal in posterior band in normal joint. Small, wedge-shaped area of bright signal (arrow) in the posterior aspect of the posterior band in a joint with normal superior disk position.

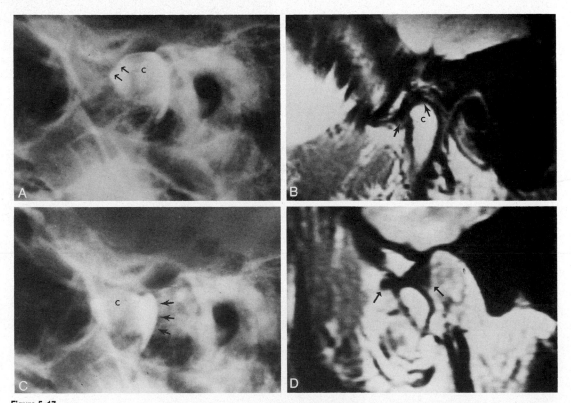

Figure 5–17
Comparison of normal lower joint space arthrogram with sagittal MR images in the same subject. A, This lower joint space arthrogram demonstrates the normal teardrop configuration (arrows) of the anterior recess of the lower joint space with the jaw closed, indicating normal anatomy. The contrast medium veils the condyle (C). B, MR image in the same patient, also with the jaw closed. The low signal intensity disk (arrows) is in the proper anatomic location between the condyle (C) and temporal bone. Notice that the disk is visualized directly by MR, whereas the position of the disk is indirectly determined with the lower joint space arthrogram. C, With the jaw maximally opened, the contrast material flows into the posterior recess of the lower joint space (arrows), indicating normal disk function and position. D, MR image at a comparable jaw position shows the bowtie configuration of the low signal intensity disk (arrows) and the proper anatomic relationship to the condyle inferiorly and the temporal bone superiorly. Note the very bright signal intensity of the tissues anterior to the disk and of the tissues immediately posterior to the disk in the region of the posterior ligament.

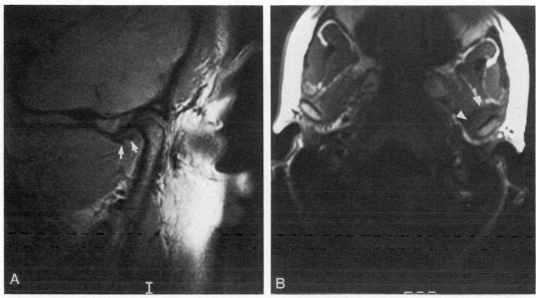

Figure 5–18
Sagittal and axial imaging showing anterior disk displacement. A, Sagittal proton density image showing anterior disk displacement. The disk is indicated by arrows. B, The axial image of the same patient demonstrates the disk (arrowheads) anterior to the condyle to the left side. In this case, the axial image confirms that the disk is anteriorly displaced without significant medial or lateral components.

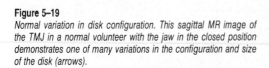

Figure 5–19
Normal variation in disk configuration. This sagittal MR image of the TMJ in a normal volunteer with the jaw in the closed position demonstrates one of many variations in the configuration and size of the disk (arrows).

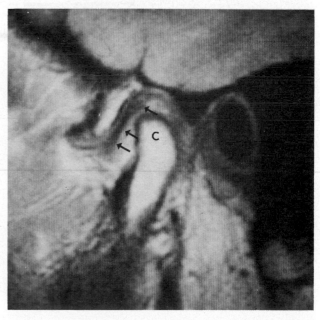

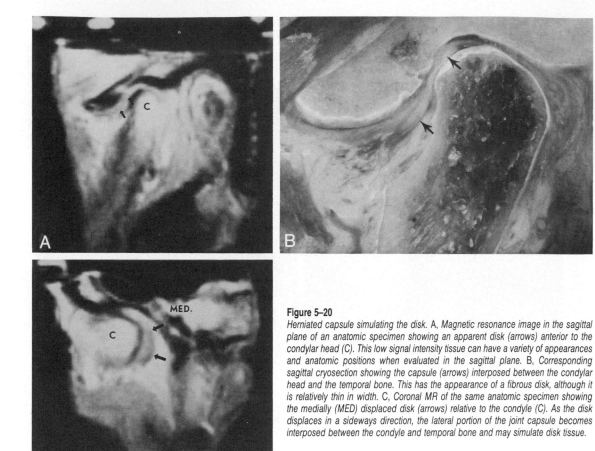

Figure 5–20
Herniated capsule simulating the disk. A, Magnetic resonance image in the sagittal plane of an anatomic specimen showing an apparent disk (arrows) anterior to the condylar head (C). This low signal intensity tissue can have a variety of appearances and anatomic positions when evaluated in the sagittal plane. B, Corresponding sagittal cryosection showing the capsule (arrows) interposed between the condylar head and the temporal bone. This has the appearance of a fibrous disk, although it is relatively thin in width. C, Coronal MR of the same anatomic specimen showing the medially (MED) displaced disk (arrows) relative to the condyle (C). As the disk displaces in a sideways direction, the lateral portion of the joint capsule becomes interposed between the condyle and temporal bone and may simulate disk tissue.

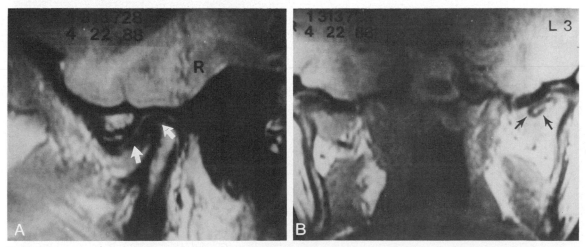

Figure 5–21
Herniated capsule simulating disk tissue interposed between the anterior surface of the condylar head and the inferior surface of the temporal bone. A, In the sagittal plane of imaging, a low signal intensity structure (arrows) is noted anterior to the condyle and underneath the posterior slope of the tubercle. This tissue cannot be distinguished from the disk. B, Coronal MR image in the same patient with the jaw closed shows the medially displaced disk (arrows) on the left side. Thus, the low signal intensity tissue noted in A represents the lateral joint capsule that has been pulled into the fossa. Since the capsule is made of fibrous tissue, it has a low signal intensity indistinguishable from that of disk tissue.

internal derangement as the etiology. The clinical presentation should include (1) the subjective component, i.e., pain and discomfort; and (2) the mechanical component, i.e., clicking and/or a range of motion abnormalities of the jaw. The two most common intra-articular abnormalities to be evaluated by MR imaging of the TMJ are (1) internal derangement due to disk displacement, and (2) degenerative arthritis, which can be a sequela of internal derangement.

In association with disk displacement, morphologic changes of the disk per se occur, as described in Chapter 2, Pathology of the TMJ. Abnormalities of disk position and configuration are effectively depicted by MR imaging.

Disk Displacement with Reduction

In the clicking jaw, commonly associated with disk displacement with reduction, the TMJ is first imaged in the closed-jaw position to determine whether or not the disk is displaced (Fig. 5–22A through D). The patient is then instructed to open the jaw beyond the opening click, and the TMJ is imaged using a syringe wrapped with gauze as a bite block (see Figure 5–10B). A comparison of MR imaging with arthrography is shown in Figure 5–22. The elongated, low signal intensity disk is easily demonstrated by MR imaging owing to the surrounding high signal intensity fat on T1- or proton-weighted images.

The configuration of the lower joint space depicted by arthrography is compared with the direct demonstration of the disk by MR imaging in Figure 5–22. These comparisons are invaluable for many reasons, but specifically they provide further insights into the subtleties of the arthrographic diagnosis. With the jaw open beyond the click, the bowtie-like configuration of the disk on MR imaging is well demonstrated (Fig. 5–22D). The condylar head is now seated properly within the concave inferior margin of the disk and likewise the convex configuration of the articular tubercle fits smoothly within the concave upper margin of the disk. In the arthrogram, there is expansion of the posterior recess of the lower joint space, indicative of a recaptured disk.

Morphologic changes of the disk might be incorrectly suspected by MR imaging if the closed-jaw position only is acquired. This may lead to an overstaging of the chronicity of the internal derangement. The actual configuration of the disk is probably more correctly assessed by examining its shape in the open-jaw position, and after it has been reduced to a normal anatomic relationship to the condyle and tubercle (Fig. 5–23). Volume averaging between the top of the condyle, the disk, and the glenoid fossa sometimes makes it difficult to evaluate the posterior band of the disk in the closed-mouth position. At open-mouth position, the tissue of the posterior disk attachment surrounds the disk, and the form can best be evaluated after reduction. A classic example of a patient with disk displacement with reduction is shown in Figure 5–24.

Frequently, the disk is not totally anteriorly displaced, but instead only partially anteriorly displaced. This implies that the lateral (Fig. 5–25) or medial (Fig. 5–26) part of the disk is displaced in an anterior direction while the other parts of the disk are still in a normal superior position. Most frequently, partial anterior disk displacement is associated with disk displacement with reduction (Fig. 5–25), but occasionally it has also been seen to be associated with disk displacement without reduction. To detect partial disk displacement and differentiate it from normal superior disk position, it is important to obtain sections all the way through the joint from lateral to medial. The joint could be normal in one part but abnormal only a few millimeters more laterally or

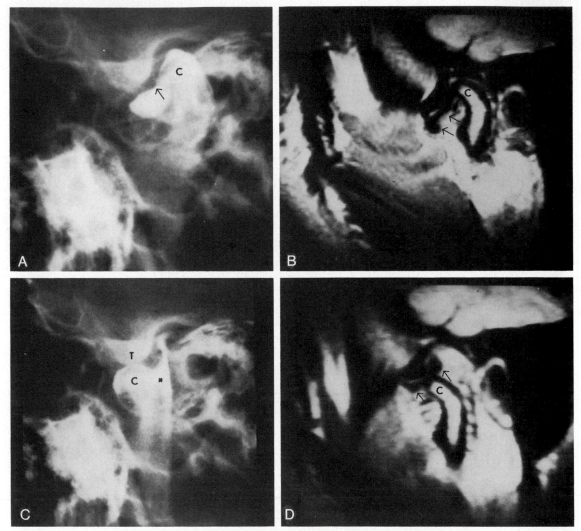

Figure 5–22

Comparison of lower joint space arthrogram and MR for disk displacement with reduction. A, This lower joint space arthrogram demonstrates that the posterior band of the disk is anterior to the 12 o'clock position of the condyle (C) and creates a concave impression (arrow) on the anterior recess of the lower joint space. B, MR image in the same patient, also with the jaw closed. The low signal intensity disk (arrows) is anterior to the 12 o'clock position of the condyle (C). The posterior band of the disk is demonstrated by the upper arrow. C, Reduction of the displacement of the disk. The jaw is now maximally opened and the condyle (C) is just beyond the margin of the apex of the tubercle (T). The disk is now reduced and the contrast material has cleared from the anterior recess of the joint space and filled the posterior recess of the joint space (*). D, Sagittal MR image depicts the disk (arrows) in the normal relationship to the condylar head (C) inferiorly and the tubercle superiorly. The bowtie-like configuration of the disk on MR is well demonstrated. The condylar head is now seated properly within the concave inferior margin of the disk and, likewise, the convex configuration of the articular tubercle fits smoothly within the concave upper margin of the disk.

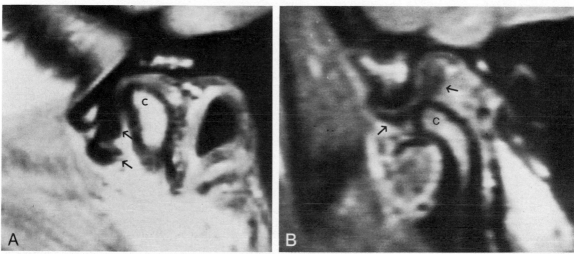

Figure 5–23

MR demonstration of configuration change of the disk before and after recapture. A, Sagittal MR image with the jaw closed and before the click. Note the apparent deformity of the disk (arrows), suggesting chronic, longstanding internal derangement. The disk is noted anterior to the condyle (C). B, Sagittal MR image in the open jaw position and beyond the clinical click. The disk (arrows) is now in a correct anatomic relationship to the condyle (C) and tubercle. Note the normal appearing, bowtie-like configuration of the disk following realignment.

Figure 5–24

Characteristic example of disk displacement with reduction. Proton density sagittal images in closed- (A) and open-mouth position (B), showing disk displacement with reduction. In the closed-mouth image (A), the disk (arrow) is located anterior to the condyle. At the maximal mouth-open image (B), the disk (arrow) is located in normal relationship to the condyle. The disk is normally biconcave.

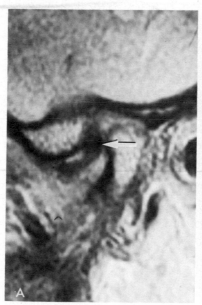
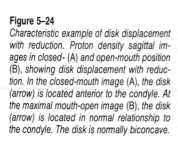
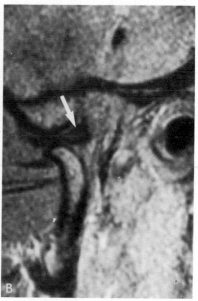

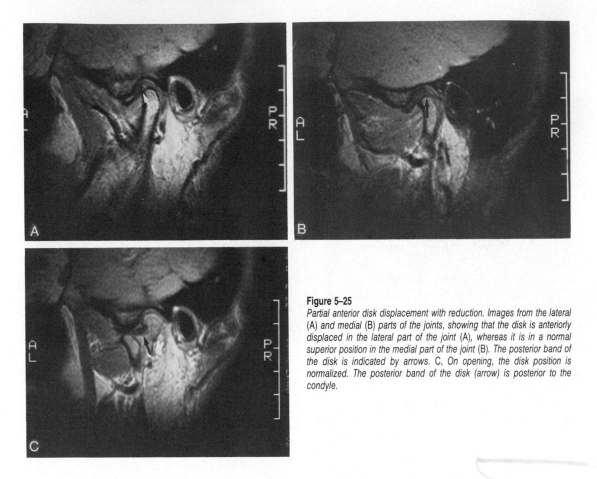

Figure 5–25
Partial anterior disk displacement with reduction. Images from the lateral (A) and medial (B) parts of the joints, showing that the disk is anteriorly displaced in the lateral part of the joint (A), whereas it is in a normal superior position in the medial part of the joint (B). The posterior band of the disk is indicated by arrows. C, On opening, the disk position is normalized. The posterior band of the disk (arrow) is posterior to the condyle.

sometimes more medially. Multiple sections are necessary to avoid a false-negative diagnosis.

MR imaging can be utilized to assess the efficacy of protrusive splint therapy that is sometimes employed in the treatment of disk displacement with reduction. Figure 5–27A through C shows the recapture of a disk with the jaw slightly protruded and stabilized by an intraoral splint. The additional imaging time with the jaw in the splint can be minimized since the position and configuration of the disk are now familiar. Utilization of a T1-weighted image sequence, in conjunction with one excitation and a 128 × 256 matrix, can provide this information in less than 2 minutes on the 1.5-T imaging system.

Disk Displacement Without Reduction

As noted in previous chapters, disk displacement without reduction is often associated with the clinical condition of "closed lock," which is the inability of the patient to open the jaw maximally and with opening deviation to the affected side. This condition is often associated with deformation of the disk and is often preceded clinically by reciprocal clicking. MR imaging is an excellent modality to depict the wide array of these complex anatomic abnormalities.

A characteristic clinical example of disk displacement without reduction is shown in Figure 5–28A and B. An example with an anatomic correlation for both MR imaging and CT is shown in Figure 5–29A through C. MR imaging

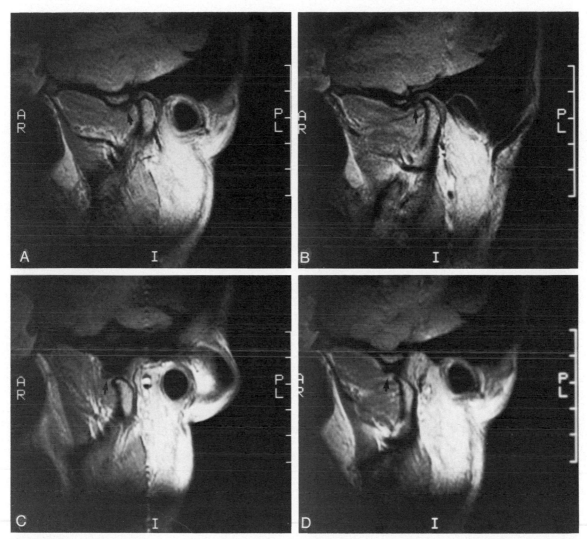

Figure 5–26
Partial anterior disk displacement without reduction. Sagittal proton density images from the central (A and C) and medial (B and D) parts of a joint with partial anterior disk displacement without reduction. In the central part of the joint (A and C), the disk (arrow) is located normally over the condyle and functions normally on opening (C). In the medial part of the joint (B and D), the disk (arrow) is anteriorly displaced at the closed- (B) and open-mouth positions (D), suggesting disk displacement without reduction. The condyle is not moving into the central thin zone.

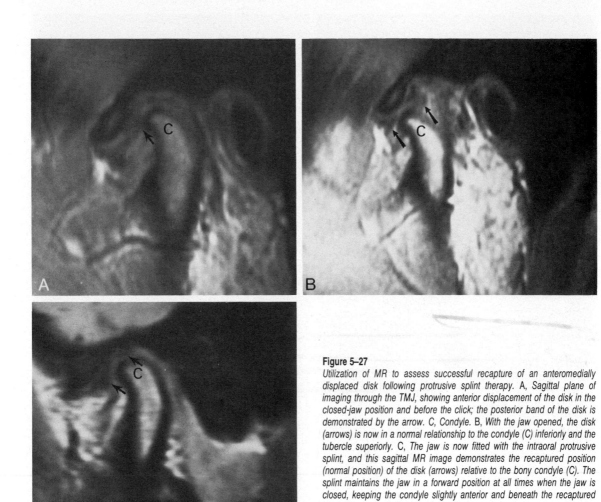

Figure 5–27

Utilization of MR to assess successful recapture of an anteromedially displaced disk following protrusive splint therapy. A, Sagittal plane of imaging through the TMJ, showing anterior displacement of the disk in the closed-jaw position and before the click; the posterior band of the disk is demonstrated by the arrow. C, Condyle. B, With the jaw opened, the disk (arrows) is now in a normal relationship to the condyle (C) inferiorly and the tubercle superiorly. C, The jaw is now fitted with the intraoral protrusive splint, and this sagittal MR image demonstrates the recaptured position (normal position) of the disk (arrows) relative to the bony condyle (C). The splint maintains the jaw in a forward position at all times when the jaw is closed, keeping the condyle slightly anterior and beneath the recaptured disk.

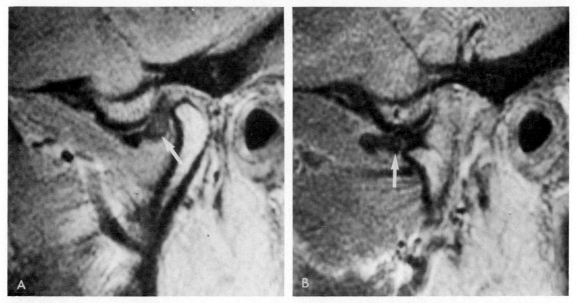

Figure 5–28
Characteristic example of disk displacement without reduction. Proton density at closed-mouth position (A) and maximal mouth opening (B), showing the disk to be anteriorly displaced in both positions. The posterior band of the disk is indicated by an arrow. There are some areas of fibrosis in the posterior disk attachment.

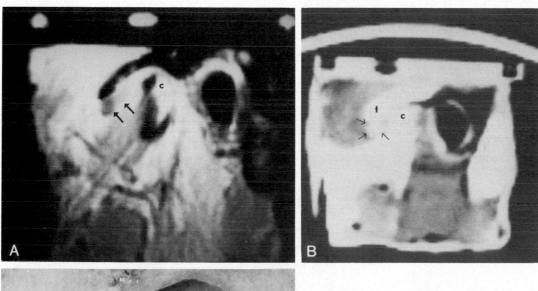

Figure 5–29
Disk displacement associated with deformation of the disk (biconvex) and degenerative joint disease, comparing MR, CT, and the corresponding anatomic specimen. A, Sagittal MR image demonstrating the displaced, deformed disk (arrows) anterior to the flattened condylar head (c). B, Sagittal CT image of the same anatomic specimen and with soft tissue settings. The relatively high attenuation disk (arrows) is noted anterior to the flattened condylar head (c). Somewhat greater anatomic detail is demonstrated by MR than by CT. C, Corresponding anatomic specimen showing the deformed, displaced disk (d) anterior to the flattened condyle (c).

shows both the soft and hard tissue anatomy with fine detail that corresponds closely to the sectioned specimen. In this example, CT is also diagnostic. The disk is of high CT attenuation, as there are mineral deposits within the substance of the disk actually composed of microscopic foci of calcification. Both modalities demonstrate degenerative arthritis manifested by flattening of the condylar head.

The outstanding anatomic soft tissue detail provided by MR imaging, compared with that provided by CT, is demonstrated in Figure 5–30A and B. In this patient with a closed lock, the high CT attenuation of the disk is noted anterior to the condylar head but with little, if any, other anatomic detail. On the other hand, the MR image in this same patient shows the actual configuration of the displaced disk, with details (Fig. 5–30A) of the thickening of the tendinous insertion of the inferior belly of the lateral pterygoid muscle to the disk, and thickening of the fascial coating of the interior belly of the lateral pterygoid muscle. These findings by MR imaging suggest that the disk has been chronically displaced.

The fine anatomic detail of the disk provided by MR imaging in this patient is worthy of additional comment. The notchlike undersurface of the disk is clearly visible and is an altered configuration that we have commonly encountered, caused by thickening of both the posterior and anterior bands. The notchlike landmark on the undersurface of the disk between the thickened posterior and anterior bands can be invaluable in determining disk displacement. Confusion in diagnosis may occur when the posterior disk attachment has undergone remodeling to become more fibrotic. Then, the clear distinction usually seen between the posterior band of the disk and the posterior disk attachment may be obscured. Figure 5–31A and B demonstrates a chronically displaced disk in association with remodeling and MR image signal change of the posterior disk attachment. In this example, it is notable that the usual sharp distinction between the low signal of the posterior band of the disk and the

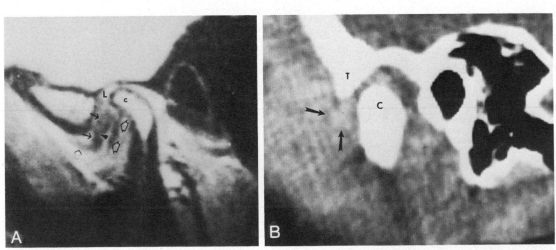

Figure 5–30
Comparison of MR imaging and direct sagittal CT imaging in a patient with disk displacement without reduction. A, Sagittal MR image following attempted maximal jaw opening in a patient with suspected disk displacement without reduction associated with the clinical closed lock. The disk (arrows) is noted to be displaced anterior to the condyle (c). The posterior disk ligament (L) is interposed between the convexity of the condyle inferiorly and the temporal bone superiorly. Deformity of the disk is noted in that the thin zone of the disk is now only a notchlike structure on the belly or undersurface of the disk (arrowhead). Thickening of the fascial coating of the inferior belly of the lateral pterygoid muscle (open arrows) is noted, along with thickening of the fascial insertion of the superior belly of the lateral pterygoid (open arrows). Outstanding anatomic detail is visible on this MR image. B, Direct sagittal CT scan in the same patient and also with attempted maximal jaw opening. The disk is recognizable only as a high attenuation area wedged between the condyle (C) inferiorly, and the tubercle (T) superiorly.

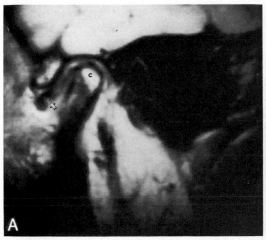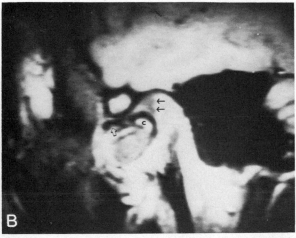

Figure 5-31
Chronically displaced disk with remodeling of the posterior disk ligament. A, Sagittal MR image with the jaw in the closed position. The disk is displaced downward and forward of the condyle (c). An identifying feature of the displaced disk is the notchlike configuration (open arrow) on the undersurface of the disk. B, Sagittal MR image of the same patient with the jaw in the maximally open position shows disk displacement without reduction, the diagnosis clarified by the demonstration of the notchlike undersurface configuration (open arrow) of the disk. Note the intermediate signal intensity tissue (arrows) interposed between the condyle (c) inferiorly and the temporal bone superiorly. The configuration of the undersurface of the disk confirms the diagnosis of disk displacement without reduction, which helps distinguish the disk from the remodeled posterior ligament.

usual bright signal of the posterior disk attachment is no longer possible to define. Yet, the notch on the undersurface of the disk clearly signifies that the disk is not in a proper anatomic location with its posterior band superior to the condyle and the central thin zone between the anterior convexity of condyle and the posterior convexity of the articular eminence. The low signal in the posterior disk attachment might indicate fibrotic changes in the attachment. However, this was not proved histologically.

Disk Deformation

A multitude of alterations of disk configuration is encountered in MR imaging of the TMJ. The first stage of the disk deformation is usually a thickening of the posterior band (Fig. 5–32). The next step is when the posterior band increases in thickness and anteroposterior length, resulting in a biconvex disk (Fig. 5–33A and B). With the open-mouth position, the configuration is rounded. A sigmoid configuration is another example of a deformed disk, shown in Figure 5–34.

Osseous Changes

With a chronically displaced, chronically deformed disk, changes in the osseous anatomy are frequently encountered. Figure 5–35 demonstrates a chronically displaced disk associated with degenerative joint disease in the sagittal imaging plane, with the jaw in the closed-mouth position. Not only are morphologic changes of the condyle demonstrated but also changes in the signal intensity of the bone marrow of the condyle. These latter changes are commonly associated with chronic internal derangement and may be present with or without actual morphologic alterations of bone. An extreme example of marrow signal changes is shown in Figure 5–36A and B, associated with

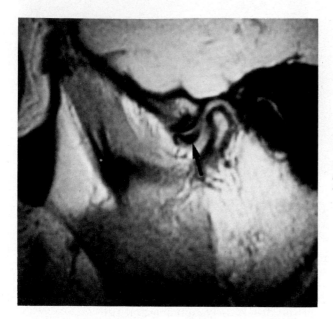

Figure 5–32
Thickening of the posterior band. Proton density sagittal MR images at the closed-mouth position. The disk is anteriorly displaced. The posterior band is thickened and enlarged (arrow). The central thin zone is folded.

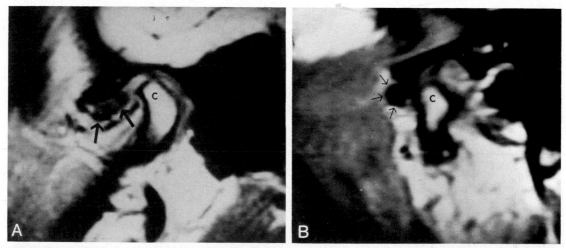

Figure 5–33
MR demonstration of marked changes in disk configuration in a patient with differing jaw positions. A, Sagittal MR image with the jaw in the closed position shows the biconvex disk (arrows) displaced anterior to the condyle (C). Note that the disk has a relatively elongated shape. B, Sagittal MR image in the same patient with the jaw maximally open, showing a rounded configuration to the disk (arrows) anterior to the condyle (C). It is a frequent finding in patients with internal derangement to note fairly significant configurational changes of the disk in association with internal derangement and at differing jaw positions.

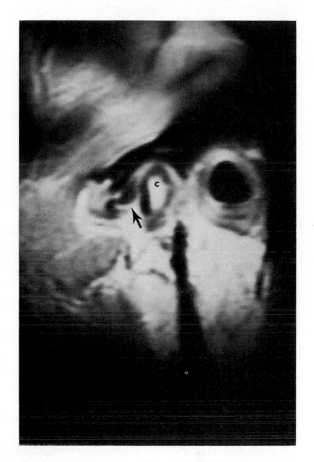

Figure 5–34
Sagittal MR image through the lateral third of the TMJ, closed-jaw position, showing a sigmoid-like configuration to the displaced disk. c, Condyle.

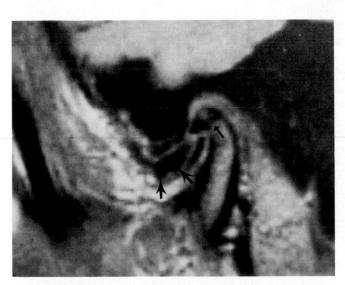

Figure 5–35
Sagittal MR image with the jaw in the closed position, demonstrating disk displacement without reduction associated with degenerative joint disease and change in the signal intensity of the marrow of the condyle. The disk (large arrows) is displaced far foward of the condyle. It has a marked alteration in its configuration, but its notchlike undersurface (between the two large arrows) is a distinguishing feature of its altered morphology. The condylar head has a beaklike anterior configuration, with changes in the marrow signal (single arrow) compatible with fibrotic (sclerotic) degeneration or remodeling. The abnormalities of the condyle were not apparent on the multidirectional tomograms acquired previously.

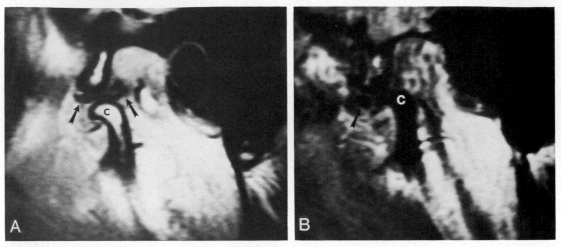

Figure 5–36
MR evaluation of a 21-year-old woman with a longstanding internal derangement, demonstrating extreme marrow signal intensity changes on the affected side secondary to internal derangement. A, Sagittal MR image on the asymptomatic side with the jaw maximally opened. Notice that the disk (arrows) is in a normal anatomic relationship to the condyle (C) inferiorly and the tubercle superiorly. The normal bright signal intensity of the marrow of the condyle is well demonstrated. B, Sagittal MR scan with the jaw maximally opened in the same patient, demonstrating not only disk displacement (arrows) without reduction but also extreme marrow signal intensity changes as a sequela. The signal intensity of the condyle (C) and condylar neck is black, indicating degeneration with probable fibrosis. The multidirectional plain film findings were suggestive of only mild sclerosis on this side.

long-standing, unilateral disk displacement without reduction in a 21-year-old woman. Figure 5–37A and B is another example of an area with low MR imaging signal intensity in the bone marrow of the condyle. This is a 57-year-old man with rheumatoid arthritis. This area of low MR signal intensity is more focal and is confined to the lateral superior third of the mandibular condyle, as seen in the coronal and sagittal images in Figure 5–36. No specific TMJ treatment was given; the patient had continued on his regular medical treatment for his rheumatoid arthritis. At the follow-up examination 2.5 years after the first scan (Fig. 5–38), an essentially unchanged status was found. The histologic background to these alterations of the bone marrow of the mandibular condyle has not been fully documented at this time. They could represent sclerosis, fibrosis, or possibly avascular necrosis.[20, 21] The clinical significance of these changes has not been established.

Another alteration that possibly could be associated with the same disease is increased bone marrow edema (see Figures 5–12 and 5–13). An increased signal from the bone marrow of the condyle is sometimes observed in the T2-weighted images. This observation has not been made in normal volunteers and is not seen in joints with asymptomatic internal derangement. The increased signal from the bone marrow of the condyle could represent bone marrow edema; in our experience, it has been seen only in painful joints with disk displacement. Increased bone marrow signal is usually associated with inflammatory reactions, reflective of joint effusion in the joint spaces. Further studies need to be done to document the histologic background and the clinical significance of these findings that might indicate bone marrow edema in the mandibular condyle. Although the histologic background of the changes seen on MR images still is lacking to a large degree, it is obvious that MR imaging represents an exciting tool to acquire unique information about the biology of the bone marrow of the mandibular condyle in a noninvasive manner that was inconceivable only a few years ago.

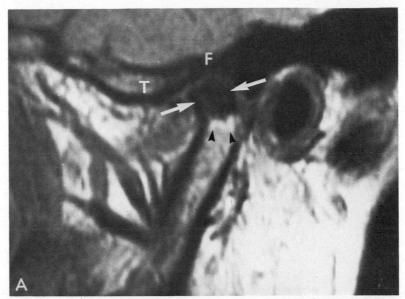

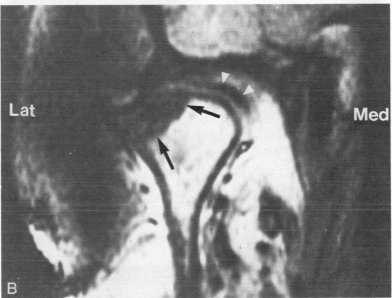

Figure 5–37
Possible avascular necrosis. A, Closed-mouth sagittal and B, MR images of the left TMJ of a 57-year-old man with a long history of rheumatoid arthritis. The fossa (F) and the tubercle (T) are indicated for orientation. An area of low signal intensity is indicated by arrows. In the sagittal image, an area of bright signal inferior to the dark area is marked with arrowheads. The disk is perforated laterally: only a small part of the disk remains medially (arrowheads in B). This image is similar to what has been described as avascular necrosis in the hip, but this was not histologically proved in this patient.

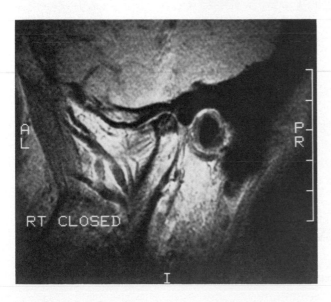

Figure 5–38
Sagittal proton density image of the joint shown in Figure 5–37, obtained 2.5 years later. The status remains unchanged, with an area of decreased signal in the upper part of the condyle but without significant breakdown or other osseous changes. The radiograph indicates this condition to be morphologically stable. No local treatment of the TMJ was undertaken.

Joint Effusion

Joint effusion can be demonstrated by the use of T2-weighted imaging sequences, as mentioned previously and shown in Figure 5–11. Joint effusion is diagnosed when there is an area of high signal on the T2-weighted images in the upper or lower joint spaces or both. The amount of joint effusion varies greatly, from a subtle, thin line along the articular surfaces (Fig. 5–39A and B) to large, significant collections (Fig. 5–40A through D). A thin layer of joint effusion (Fig. 5–39) has been seen in both normal asymptomatic and pathologic and painful joints. A thin layer of joint effusion is probably of no clinical significance. A collection of joint effusion, on the other hand, is seen much more often in abnormal joints and is probably a reflection of the inflammatory component of the disease process.[20, 21] It has been our experience that joint effusion is strongly associated with joint pain.[22] This is also supported by another series of work in which 88 per cent of painful joints showed MR evidence of joint effusion.[23] Thus, joint effusion, if seen as a collection, is a strong indication that the patient's pain symptoms are emanating from the joint. This is important diagnostic information because it is frequently difficult with the clinical examination to determine whether the pain is coming from the joint or from the muscles of mastication.

When diagnosing joint effusion on T2-weighted images obtained in the open-mouth position, one has to be aware that the posterior disk attachment normally has a high MR signal owing to its high vascularity in the open-mouth images (Fig. 5–41A through C). High signal of the posterior disk attachment at open-mouth must not be confused with joint effusion. This is seen in both normal and abnormal joints and does not seem to separate painful from pain-free joints.

Perforation

A disadvantage of MR imaging in the depiction of disk displacement is its inability to demonstrate perforations consistently. Figure 5–42A and B is an

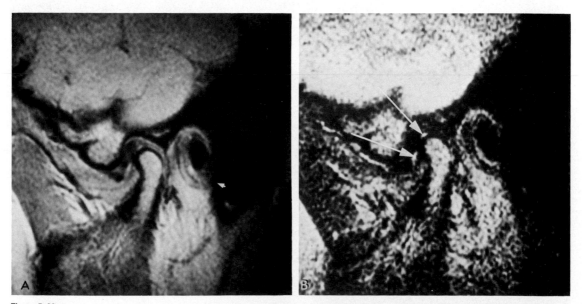

Figure 5–39
Joint effusion. A, Proton density and B, T2-weighted image of a joint with slight anterior disk displacement and a minimal amount of joint effusion (arrows in B) in the lower joint space. This small amount of joint effusion is seen in both normal and abnormal joints and is probably of no clinical significance.

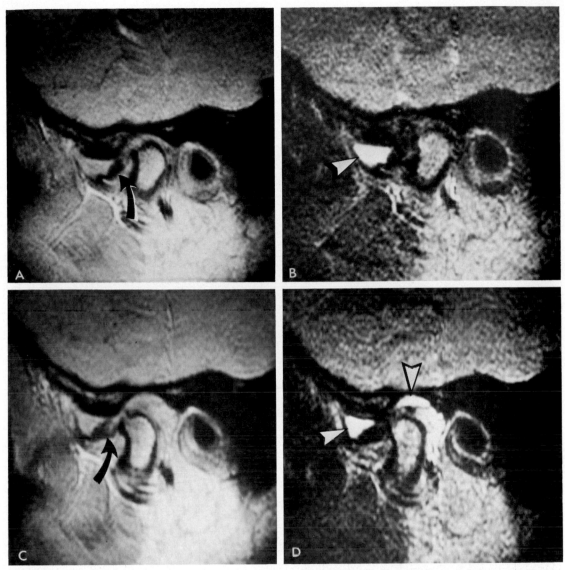

Figure 5–40
Large joint effusion. Sagittal closed-mouth images (A and B) and open-mouth MR images (C and D), showing anterior disk displacement without reduction. The position of the disk is indicated by arrows in A and C. The joint effusion (arrowheads in B and D) is seen to change distribution on the open-mouth images.

example of a chronically displaced disk that is associated with a perforation demonstrated by arthrography but not by MR imaging. This is the most comon situation in which MR imaging cannot demonstrate perforations. However, there is a high likelihood of perforation when there is a clear bone-to-bone contact between the mandibular condyle and the temporal component, associated with advanced degenerative joint disease, and only remnants of the disk are seen in the periphery of the joints, and MR imaging can diagnose this indirectly. Occasionally, with T2-weighted images and in the presence of joint effusion, it is possible with MR imaging to demonstrate the presence of perforations in the posterior disk attachment. Figure 5–43 is an example of a joint with late-stage degenerative joint disease, deformation of the disk, and a perforation in the posterior disk attachment. In the T2-weighted image in Figure 5–43, the perforation between the disk and the posterior disk attachment can be seen owing to the arthrographic effect of the joint effusion. It has been

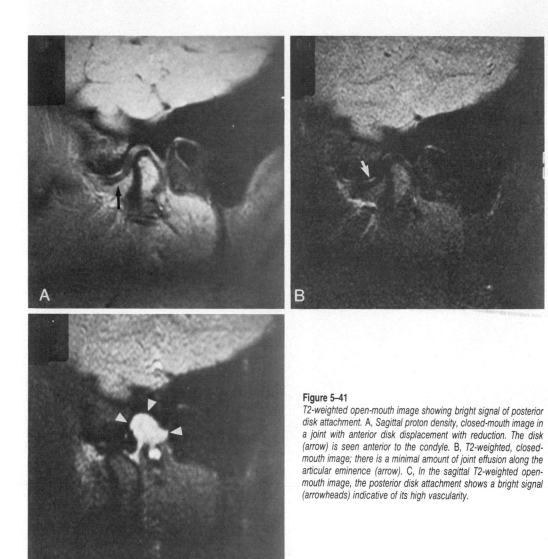

Figure 5–41
T2-weighted open-mouth image showing bright signal of posterior disk attachment. A, Sagittal proton density, closed-mouth image in a joint with anterior disk displacement with reduction. The disk (arrow) is seen anterior to the condyle. B, T2-weighted, closed-mouth image; there is a minimal amount of joint effusion along the articular eminence (arrow). C, In the sagittal T2-weighted open-mouth image, the posterior disk attachment shows a bright signal (arrowheads) indicative of its high vascularity.

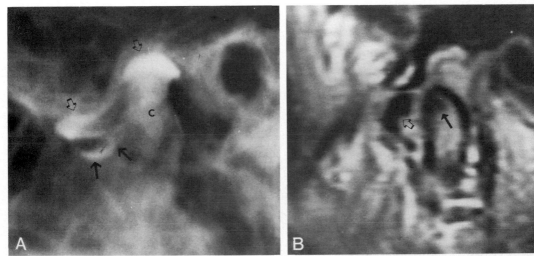

Figure 5–42

Correlation of arthrogram and MR scan in a patient with disk displacement without reduction associated with perforation or tear in the posterior disk ligament. A, The contrast material was injected into the lower joint space (arrows), demonstrating disk displacement without reduction and filling of the upper joint space (open arrows), indicating perforation. The arthrogram is an indirect assessment of disk position anterior to the condyle (C). B, Sagittal MR scan in the same patient also demonstrates disk displacement without reduction. Both the arthrogram and the MR scan were obtained at maximal jaw opening. The groove or notchlike landmark on the undersurface of the deformed disk is depicted (open arrow). There are signal intensity changes in the marrow of the condyle (arrow) indicating degeneration or remodeling. The multidirectional plain film tomogram of the condyle was normal. Although the tear in the posterior disk ligament was correctly suspected on the arthrogram, it could not be diagnosed on the MR scan.

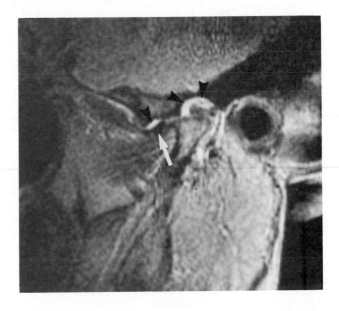

Figure 5–43

Perforation of posterior disk attachment diagnosed with T2-weighted image. The disk (arrow) is anteriorly displaced in this joint with severe degenerative joint disease. The joint effusion (arrowheads) seen around the disk and the remnants of a posterior disk attachment outlines a perforation between the disk and the posterior disk attachment.

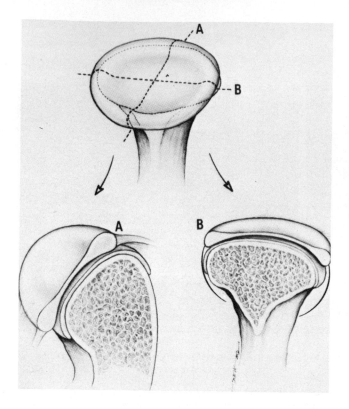

Figure 5–44
Sagittal (A) and coronal (B) diagrams of the normal disk and condyle. In the sagittal plane, the posterior band of the disk is at the 12 o'clock position relative to the condylar head, and in the coronal plane of imaging the lateral and medial margins of the disk are adjacent to the lateral and medial poles of the condyle.

our experience that this limitation of MR imaging is not as important as it may appear initially. First, perforations often may be suspected based on indirect signs on the MR images. Second, perforation is not a salient characteristic of internal derangement that dictates treatment options in most cases. Whether or not the disk is displaced and whether or not the disk is deformed seem to be the major parameters driving the various treatment protocols.

Rotational and Sideways Disk Displacements

The multiplanar imaging capability of MR imaging has recently expanded our understanding of the three-dimensional coordinates of disk position[16] (Fig. 5–44A and B). Studies in cadaver specimens and comparisons with the clinical condition have led us to a more detailed classification of anatomic disorders. We have devised a general classification scheme (Table 5–9) that places in subgroups the various disk positional conditions: (1) superior, or 12 o'clock (normal); (2) anterior; (3) anteromedial; (4) anterolateral; (5) medial; and (6) lateral.

Table 5–9
TERMINOLOGY FOR DESCRIBING THE POSITION OF THE DISK

Normal:	Superior
Abnormal:	Anterior
	Anteromedial rotational displacement
	Anterolateral rotational displacement
	Medial sideways displacement
	Lateral sideways displacement

Diagrams in the sagittal and coronal planes in the normal, sideways, and rotational disk displacements are shown in Figures 5–44A and B and 5–45A and B. Sideways disk displacement is defined as a displacement that is either lateral (Fig. 5–46A through C) or medial relative to the long axis of the condyle without an anterior component. Rotational disk displacement represents those disks that are displaced anteriorly in association with either a medial or lateral component (Fig. 5–47A and B) to the displacement. By far the most common types of disk displacements are anterior, anteromedial, and anterolateral (Fig. 5–47). The value of coronal imaging is demonstrated in Figure 5–48A through D in a case with anterior medial disk displacement with reduction.

A suspicion of a sideways or rotational displacement arises if the disk is not well-defined in all the sagittal images. If the disk is not well seen in the lateral part of the joint, this is termed "empty fossa"; typical examples are shown in Figures 5–49A and B and 5–50A and B. In these patients the conventional sagittal images do not clearly depict the position and configuration of the disk, but the coronal images do show rotational and sideways displacements out of the glenoid fossa. A lateral disk displacement is shown in Figure 5–51.

Studies have suggested that sideways disk displacement could be diagnosed with lower compartment arthrography as well.[24] The investigators suggested that the "edge-sign" was an indication of a lateral disk displacement. The edge-sign is defined as a horizontal contrast medium margin passing over the lower part of the condyle, as seen in Figure 5–52A through D. Correlation between coronal cryosections of cadaver specimens and arthrography also has suggested that the edge-sign may indicate sideways disk displacement.[25] However, sideways disk displacement was seen in a significant number of joints that did not show the edge-sign. False-positives also frequently occur, lowering the reliability of this finding.

The coronal plane of imaging is also valuable for the depiction of abnormalities of the bone. Examples of osseous abnormalities are clearly shown by MR imaging in the coronal plane, as indicated in Figures 5–53 and 5–54.

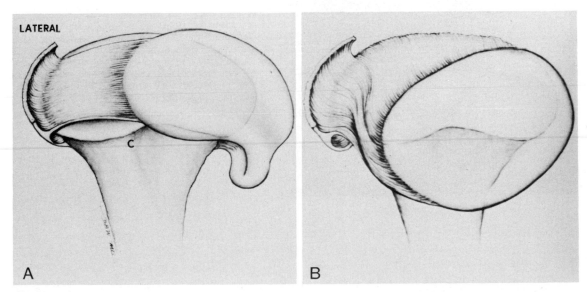

Figure 5–45
Sideways and rotational disk displacement. A, This diagrammatic depiction shows a side-to-side displacement of the disk relative to the condyle (C). It is termed a sideways displacement as there is no anterior component to the abnormal position. B, Depiction of a rotational displacement that shows both anterior and sideways components to the displacement. The disk appears to rotate anteromedially owing to a loose lateral capsular attachment and posterior disk attachment. The disk may remain attached to the medial capsular attachment and medial neck of the condyle.

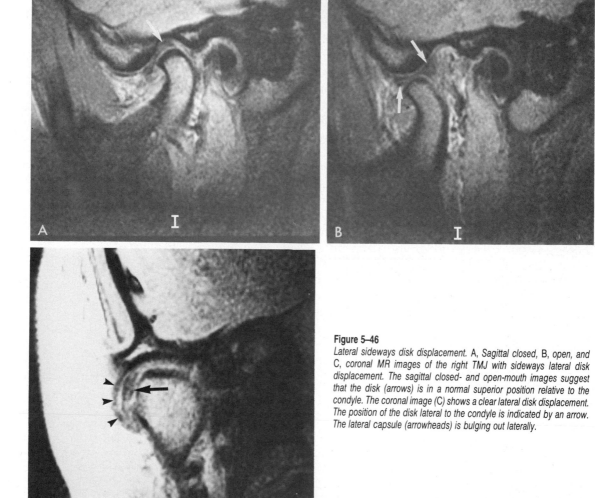

Figure 5–46

Lateral sideways disk displacement. A, Sagittal closed, B, open, and C, coronal MR images of the right TMJ with sideways lateral disk displacement. The sagittal closed- and open-mouth images suggest that the disk (arrows) is in a normal superior position relative to the condyle. The coronal image (C) shows a clear lateral disk displacement. The position of the disk lateral to the condyle is indicated by an arrow. The lateral capsule (arrowheads) is bulging out laterally.

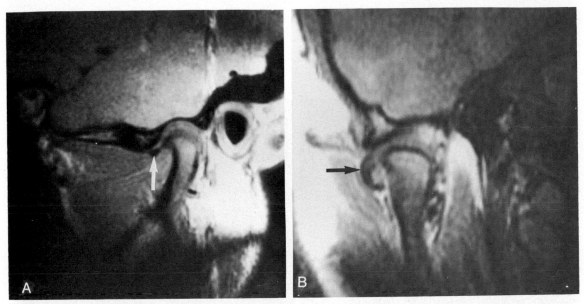

Figure 5–47
Lateral rotational disk displacement. A, Sagittal and B, coronal proton density MR images of the right TMJ showing the disk (arrows) to be anterior to the condyle in the sagittal plane and lateral to the condyle in the coronal plane.

Posterior Disk Displacement

Debates continue in the literature as to whether or not posterior displacement of the disk does occur. In well over ten thousand TMJ arthrograms and MR scans, we have encountered a few joints with MR or arthrographic findings compatible with a posterior disk displacement. Surgical confirmation is not available because the patient's clinical status in these cases has not justified invasive treatment. An example of an MR scan that indicates posterior disk displacement is shown in Figure 5–55. Another form of posterior disk displacement occurs with subluxation of the condyle far beyond the bony tubercle. When the condyle translates well anterior to the articular eminence, it sometimes also translates anterior to the anterior band of the disk (Fig. 5–56A and B). In these cases, the patient can get an open lock, in which the condyle is prevented from moving posteriorly by the tubercle or by the disk.

Joint Capsule

With improvement of the quality of MR images, the joint capsule is now frequently well visualized in the coronal images (see Figures 5–15C, 5–46, 5–57, and 5–58A and B). In the normal joint the capsule is seen as a thin, relatively smooth dark line lateral to the condyle. In the abnormal joint, we have frequently encountered bulging of the capsule in a lateral direction (Fig. 5–57 and 5–58A and B). In joints with lateral disk displacement, we also frequently have seen thickening of the joint capsule (Fig. 5–58). In some patients with lateral joint tenderness and swelling, the T2-weighted images in the coronal plane have shown increased joint fluid in the capsule, suggestive of capsular edema. All the observations are suggestive of capsulitis (Fig. 5–59A and B), although not histologically proved at this time. An example of increased signal from the capsule anteriorly is shown in Figure 5–60A and B. This is suggestive, but not surgically confirmed, as evidence of capsulitis.

Text continued on page 219

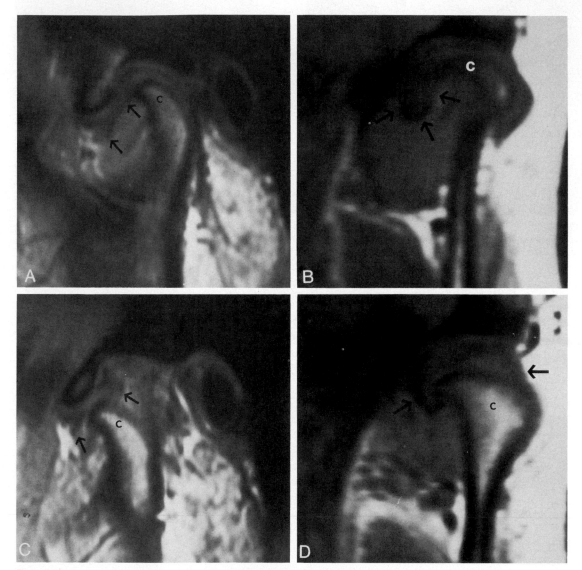

Figure 5–48
Value of coronal MR images in a patient with left-sided anteromedial disk displacement with reduction. A, Sagittal MR image with the jaw in the closed position shows the disk (arrows) in a slight anterior position relative to the condyle (C) in a patient with painful clicking. B, Coronal image in the same patient with the jaw closed, showing the medial component to the anterior displacement—thus representing anteromedial disk displacement. The disk (arrows) is of low signal intensity and is noted medial to the medial margin of the condyle (C). C, Sagittal MR image in the same patient with the jaw opened to beyond the click, showing recapture of the disk (arrows). Notice the bowtie-like configuration of the disk, indicating normal configuration. C, Condyle. D, Coronal MR image following reduction of the displacement of the disk (arrows) relative to the condyle (C), and in a normal anatomic relationship compared with Figure 5–48B.

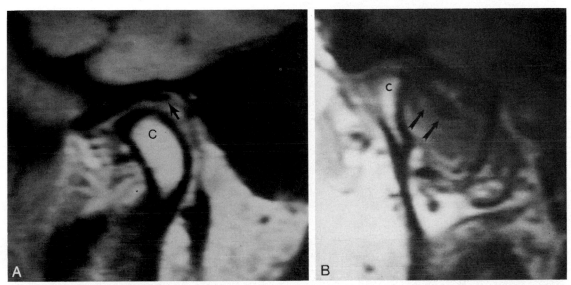

Figure 5–49

MR images of the "empty fossa." A, Sagittal MR scan of the right TMJ with the jaw in the closed position shows the condyle (C) and fossa but without visualization of the disk. A sliver (arrow) of low signal intensity tissue is noted near the roof of the glenoid fossa, probably representing a small portion of the herniated joint capsule. B, Coronal MR image in the same patient with the jaw in the closed position shows the far medial displacement of the disk (arrows) relative to the condyle (C). Absence of recognizable disk tissue within the fossa should raise the suspicion of a rotational or sideways disk displacement.

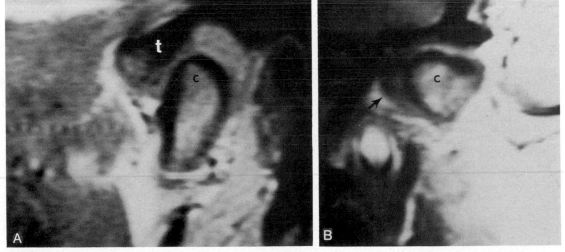

Figure 5–50

MR demonstration of "empty fossa" associated with sideways disk displacement. A, Sagittal MR image of the left TMJ with the jaw slightly opened and with inability to demonstrate disk tissue either above or anterior to the condyle (C). The tubercle (t) is also well-defined but without recognizable disk tissue. B, Coronal image in the same patient showing a medial disk (arrow) relative to the condylar head (C). Note the bright signal intensity tissue superior to the condyle and between the condyle and tubercle, which explains the relatively bright signal noted in the fossa in the sagittal image.

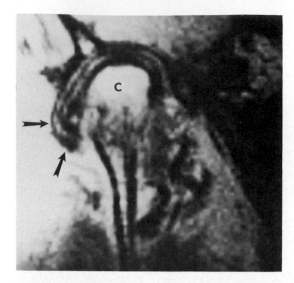

Figure 5–51
Coronal MR image depicting a lateral disk (arrows) displacement of the right TMJ. The coronal plane of imaging is valuable in demonstrating this type of abnormality. C, Condyle.

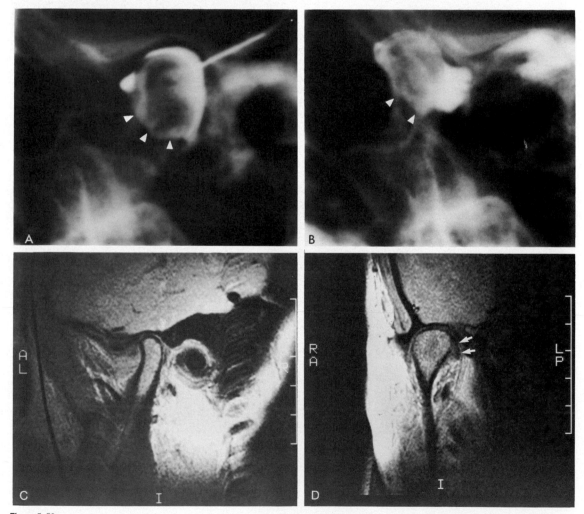

Figure 5–52
Sideways disk displacement with arthrography and MR imaging. Transcranial lower compartment arthrogram in the A, closed- and B, open-mouth position of the right TMJ. C, Sagittal MR scan and D, coronal MR scan of the same joint. A, A horizontal contrast medium margin (arrowheads) is passing over the lower part of the condyle. This is also seen in B (arrowheads). This is termed the edge-sign and indicates a medial disk displacement. In C, the disk is not well visualized. In D, the disk (arrows) is seen to be medially displaced in relation to the condyle.

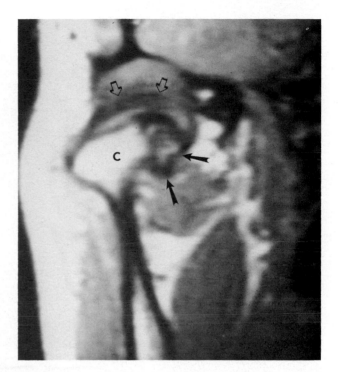

Figure 5–53
MR coronal image depicting medial condylar (C) hyperplasia of the right TMJ appearing as osteophyte (arrows) of low signal intensity. This abnormality was not demonstrable by plain film tomographic radiography, arthrography, or sagittal MR imaging. Note that the disk (open arrows) is in a normal relationship to the condyle and is thus not displaced.

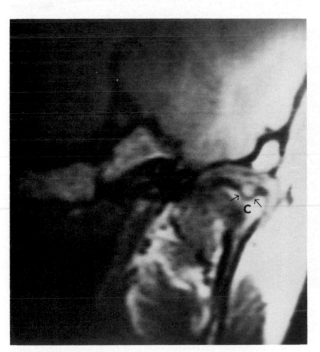

Figure 5–54
Coronal MR image in a patient with chronic left TMJ pain, demonstrating a deep groove (arrows) in the midportion of the condyle (C). This was not demonstrable by plain tomographic radiography or on the sagittal MR images. This abnormality might represent evidence for an old, healed condylar fracture or a defect from cartilaginous injury.

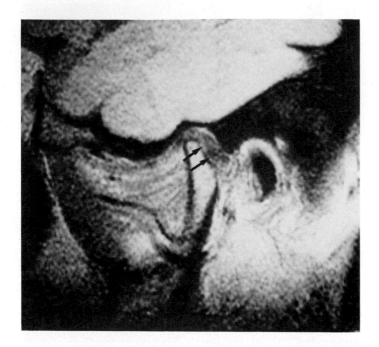

Figure 5–55
Posterior disk displacement. Sagittal proton density MR scan from the central-medial part of the joint, showing low attenuation tissue (arrows) posterior to the condyle. This was interpreted as evidence of posterior disk displacement, although surgical correlation was not available in this case.

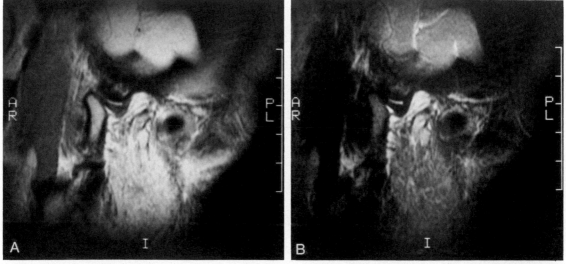

Figure 5–56
Subluxation. A, Sagittal proton density, and B, T2-weighted images, showing the condyle anterior to the articular eminence and anterior to the anterior band of the disk in a patient with clinical symptoms of subluxation.

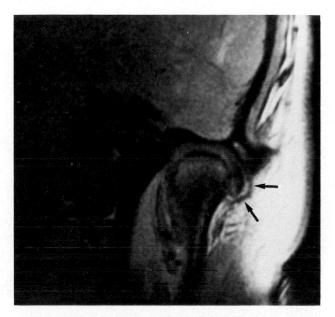

Figure 5–57
Thin lateral capsule. A lateral disk displacement and distention of the lateral capsule (arrows) are seen in this coronal proton density image of the left TMJ. The capsule is thin.

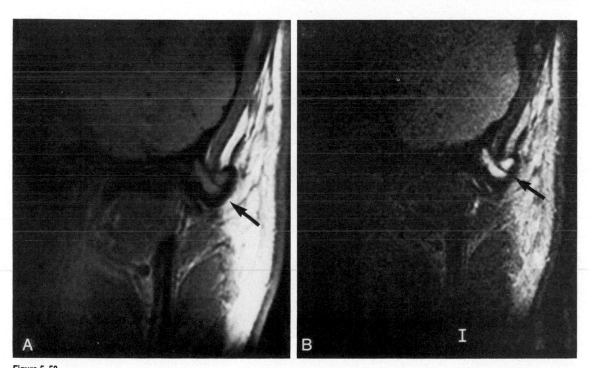

Figure 5–58
Thickening and fibrosis of lateral joint capsule of the left TMJ. A, Proton density and B, T2-weighted coronal MR images show the lateral capsule (arrows) to be bulging laterally and being thickened. The signal from the capsule is low on both images, which is suggestive of fibrosis. A small amount of joint effusion is seen in both upper and lower joint spaces.

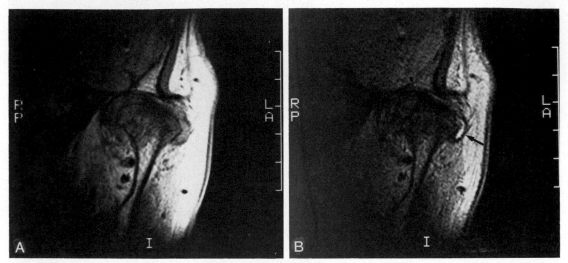

Figure 5–59
A, *Coronal proton density, and* B, *T2-weighted images of the left TMJ, showing increased signal in* B *in the lateral capsule wall, suggestive of capsular edema (arrow).*

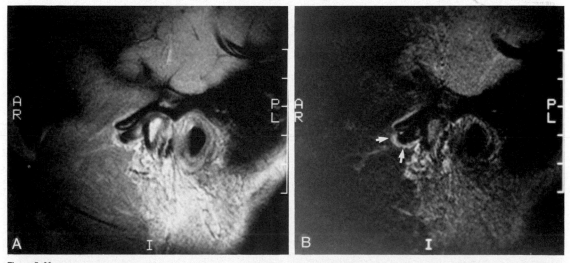

Figure 5–60
Capsular edema in anterior capsule. A, *Proton density, and* B, *T2-weighted images in the sagittal plane, showing an increased signal intensity from the anterior capsule (arrows) suggestive of capsulitis.*

Postoperative Imaging

MR imaging is an important modality for the evaluation of postsurgical changes. These findings are discussed in depth in Chapter 7. An example of a patient with a failed Teflon-proplast implant is shown in Figure 5–61, which demonstrates the remarkable image detail of both the implant and the associated granulation tissue.

FUTURE PERSPECTIVES

Further developments in the radiologic assessment of internal derangement of the TMJ will probably continue to focus on improved understanding and depiction of the normal and pathologic anatomy, utilizing multiplanar and three-dimensional imaging techniques. As with degenerative disk diseases of the spine, it is possible that MR imaging spectroscopic analysis may be helpful in evaluating metabolic and biochemical changes. Previous reports have suggested abnormalities of lactate accumulation and intervertebral and diskal (of the spine) pH parameters in the presence of degeneration and herniation.[26, 27] Growing evidence also suggests significant changes in histopathology of the TMJ disk and the posterior ligament in association with internal derangement.[28–31]

The dynamics of TMJ internal derangement are an important component in the pathophysiology of the disease, and thus cine MR imaging techniques will provide a valuable tool if image acquisition times can be decreased to the millisecond range.[32] The acute effect of muscle stress with exercise on high-energy phosphates, via MR imaging spectroscopy, is also an important area for future research. Comparisons of high and midfield magnetic strength systems are of practical importance for diagnostic accuracy, but only preliminary insights have been acquired.[11] MR imaging is an excellent modality to follow up various types of surgical and nonsurgical treatment of TMJ disorders, since there is no known biologic harm or patient discomfort. For the first time, we do have a noninvasive tool at hand that depicts the soft tissue components of the joint. It

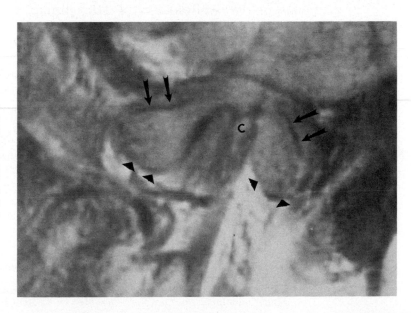

Figure 5–61
Sagittal MR image in a patient with Teflon-proplast TMJ implant. The implant (arrows) is noted to be placed within the glenoid fossa and above the markedly flattened condyle (C). The Teflon-proplast implant is poorly visualized, suggesting fragmentation. Exuberant foreign body reaction with granulation tissue (arrowheads) is noted anterior and posterior to the condylar head. No other imaging modality is capable of depicting all these findings as accurately as MR.

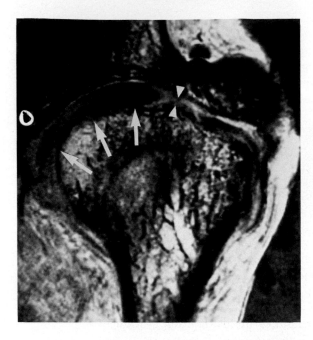

Figure 5–62
Coronal high-resolution MR image showing exquisite anatomic details. This image of the left TMJ was obtained using a 1.5-mm slice thickness, a matrix of 256 × 256, four excitations, and a field of view of 4 cm. The disk (arrows) is clearly visualized medial to the perforation (arrowheads). There is a superiorly directed osteophyte on the condyle filling in the perforation. The image is of a cadaver specimen.

is now possible to image frequently after treatment, and it should be possible to acquire significant information about the morphologic results of different forms of treatment and correlate these to patient symptomatology.

Thinner-section MR scans probably will be clinically useful in the near future. Since the joint has such a small dimension, especially in its anteroposterior dimension, the reduction of volume average by using thinner slices will be an important step toward refining the diagnosis. An example of a very high resolution, thin-section coronal MR scan of a cadaver specimen is shown in Figure 5–62*A* and *B*. This image was obtained with 1.5-mm slice thickness, 4-cm FOV, and a matrix of 256 × 256, using four excitations. There are exquisite details of the osseous anatomy, and the defect in the lateral part of the disk is clearly visualized. We are convinced that high-quality, thin-section MR scans close to this quality will be available for clinical use in the near future. Thereby some of the disadvantages of MR imaging, such as the inability to detect perforations, will be overcome.

The development of MR angiography has given some promising initial results.[32] The vascular anatomy can be depicted without the use of invasive techniques or contrast agents. This technique is exciting, but it still has a long way to go before it can be applied to the fine vascular structures of the TMJ. However, judging by the rapid development that occurs in this area, probably in not too many years we will be able to study this vascular anatomy of the joint and its surrounding soft tissue with noninvasive MR angiography.

Magnetic resonance imaging, as both a diagnostic and research instrument, will continue to advance our understanding of the pathophysiology of this multifaceted and widely prevalent joint disorder.

References

1. Harms SE, Wilk RM, Wolford LM, et al: The temporomandibular joint: Magnetic resonance using surface coils. Radiology 1985;*157*:133–136.
2. Katzberg RW, Schenck J, Roberts BA, et al: Magnetic resonance imaging of the temporomandibular joint meniscus. Oral Surg Oral Med Oral Pathol 1985;*59*:332–335.

3. Katzberg RW, Bessette RW, Tallents RH, et al: Normal and abnormal temporomandibular joint: MR imaging with surface coil. Radiology 1986;*158*:183–189.

4. Katzberg RW: Temporomandibular joint imaging. Radiology 1989;*120*:297–307.

5. Schellhas KP, Wilkes CH, Omlie MR, et al: The diagnosis of temporomandibular joint disease: Two-compartment arthrography and MR. AJR 1988;*151*:341–350.

6. Kaplan PA, Helms CA: Current status of temporomandibular joint imaging for the diagnosis of internal derangements. AJR 1989;*152*:697–705.

7. Jacobson HG: Counsel on Scientific Affairs: Musculoskeletal applications of magnetic resonance imaging. JAMA 1989;*262*:2420–2427.

8. Elster AD: Magnetic Resonance Imaging: A Reference Guide and Atlas. Philadelphia, JB Lippincott, 1986, pp 1–56.

9. Balter S: An introduction to the physics of magnetic resonance imaging. Radiographics 1987;*7*:371–383.

10. Lauterbur PC: Image formation by indirect local interactions: Examples employing nuclear magnetic resonance. Nature 1973;*242*:190–191.

11. Hansson L-G, Westesson P-L, Katzberg RW, et al: MR imaging of the temporomandibular joint: Comparison of images of autopsy specimens made at 0.3T and 1.5T with anatomic cryosections. AJR 1989;*152*:1241–1244.

12. Musgrave MT, Westesson P-L, Tallents RH, et al: Improved magnetic resonance images of the temporomandibular joint by oblique scanning planes. Oral Surg Oral Med Oral Pathol 1991;*71*:525–528.

13. Westesson P-L, Kwok E, Barsotti JB, et al: Temporomandibular joint: Improved MR image quality with decreased section thickness. Radiology 1992;*182*:280–282.

14. Westesson P-L, Katzberg RW, Tallents RH, et al: Temporomandibular joint: Comparison of MR images with cryosectional anatomy. Radiology 1987;*164*:59–64.

15. Westesson P-L, Katzberg RW, Tallents RH, et al: CT and MR of the temporomandibular joint: Comparison with autopsy specimens. AJR 1987;*148*:1165–1171.

16. Katzberg RW, Westesson P-L, Tallents RH, et al: Temporomandibular joint: MR assessment of rotational and sideways disk displacement. Radiology 1988;*169*:741–748.

17. Schellhas KP, Fritts HM, Heitoff KB, et al: Temporomandibular joint: MR fast scanning. J Craniomandib Pract 1988; *6*:209–216.

18. Burnett KR, Davis CL, Read J: Dynamic display of the temporomandibular joint meniscus using "fast scan" MR imaging. AJR 1987;*149*:959–962.

19. Conway WF, Hayes CW, Campbell RL: Dynamic magnetic resonance of the temporomandibular joint using FLASH sequences. J Oral Maxillofac Surg 1988;*46*:930–937.

20. Schellhas KP, Wilkes CH: Temporomandibular joint inflammation: Comparison of MR to fast scanning with T_1- and T_2-weighted imaging techniques. AJR 1989;*153*:93–98.

21. Schellhas KP, Wilkes CH, Fritts HM, et al: MR of osteochondritis dissecans and avascular necrosis of the mandibular condyle. AJNR 1989;*10*:3–12.

22. Westesson P-L, Brooks SL: Temporomandibular joint: Magnetic resonance evidence of joint effusion relative to joint pain and internal derangement. AJR 1992; *159*:559–563.

23. Schellhas KP, Wilkes CH: Temporomandibular joint inflammation: Comparison of MR fast scanning with T1- and T2-weighted imaging techniques. AJR 1989;*153*:93–98.

24. Khoury MB, Dolan E: Sideways dislocation of the temporomandibular joint meniscus: the edge sign. AJNR 1986;*7*:869–872.

25. Liedberg J, Westesson P-L, Kurita K: Sideways and rotational displacement of the temporomandibular joint disk. Diagnosis by arthrography and correlation to cryosectional morphology. Oral Surg Oral Med Oral Pathol 1990;*69*:757–763.

26. Digmant B, Karlsson J, Nachenson A: Correlation between lactate levels and pH in discs with lumbar rhizopathies. Experientia 1968;*24*:1195–1196.

27. Nachenson A: Intradiscal measurements of pH in patients with lumbar rhizopathies. Acta Orthop Scand 1969;*40*:23–42.

28. Piper M: Associated anatomical findings with avascular necrosis of the mandibular condyle. American Association of Oral Maxillofacial Surgery Annual Meeting, September 14, 1990.

29. Paz M, Katzberg RW, Tallents RH, et al: CT assessment of temporomandibular joint meniscus density in internal derangements. Oral Surg Oral Med Oral Pathol 1988;*66*:519–524.

30. Kurita K, Westesson P-L, Sternby NH, et al: Histologic features of the temporomandibular joint disk and posterior disk attachment: Comparison of symptom-free persons with normally positioned disks and patients with internal derangements. Oral Surg Oral Med Oral Pathol 1989;*67*:635–643.

31. Schellhas KP, Piper MA, Omlie MR: Facial skeleton remodeling due to temporomandibular joint degeneration: An imaging study of 100 patients. AJNR 1990;*11*:541–551.

32. Higgins CB: MR of the heart: Anatomy, physiology, and metabolism. AJR 1988;*151*:239–248.

Miscellaneous Modalities: Computed Tomography, Single Photon Emission Computed Tomography, and Sound Analysis

This chapter provides an overview of unrelated technologies that have specific but differing capabilities in the assessment of the temporomandibular joint (TMJ). These modalities are computed tomography (CT), radionuclide imaging with special attention to single photon emission computed tomography (SPECT), and the evolving technology of joint sound analysis ("sonography").

CT as a primary imaging modality for internal derangement of the TMJ has fallen into disfavor because of the superiority of magnetic resonance (MR) imaging,[1–3] but it does have specialized imaging capabilities for bone detail,[4–7] disk density measurements,[7–13] and three-dimensional assessment of congenital, traumatic, and postsurgical conditions involving the TMJ.[14–16] Radionuclide imaging is the most sensitive modality in the assessment of both destructive and reparative bony remodeling.[17–19] The emerging technology of joint sound analysis offers a potentially noninvasive and inexpensive clinical screening technique to define and categorize subgroups of internal derangement based on an analysis of the joint sounds that might be associated with various stages of internal derangement.[20–23]

COMPUTED TOMOGRAPHY

CT has been used extensively in the past to study the complex anatomic structures of the TMJ. Direct sagittal and axial images of the TMJ have allowed a noninvasive technique of imaging of both osseous and soft tissue abnormalities related to disk damage and dysfunction. The diagnostic accuracy of CT has been correlated with TMJ cadaver anatomic sections,[4, 7] arthrography,[4, 24] and surgery.[8–11] High-resolution CT can depict bony and soft tissue changes not detectable by conventional radiography. CT attenuation values have been used as a diagnostic approach to delineate tissues of different densities.[8–13] Since mineralization of the soft tissue elements of the TMJ alters their x-ray attenuation, CT has been used as a modality to assess this aspect of internal derangement.[13]

For the assessment of bone detail, CT is a superior imaging method since it is not subject to the projectional limitations of conventional radiography.

Multiplanar reconstructions give superior morphologic analyses of the osseous joint structures. Computer-generated analysis and displays of three-dimensional imaging data are now routinely available in conjunction with CT scanning.[14–16]

Though CT has been largely displaced as the primary imaging modality for internal derangement, it does have powerful capabilities that should be considered in specialized clinical circumstances when the primary interest is in osseous abnormalities.

Scanning Technique for CT Assessment of Internal Derangement of the TMJ

Two techniques have been described as useful in the assessment of TMJ internal derangement. One is the direct sagittal technique described by Manzione and associates[4, 25, 26] (Fig. 6–1) and the other is the axial technique with parasagittal reconstruction described originally by Helms and colleagues (Fig. 6–2).[8–10] Reports of the accuracy of both techniques have compared well with arthrography, surgical observations, and magnetic resonance imaging.[4, 6–11, 24–27]

For the direct sagittal technique, the patient lies supine on a stretcher placed lateral to the scanner gantry at a 45° or 90° angle to the scanner trolley (Fig. 6–1).[4, 25, 26] The head is positioned facing upward in the gantry in a lateral orientation. Scanning begins laterally, and as the patient is moved through the gantry, the medial portion of the TMJ is examined. Each TMJ is studied separately using 1.5- to 2-mm collimation and 1- to 2-mm table increments. Five to ten scans through the TMJ are obtained in both the open- and closed-mouth positions. Machine parameters are given in Table 6–1. The estimated maximal skin dose is 2.9 rads (0.029 Gy) per scan or 5.8 rads (0.058 Gy) per study.[11] All studies are filmed at both soft tissue and bone windows.

The axial technique has been described both with the General Electric 8800 and with the General Electric 9800 Quick by Helms and associates[8–10] and Christiansen and colleagues.[12] The patient's head is stabilized on a head rest, and a lateral digital scout view is acquired to ensure proper patient alignment. Line cursors prescribing the upper and lower limits of the scan are placed parallel to Reid's base line, which is represented by a line from the inferior margin of the orbit to the superior margin of the auditory meatus. Imaging in

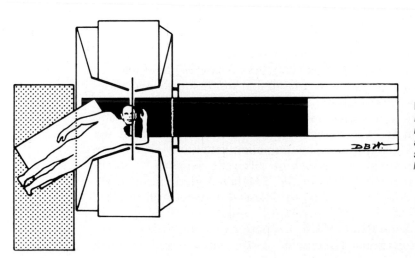

Figure 6–1
Patient positioned for direct sagittal CT scanning. The patient lies supine on a stretcher and wooden board so that the head is positioned facing up in the gantry and in a lateral orientation.

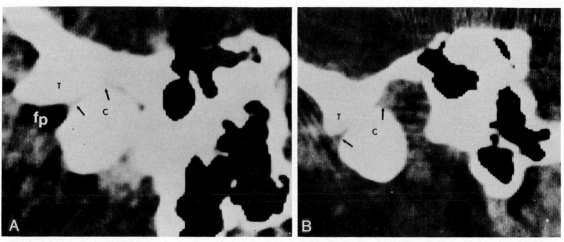

Figure 6–2
Direct sagittal CT scan through a normal TMJ. A, In the closed-jaw position the low density area in the angle between the condyle (C) and articular tubercle (T) is the lateral portion of the fat pad (fp). The disk (arrows) is noted to be a higher density structure (approximately 70 HU) interposed between the condyle and tubercle. B, The open-jaw position shows the condyle (C) to have translated anteriorly beneath the tubercle (T). The disk (arrows) is noted to be normally positioned between the two bony structures of the articulation.

the axial plane utilizes 1.5-mm thick sections acquired each 1.0 mm. Scan parameters are given in Table 6–1. During scanning the gantry angle is 0°. Utilizing this technique, approximately 20 sections are acquired for each of the two scan sequences with the jaw closed and open. The prospective soft tissue sections are enlarged with a field of view of 16 cm². The raw data are then retrospectively "ReViewed" for bone detail. The scan data are then manipulated by the "Arrange" software program to obtain vertically reformatted images in sagittal and coronal planes.

Interpretation of CT Images

Disk Position

For the assessment of internal derangement, the angle between the condylar head and glenoid fossa is closely examined on each scan (Figs. 6–2 through 6–

Table 6–1
MACHINE PARAMETERS IN CT ASSESSMENT

	Siemens Somatom DR2*	General Electric† 9800
Scan plane	Sagittal	Axial
Jaw position	Closed/open	Closed/open
Number of slices/jaw position	5	20
Slice thickness	2 mm	1.5 mm
Table incrementation	2 mm	1 mm
kVp	125	120
mAs	350	200
Scan time	1.4 sec	2 sec
Matrix	256 × 256	256 × 256

*Iselin, New Jersey
†Milwaukee, Wisconsin

7).[3–12] The soft tissue that normally fills this angle is composed of both the superior and inferior bellies of the lateral pterygoid muscle, separated by a margin of intervening fatty connective tissue (Fig. 6–2A and B). This has been termed the "lateral pterygoid fat pad" that extends laterally to fill completely the space between the bony margins.[4] Increased density beyond approximately 70 HU is interpreted as anterior displacement of the disk (see Figs. 6–3, 6–5, and 6–6). This angle can be assessed subjectively by visual inspection or by utilizing the "blink mode" technique available to enhance subtle differences in density between the fibrocartilaginous disk and adjacent low-density soft tissue.[8–10] The soft tissues anterior to the condyle and the articular tubercle are then assessed in the same way, with the jaw in the maximal open position.

The ability of direct sagittal CT to evaluate osseous structures is an important advantage of this technique.[1–11] Osteoarthritis is a common disease of the TMJ and is often associated with disk derangement.[28–30] The diagnosis of degenerative joint disease is based on the criteria of bone erosion, eburnation, fragmentation, remodeling of the articular eminence or condylar head, and osteophyte formation.[28]

Calcifications in the Disk

MacAlister first reported the presence of areas of calcific degeneration within the substance of the disk in postmortem human TMJs.[31] Several workers have associated the appearance of calcifications and other metaplastic changes in the disk structure with pathologic change.[10–13, 32] CT has been shown to have a high sensitivity to density changes and has been proved to be reliable in detecting the presence and amount of calcium concentration within many different tissues, an example being benign pulmonary nodules.[33, 34] A study by Paz and coworkers showed a significant difference in CT attenuation values of the TMJ disk, in large measure correlating with the presence of calcification.[35]

Text continued on page 231

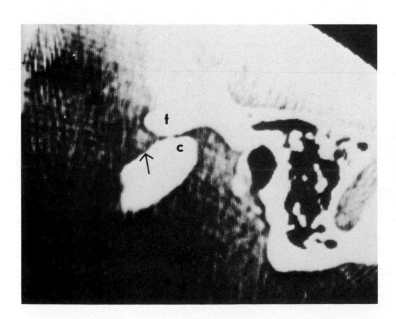

Figure 6–3
Disk displacement without reduction. This is the maximal open-jaw position, and it demonstrates a focal area of increased density within the anterior portion of the angle between the condyle (c) and the tubercle (t). This focal area of increased density (arrow) represents the displaced disk.

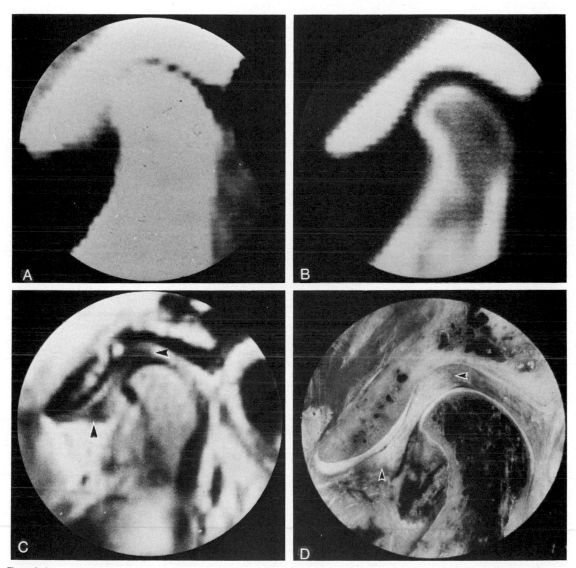

Figure 6–4
A, *Soft-tissue, and* B, *bone CT settings;* C, *MR, and* D, *corresponding cryosection of normal TMJ. The disk is biconcave and located in the superior position. Diagnosis of a superior disk position was correctly made in both CT and MR images. Anterior and posterior margins of the disk are indicated by arrowheads in C and D. Bone in this section was correctly diagnosed as normal with CT and MR.*

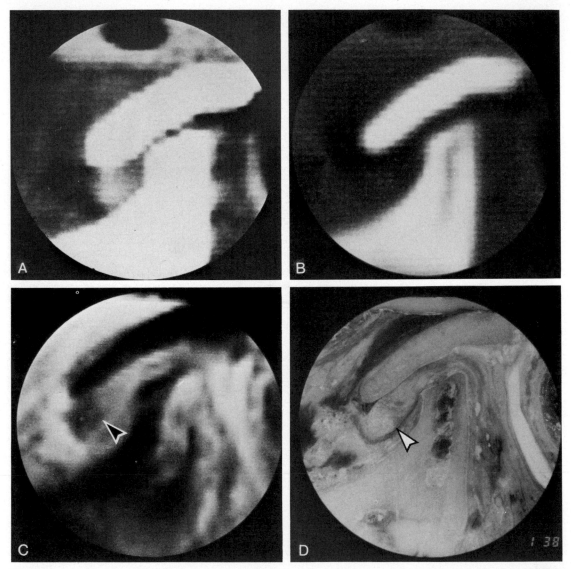

Figure 6–5
A, *Soft-tissue, and B, bone CT settings; C, MR, and D, corresponding cryosection of a TMJ with a deformed disk in the anterior position (arrowheads in C and D). A displaced disk was correctly diagnosed in both CT and MR images. The flattened tubercle and condyle were also correctly diagnosed with both methods.*

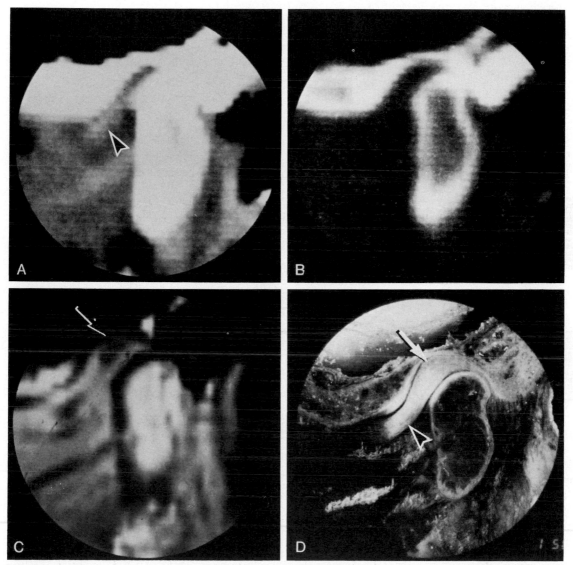

Figure 6–6
A, Soft-tissue, and B, bone CT settings; C, MR, and D, corresponding cryosection of TMJ with a biconcave disk in the superior position. High attenuation tissue inferior to the tubercle (arrowhead in A) was incorrectly interpreted as a displaced disk, resulting in a false-positive CT diagnosis. In cryosection, high attenuation tissue was the anterior band of the disk (arrowhead in D). The posterior band (arrows in C and D) was in a superior position but could not be visualized on CT, leading to a false interpretation of a displaced disk. In the MR image, the disk position was correctly diagnosed as superior.

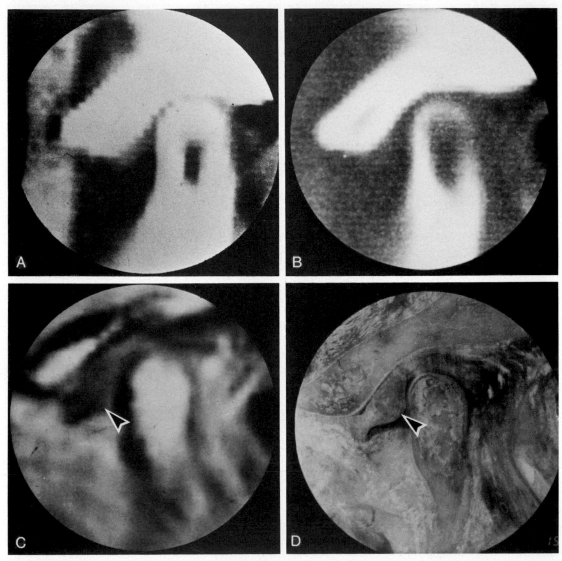

Figure 6–7
False-negative CT diagnosis. A, Soft-tissue, and B, bone CT settings; C, MR, and D, corresponding cryosection of the TMJ with anterior disk displacement. The posterior band of the disk (arrowheads in C and D) is located anterior to the condyle. This was correctly diagnosed in the MR image (C) but was not seen in the CT scans (A and B).

Value of Using CT Attenuation Numbers

Manco and colleagues studied 454 TMJ patients with direct sagittal CT and suggested that in joints with chronic displacement and long-standing symptoms the disk density was usually greater than 60 HU on the Siemens Somatom DR2, making the disk easily separable from the surrounding muscle, fat, and connective tissue structures.[11] Christiansen and colleagues reported an average CT number for the disk of 100 HU on the General Electric 9800.[12] The study by Paz and associates, also on the General Electric scanner, showed that the mean disk density values for patients with internal derangement were 104.31 HU in disk displacement without reduction, 99.99 HU in disk displacement with reduction, and 72.24 HU in symptomatic normal subjects (Table 6–2).[13] The internal derangement group had significantly higher CT attenuation values than did the symptomatic normal group.

A subsequent study that assessed CT attenuation values in cadaver specimens was correlated with the histopathologic findings. A correlation existed between extensive histologic alterations, which included foci of calcifications within the displaced disks, and the high CT attenuation numbers.[35] Lower CT attenuation numbers were noted in the cadaver specimens with normal disk position and histology.

CT numbers for the specific identification of the disk must be used with caution, since these values may differ from scanner to scanner: the relative rather than the absolute CT numbers are most important. Wide ranges in standard deviations in attenuation values of the disk, surrounding tendon, muscle, and fat have been reported.[12] Another potential difficulty in using measurements is that there is little difference in the densities of the ligamentous insertion of the superior belly of the lateral pterygoid muscle and normal articular disk (Fig. 6–6).[12] Thus, it is possible that the insertion of the lateral pterygoid muscle will be confused with the articular disk, particularly when the disk displaces anteromedially. When the disk is thinned, diagnosis with CT number highlighting alone will be even more difficult.

Comparison of CT and Magnetic Resonance (MR) for Diagnosis of TMJ Internal Derangement

A direct comparison between CT and magnetic resonance (MR) imaging for TMJ imaging was described by Westesson and associates.[7] Direct sagittal CT and sagittal MR on 15 fresh TMJ autopsy specimens were acquired and compared with the cryosectional findings in a blind fashion. No statistically significant difference was found between these procedures in detecting bony

Table 6–2
AVERAGE DISK CT DENSITY VALUES VERSUS STATUS OF THE JOINT

Status of the Joint	N	Mean (HU)	Standard Error
Normal	24	72.24	±3.34
Disk displacement with reduction	23	99.99	±5.59
Disk displacement without reduction	29	104.31	±3.98

Data from Paz ME, Katzberg RW, Tallents RH, et al: CT assessment of TMJ meniscus density in internal derangements. Oral Surg Oral Med Oral Pathol 1988;66:519–524.

abnormalities or disk position (Table 6–3). However, a side-by-side comparison of the CT and MR images demonstrated that MR depicted the soft tissue anatomy of the joint with greater detail than did CT (Figs. 6–4 through 6–7). MR clearly displayed the disk when it was positioned either superiorly or anteriorly, whereas CT showed the disk adequately only when it was positioned anteriorly. MR demonstrated the configuration of the disk and its borders, which were not adequately depicted on the CT images. MR was adequate for the evaluation of the osseous structures but did not equal the accuracy of CT.

The false-positive diagnoses by CT in the cadaver study resulted from increased attenuation of the soft tissues underneath the bony tubercle in the medial and central regions of the joint (Fig. 6–6). This is the area of attachment of the lateral pterygoid muscle, and increased density of this muscle attachment is the probable cause of the false-positive CT diagnoses, as reported by Christiansen and coworkers.[12] False-negative CT diagnoses tend to occur when there is partial anterior disk displacement and the exact margins of the disk cannot be determined with adequate precision (Fig. 6–7).

The errors that occurred by MR were the result of the inability to differentiate the disk from the joint capsule when assessed in the sagittal plane only. However, when combined sagittal and coronal planes of imaging were assessed, this error was readily recognized.[7]

The growing consensus is that MR is a superior modality for the evaluation of internal derangement of the TMJ (see Chapters 5 and 12).[1–3] CT scanning, however, is valuable when imaging of the bone structure is essential. An example is the elongated coronoid process, which could interfere with the zygomatic process of the maxilla on opening, causing limitation of opening. This is usually seen in adolescent males and can clinically be misinterpreted for disk displacement without reduction. A clear example is shown in Figure 6–8; the elongated coronoid process of the mandible is interfering with the zygomatic process of the maxilla.

Three-Dimensional CT Scanning of the TMJ

Refinements in the software capabilities of three-dimensional CT scanning have reduced processing times and increased resolution dramatically. A technique that has been useful in our assessment of the three-dimensional characteristics of TMJ abnormalities utilizes either the General Electric 8800 or 9800 scanner.[15] The patients are placed in a supine position, and axial images are obtained with the x-ray beam projecting at a 10° angle to Reid's base line. Slices of 5-mm thickness are utilized, with an overlap of 3 mm from the sella turcica to the chin. This represents an average of 45 slices and a scan time of between 5 and 25 minutes, depending on the type of scanner and the kVp, mAs, and

Table 6–3
DIAGNOSTIC ACCURACY OF CT AND MR FOR POSITION OF THE DISK

Method (N = 15)	Diagnosis				Accuracy* (%)
	True-Negative	False-Negative	True-Positive	False-Positive	
CT	4	1	6	4	67
MR	5	1	6	3	73

*Number of correct diagnoses out of all diagnosed joints.

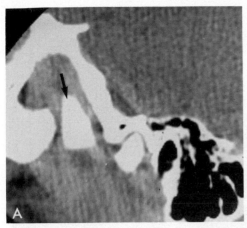 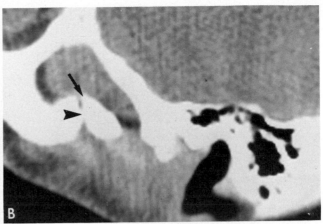

Figure 6–8
Elongated coronoid process interfering with the zygomatic process of the maxilla on maximal mouth opening. A, In the closed-mouth position, the elongated coronoid process (arrow) is clearly seen. B, On opening, the coronoid process (arrow) is interfering with the zygomatic process of the maxilla (arrowhead), restricting the maximal mouth opening.

pulse settings. If greater detail is needed, thinner slices—down to 1.5 mm—may be used. The imaging data are then transferred to an independent computer console for the purpose of generating three-dimensional reconstructions. Our software utilizes standard CT data by identifying surface areas and structures and then by rotating these data around the X, Y, and Z axes. The images are displayed on a computer screen, at which time different window and level settings are utilized to best depict the hard and soft tissue components.

Figure 6–9A through C depicts a 6-year-old boy with a craniofacial asymmetry known as hemifacial microsomia. The patient illustrated with three-dimensional CT in Figure 6–10A and B was assessed because of a facial asymmetry and limitation of mandibular opening following mandibular trauma 2 years previously. Fracture of the neck of the condyle was determined at the time of injury, and the current examination depicted the healed fracture. The spatial relationships of the condylar head, neck, and body of the mandible are well shown. These images allow a rapid assessment of the complex spatial relationships that must otherwise be mentally synthesized from numerous cross-sectional image sets.

Postsurgical assessments employing three-dimensional CT are shown in a patient with a large Silastic implant inserted into the left TMJ following diskectomy (Fig. 6–11A and B). The three-dimensional CT images confirm satisfactory relationships between the implant and the contiguous osseous anatomy. A thinner Silastic implant also can be well visualized (Fig. 6–12).

An idiopathic bony protuberance was suspected to be a loose joint body on plain films. A three-dimensional CT scan (Fig. 6–13) showed it to be external to the joint space and rising from the temporal bone.

RADIONUCLIDE SKELETAL IMAGING AND SINGLE-PHOTON EMISSION COMPUTED TOMOGRAPHY

Arthrosis of the TMJ is often associated with internal derangement related to disk dysfunction (see Chapter 2, Pathology).[28–30] Conventional radiographic imaging, such as multidirectional tomography or transcranial radiographs, can

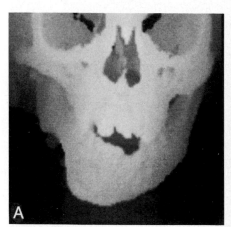

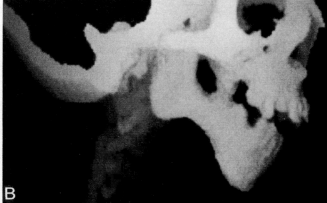

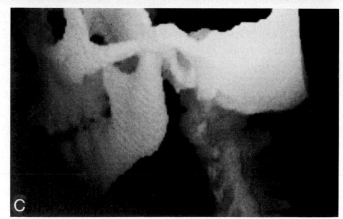

Figure 6–9

A six-year-old boy presented with craniofacial asymmetry and was evaluated with three-dimensional (3-D) CT imaging. The history revealed a deformity of the first and second branchial arches, representing a unilateral major facial deformity defined as a craniofacial microsomia. This syndrome is also known as hemifacial microsomia, lateral facial dysplasia, and oculoauriculovertebral dysplasia. A, The frontal 3-D image indicates that the affected side is considerably smaller. In the midface, on the right side the malar bone, zygomatic arch, and maxilla were involved. The deformity was also evident in the right mandible. B, The lateral 3-D image of the affected side shows absence of the external auditory canal and indicates lack of mandibular development, which includes incomplete formation of the condylar head and neck, ramus, and body and incomplete development of the zygomatic arch. C, The lateral 3-D image of the left (normal) side shows the presence of an auditory canal and a more normal development of the condylar head and neck, ramus, and body.

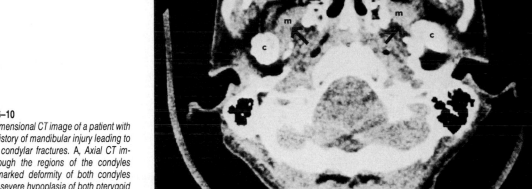

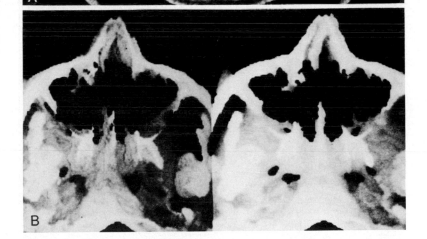

Figure 6–10
Three-dimensional CT image of a patient with a prior history of mandibular injury leading to bilateral condylar fractures. A, Axial CT image through the regions of the condyles shows marked deformity of both condyles (c), with severe hypoplasia of both pterygoid muscles (m; arrows). B, Three-dimensional CT image reconstruction in the same patient shows gross deformity of both condylar heads, with a "cauliflower" type of configuration. The 3-D image gives an excellent depiction of the spatial anatomy of the deformities.

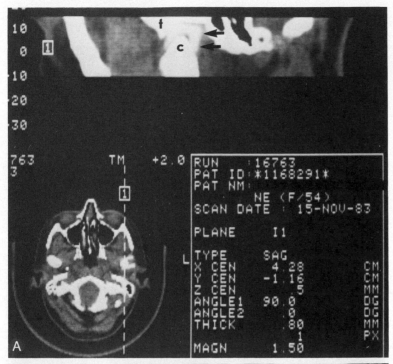

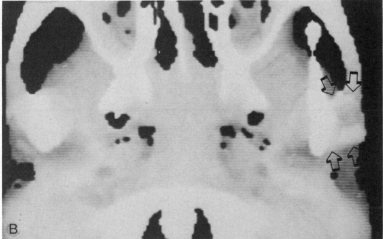

Figure 6–11
Axial CT image with parasagittal reconstruction and 3-D CT reconstruction in a postsurgical patient with a Silastic cap interposed between the condylar head and fossa. A, The Silastic cap (arrows) is noted interposed between the condylar stump (C) and temporal bone (T). B, The 3-D reconstruction allows a clearer spatial determination of the relationship of the Silastic cap (arrows) versus the condyle and fossa of the TMJ.

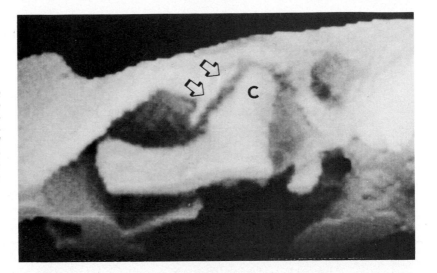

Figure 6–12
Three-dimensional CT in a patient with a Silastic disk implant postdiskectomy. The arrows demonstrate the satisfactory position of the 2-mm thick Silastic interpositional implant between the condylar head (C) and temporal bone. Confirmation of the normal anatomic relationship of the Silastic implant versus the osseous structures is well depicted by 3-D CT reconstructions.

detect osseous disease only when the subarticular cortical bone becomes severely damaged.[28] As a result, this disease process may be long-standing before it becomes evident on standard radiographs. For example, it is estimated that one must remove 40 to 50 per cent of the calcium content of a single lumbar vertebral body before decalcification will be evident radiographically.[17] On the other hand, skeletal imaging with radionuclides depicts the current activity of bone metabolism and blood flow and, in comparison, can detect as little as a 5 per cent change in bone content.

Nuclear medicine instrumentation has advanced from the fairly crude rectilinear scanner to the scintillation camera, which is more suitable for dynamic and static imaging. The latter consists of a gamma detector (crystal), 280 to 380 mm in diameter and 6 to 15 mm thick, which detects the gamma ray emissions of isotopes such as ^{99m}technetium. The image obtained on such a system is usually referred to as a "planar" or "routine" skeletal image.

Recent innovative developments have allowed the application of computed tomographic principles through radionuclide imaging by moving the detector, such as a scintillation camera, about the patient. This allows a tomographic "slice" ranging in thickness from the 2 to 16 mm to be obtained through an

Figure 6–13
Three-dimensional CT reconstruction in a patient with an idiopathic bony protuberance noted on a Panorex radiograph. It was unclear whether this bony protuberance represented an abnormality attached to the temporal bone or a loose joint body within the joint space. The 3-D CT scan showed this mass (arrows) to be a protuberance from the temporal bone rather than an intra-articular abnormality. The coronoid process is shown anterior and inferior to the bony protuberance, which was anterior to the fossa.

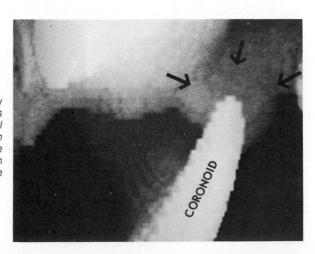

organ system. Organ systems may be studied in multiple planes, mainly transverse (axial), coronal, and sagittal.[18, 19] This has resulted in improved spatial resolution of structures, since over- and underlying soft tissues and bones are in effect removed and only features lying in the plane of interest are seen in the image, such as a transverse or coronal scan that separates the TMJ from the remainder of the skull. This type of imaging system is referred to as single-photon emission computed tomography (SPECT).

Methodology

The most widely used radiopharmaceutical agent for bone scintigraphy is one of the ^{99m}Tc-labeled phosphate complexes. On the morning of the imaging procedure, the patient is given an intravenous injection of 15 to 20 mCi (555 to 740 MBq) of ^{99m}Tc-MDP (^{99m}technetium methylene diphosphonate) (Table 6–4). The patient is then studied with a "three-phase" technique: (1) a 30-second perfusion study in which analog images are obtained every 3 seconds, with computed analysis of perfusion; (2) immediate soft tissue views of the head and anterior and both lateral projections with the mouth open and closed; and (3) delayed views of the TMJ in anterior, posterior, and both lateral projections with the mouth open and closed.[18, 19] The delayed views include planar nuclear medicine images and single-photon emission computed tomography images (Fig. 6–14A through D).

Improved spatial resolution is possible through the use of SPECT. Multiple images are obtained at different angles by rotating the detector around the subject. The gamma camera with a high-resolution collimator is used to obtain 64 projections over 360° of rotation, with each image acquired for 20 seconds per projection in a 64 × 64 matrix. Data processing, including uniformity correction, smoothing, and reconstruction by filtered-back projection, is used to produce images representing slices of 2 mm or more in thickness. The information is reconstructed in different planes, usually sagittal, coronal, and transaxial (Fig. 6–14C). Additional planes at different angles may be obtained through the use of different computer reconstruction programs.

The localization of the radiopharmaceutical agent at sites of bone pathology depends on blood flow, bone remodeling, capillary or membrane permeability, and other physical-chemical mechanisms and physiologic modifying influences beyond the scope of this discussion. Blood flow transports the radiopharmaceutical agent to the surface of the apatite crystal in the affected area. Increased microscopic blood flow is a normal response to disease or trauma and serves to increase the amount of nutrient materials provided to the bone surface undergoing repair. Increased osteoblastic activity is also a reparative process of bone in response to injury of any kind. The increased osteoblastic activity results in an increased deposition of the radiopharmaceutical agent through

Table 6–4
RADIONUCLIDE IMAGING OF THE TEMPOROMANDIBULAR JOINT

Radiopharmaceutical	^{99m}Tc-labeled phosphate complex
Dose	15–20 mCi
"Three-phase" imaging	
Perfusion images (0–30 sec)	Images every 3 sec × 30 sec
Immediate (at 30 sec)	Images of both temporomandibular joints with jaw open and closed
Delayed (at 2–3 hr) (planar and SPECT)	Images of both temporomandibular joints with jaw open and closed

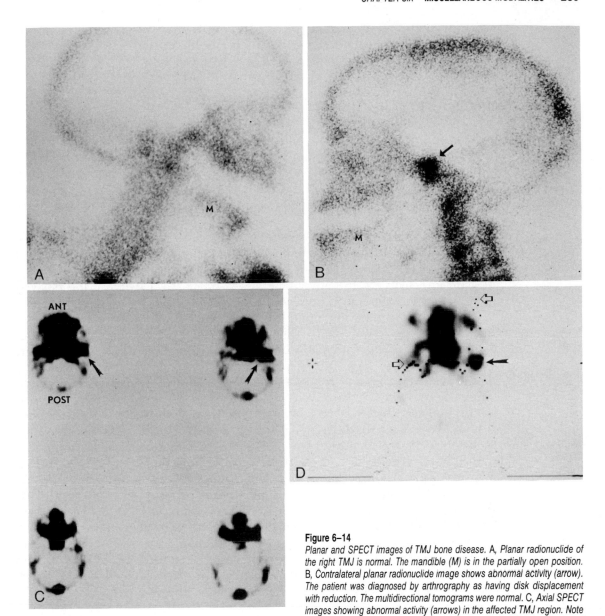

Figure 6–14
Planar and SPECT images of TMJ bone disease. A, Planar radionuclide of the right TMJ is normal. The mandible (M) is in the partially open position. B, Contralateral planar radionuclide image shows abnormal activity (arrow). The patient was diagnosed by arthrography as having disk displacement with reduction. The multidirectional tomograms were normal. C, Axial SPECT images showing abnormal activity (arrows) in the affected TMJ region. Note that the medial aspect of the joint can be imaged here but not in the planar scan. D, Count-rate profile illustrating abnormal ^{99m}Tc-MDP localization of the right TMJ superimposed on a transaxial SPECT scan. An abnormal condyle is demonstrated by a solid arrow, and the count rate profile of the right and left TMJs is indicated by open arrows.

the affected area in comparison with the nearby or contralateral normal osseous tissues.[17]

The perfusion of the TMJ may be evaluated by observing the arrival of radionuclide activity at the TMJ. This is established by imaging the patient from the anterior projection and obtaining serial images at 1- to 3-second intervals following intravenous injection of the phosphate complex. The perfusion will be increased to areas where there is inflammation or extensive osteoblastic activity. Regions of interest can be created and histograms generated (Fig. 6–14D) that plot the amount of activity in an area and allow comparison with other osseous areas. Immediate views are then obtained from the anterior and in the right and left lateral projections for evaluation of blood pool activity, which is useful in evaluating soft tissue involvement. We have found the perfusion and immediate image not to be useful in the evaluation of TMJ disease but helpful in defining other causes of facial pain.[19]

Interpretation of Radionuclide Images

In the normal subject, the perfusion is symmetric in the TMJ regions. On the immediate images there should be no evidence of increased radionuclide activity in the area of the TMJ. Delayed images demonstrate a similar amount of activity in the region of the TMJ and in the area of the base of the skull; the latter is used as a reference point. Tomographic studies should demonstrate no asymmetry in any projection.

Abnormal activity in the flow studies in the TMJ is seen in patients whose disease has an inflammatory component and reflects increased perfusion and hyperemia in the joint.[18] These patients usually will also have an abnormal increase in activity on the immediate views. Increased activity on the delayed views may vary from mildly increased to markedly increased.

In a study comparing multidirectional tomography, arthrography, and SPECT, a higher sensitivty of radionuclide imaging was demonstrated.[18] From a study of 51 patients with complaints of facial pain, 27 TMJs were diagnosed by arthrography to have disk displacement with reduction.[19] Multidirectional tomograms were positive for osseous changes in five (18 per cent) of these joints, whereas SPECT scans were positive in nine (70 per cent) affected joints. Twenty subjects (20 TMJs) had an arthrographic diagnosis of disk displacement without reduction. Multidirectional tomograms of the 20 joints were positive for osseous changes in 14 (70 per cent) joints, and SPECT scans were positive in 16 (80 per cent) joints. Five (56 per cent) of nine subjects who had normal arthrograms and normal tomograms had positive SPECT scans.

Collier's group studied a total of 23 adult patients with unilateral TMJ symptoms and 13 patients with bilateral TMJ symptoms.[18] The sensitivity of SPECT imaging for disk displacement was reported to be 94 per cent, which was similar to that of TMJ arthrography, which had a sensitivity of 96 per cent in their series. Planar radionuclide imaging demonstrated a 76 per cent sensitivity compared with the perfusion phase of the radionuclide scan, which had a 35 per cent sensitivity. Conventional radiography had a sensitivity of 4 per cent.

Positive radionuclide scans observed in symptomatic patients with both normal multidirectional tomograms and normal arthrograms or magnetic resonance images are not readily explainable.[19] It is possible that these patients, though not suffering from internal derangement, may be suffering from an inflammatory arthrosis of the joint capsule not detectable by any other imaging modality. This theory awaits further study.

The false-negative radionuclide images can occur because of symmetrically abnormal TMJs, or in the setting of long-standing internal derangement. In the latter condition, the disease process may be in a "burned-out" stage, as the plain films would be positive but the bone scans negative.

The differential diagnosis of TMJ pain and dysfunction is not always easy to analyze on clinical findings alone. Many different diseases can produce pain in and around the TMJ region that are not related to internal derangement (Fig. 6–15). Among these causes are sinusitis, fractures, osteomyelitis, dental problems, and cervical spine disease. Fortunately, these diseases have a rather

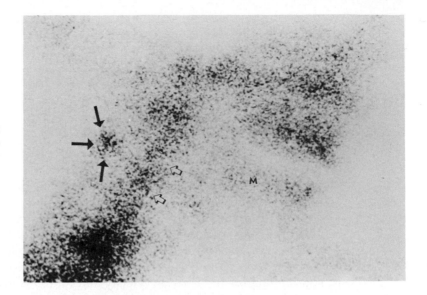

Figure 6–15
Planar radionuclide image of the right facial and neck region demonstrating degenerative disease of the posterior articulating facets (arrows) of the cervical spine (open arrows). M, Mandible.

typical appearance on either planar or SPECT bone scintigraphy. Thus, bone scintigraphy has an important potential as a screening modality.

ANALYSIS OF TEMPOROMANDIBULAR JOINT SOUND

TMJ sounds are the most frequent findings in both epidemiologic[36–39] and clinical investigations of patients with TMJ disorders.[40–42] Thus, clicking has been found to occur in as much as 44 per cent of the populations examined. Clicking has been ascribed to a variety of mechanisms, such as disk displacement, condylar subluxation, deviations in form of the articular surfaces, loose bodies, bands or adhesions in the joint space, and a vacuum phenomenon (Table 6–5) (see also Chapters 2 and 4).[1, 21–23, 43–47]

Crepitation is defined as a continuous grinding or scraping sound. The incidence of crepitation in the medical literature varies between 10 and 24 per cent.[37–39, 48] Crepitation has been considered to indicate structural damage to the articular surfaces or more specifically a sign of arthritis. However, it actually may disappear during the course of degenerative disease. Crepitation is not always a reliable sign of arthrosis.

Clicking is defined as a distinct cracking or snapping sound. "Reciprocal click" is one that occurs during mandibular retrusion and also again during mandibular opening.[49–52] The opening and closing clicks do not occur at the

Table 6–5
INTRA-ARTICULAR CHANGES ASSOCIATED WITH TEMPOROMANDIBULAR JOINT CLICKING

Common	Disk displacement with reduction
	Jaw subluxation, eminence impediment
	Deviation in the form of the articulating surfaces
Uncommon	Disk displacement without reduction
	Adhesions
	Loose joint bodies
	Vacuum phenomenon

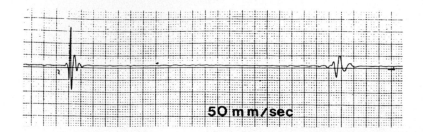

Figure 6–16

A strip chart recording in a patient with a reciprocal opening and closing click as diagnosed arthrographically. The opening click (left) generally contains higher frequency components or oscillations than the closing click. Arthrography showed anterior disk displacement with reduction.

same point on the condylar path. Single clicking implies clicking during opening only or closing only.

Clicking may be associated with pain and limitation of jaw opening and is an important accompanying sign of internal derangement.[1–3, 40, 49–52] Clicking during opening has been classified with respect to its occurrence during the early, intermediate, or late stage of jaw movement.[1] It is associated with a sudden change in condylar velocity and an inferiorly directed deflection in the condylar path.[1, 44–52] The clicking sound has been shown to be caused by the condyle hitting the disk and temporal components of the skull after having passed rapidly under the posterior band of the disk.[45, 46]

Analysis of TMJ Acoustical Patterns

The term *sonography* has been coined to describe the technique of recording and interpreting joint sounds.[20, 23, 53] A number of investigators have used sonography to study the diverse sounds emitted from the TMJ in patients with facial pain and masticatory dysfunction. Recording TMJ sounds was first discussed by Ekensten in 1952.[54] Ouellette, using a cassette recording and an audiofrequency analyzer, suggested a classification of four joint sound groups: (1) low frequency; (2) low and high frequency; (3) irregular bursts of sound energy in high or low frequency; and (4) joints with a relative absence of sound energy.[55] Watt used a recorder and stereo stethoscope to record and study the sounds of 110 patients.[53] He proposed a classification of joint sounds with attention to the nature, quality, and timing of these sounds.

Oster and group analyzed sound patterns in 67 patients by using a standard condenser microphone, ¾-inch videotape recorder, and stethoscope.[21] Patients with arthrographically demonstrated disk displacement with reduction had higher frequency acoustical oscillations associated with the opening click than with the closing click (Fig. 6–16). Patients with disk displacement without reduction, on the other hand, were shown to have multiple opening and closing low-amplitude vibrations (Fig. 6–17). The investigators also described an acous-

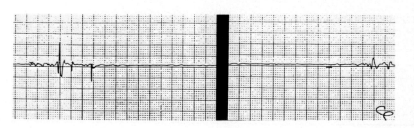

Figure 6–17

A strip chart recording in a patient with degenerative joint disease. Note the sharp peak in amplitude during the opening phase, which, although to some extent similar to the high-amplitude sound recording of Figure 6–16, is associated with multiple additional vibrations of low amplitude and high frequency. The closing phase of the sound recording (right) manifests low-amplitude vibrations.

tical pattern resulting from the "eminence click" associated with a low-amplitude oscillation during maintenance of an apparently normal condyle-disk-fossa relationship but with incoordination of the condyle and bony eminence.

In a continuation of the work of Oster and coworkers,[21] Hutta and associates[47] and Heffez and Blaustein[23] adapted a digital DSP-200 stethoscope (International Acoustics, Incorporated, Palatine, Illinois) for the purpose of auscultation and recording of TMJ sounds. This instrument contains a microprocessor, an A/D converter, and an internal memory sufficient to hold approximately 20,000 data points, which corresponds to 10 seconds of data collection time. Digital data are transferred into a computer (Compaq Disk Pro) equipped with a software package (International Acoustics) designed to present graphically the recorded sound wave forms. In addition to displaying the time-domain wave forms (amplitude versus time), this software can display a power spectrum analysis of selected portions of the time-domain wave forms (Fig. 6–18A and B). This analysis provides the capability to examine quantitatively the distribution of sound energy as a function of sound frequency. The resulting power spectra can then be used to compare TMJ sounds quantitatively between patients and between disorders.

The quantitative comparison of the sound-power spectra is facilitated by defining specific parameters associated with each power-spectrum wave form.[47] The power spectra can be subdivided into low-frequency (0 to 300 Hz) and high-frequency (301 to 600 Hz) ranges, with computations of the relative amounts of sound energy present in each particular range, along with ratios of high-frequency to low-frequency energy. The frequency at which the highest energy level occurs is defined as the "peak frequency."

The power-spectrum wave forms for gross differences in the degree of smoothness and number of energy peaks present also were found useful in the analysis. Sound emitted from patients with disk displacement without reduction have nearly fourfold more energy above a frequency of 300 Hz than either the symptomatic normal or disk displacement with reduction patients. The ratio of the frequency bands (less than 300 Hz:more than 300 Hz) in the patients who had disk displacement without reduction was significantly greater than in the patients who were symptomatic normal or had disk displacement with reduction. The frequency at which the highest energy level was obtained (peak frequency) had a numerical progression from symptomatic normal patients (48 Hz), disk displacement with reduction patients (112 Hz), and disk displacement without reduction groups (205 Hz). The results suggest that the peak acoustical frequency increases with the progression of TMJ intracapsular disease.[47]

When a qualitative rating scale of the power-spectrum wave forms was devised, the power spectra showed that 71 per cent of the disk displacement with reduction acoustical patterns could be classified as "smooth," compared with 10 per cent of the symptomatic normal and 5 per cent of the disk displacement without reduction acoustical patterns. The number of energy peaks present in the power spectra indicated that the disk displacement with reduction sounds had predominantly one energy peak, whereas the symptomatic normal and disk displacement without reduction sounds consistently had greater than one energy peak.

Heffez and Blaustein defined four wave patterns (Fig. 6–19): (1) crescendo-decrescendo, (2) crescendo, (3) coarse continuous, and (4) fine continuous.[23] These workers found that the most common combination of joint sounds emitted was an opening crescendo-decrescendo and closing crescendo or coarse continuous pattern. There was no consistent wave pattern in the symptom-free

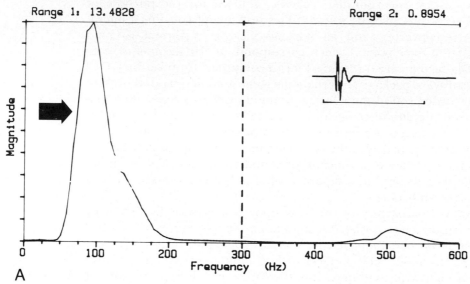

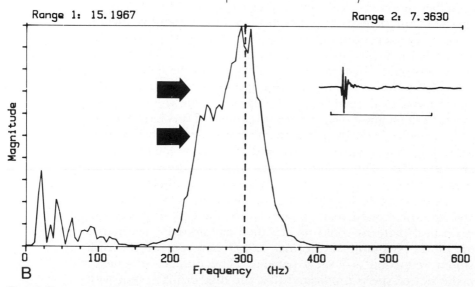

Figure 6–18
Sonographic evaluation of TMJ internal derangement. A, Sound power spectrum analysis of disk displacement with reduction, and B, of disk displacement without reduction associated with crepitation. The salient feature is a shift to the right of the power spectrum in B (arrows) compared with A (single arrow). Plots depict the magnitude versus frequency in Hertz (Hz), and a window insert in the top righthand corner displays a time-domain wave formed for the opening sounds, showing amplitude versus time. The range 1 value of 13.4828 is the amount of energy below the number of 300 Hz. The range 2 value of 0.8954 is the amount of energy above 300 Hz. In each power spectrum plot, the largest magnitude is always normalized to 1, which is located at the top of the magnitude scale.

Figure 6–19
Four wave patterns have been described and are depicted here. 1, Crescendo-decrescendo; 2, crescendo; 3, coarse continuous; and 4, fine continuous. The most common combination of joint sounds emitted was an opening crescendo-decrescendo and closing crescendo or coarse continuous pattern. (From Heffez L, Blaustein D: Advances in sonography of the temporomandibular joint. Oral Surg Oral Med Oral Pathol 1986;62:486–495.)

1.	CRESCENDO - DECRESCENDO	
2.	CRESCENDO	
3.	COARSE CONTINUOUS	
4.	FINE CONTINUOUS	

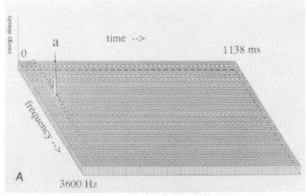

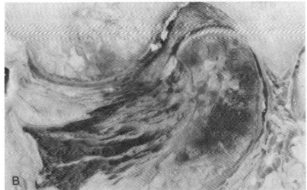

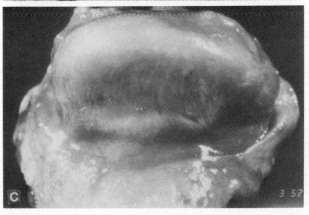

Figure 6–20
A, Joint sound recording; B, sagittal cryosection; and C, superior view of normal joint without joint sound. The peak indicated by the letter a in A is a control sound.

patients manifesting joint sounds. Heffez and Blaustein found that power-spectral analysis of the frequency of sounds emitted provided important information that ultimately might provide "acoustical signatures" for specific disease states confirmed clinically and radiographically.[23]

Widmalm and associates recorded joint sounds from anatomic specimens and correlated findings to joint morphology at dissection.[56] They showed that joint sounds indicated joint abnormality, but the absence of joint sound did not exclude intra-articular pathosis. They also showed that a higher frequency of the joint sound was associated with more advanced disease. Examples with time-frequency distribution of recordings from a normal joint without joint sound are shown in Figure 6–20. A joint with clicking is shown in Figure 6–21, and a joint with crepitation in Figure 6–22.

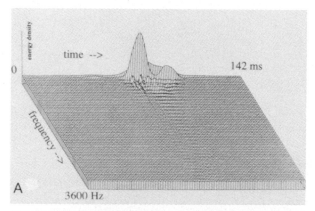

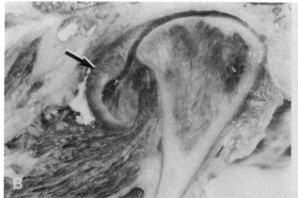

Figure 6–21
Clicking in a joint with medial disk displacement and perforation. A, Time frequency distribution of sound. B, The disk (arrow) is medially displaced. C, There is a perforation of the disk and posterior attachment in the lateral aspect of the joint (arrows). (From Widmalm SE, Westesson PL, Brooks SL, et al: Temporomandibular joint sounds: Correlation to joint structure in fresh autopsy specimens. Am J Orthod Dentofac Orthop 1992;101:60–69.)

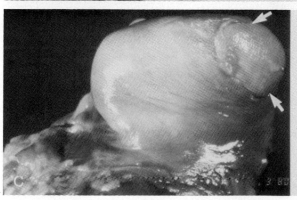

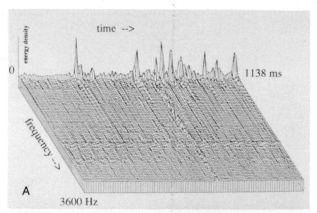

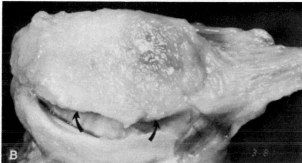

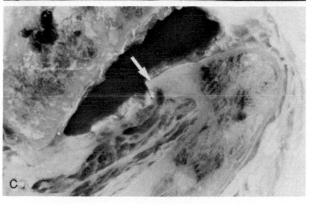

Figure 6–22
Joint with crepitation and advanced arthrosis. A, Time frequency distribution shows multiple energy peaks during recording. B, The superior surface of the condyle shows irregularity and a large perforation of the disk. On the anterior edge of the condyle is an osteophyte (arrows). C, Sagittal cryosection demonstrates the advanced osseous and soft-tissue changes, with irregularities of the joint surfaces and a large anterior osteophyte (arrow) of the condyle. (From Widmalm SE, Westesson PI, Brooks SL, et al: Temporomandibular joint sounds: Correlation to joint structure in fresh autopsy specimens. Am J Orthod Dentofac Orthop 1992;101:60–69.)

Sound power-spectrum analysis as a screening modality to differentiate patients with TMJ internal derangement could contribute significantly to the clinician's decision to treat or to request additional diagnostic studies. Determination of the degree of specificity must be clearly established for this modality for it to be accepted. We await future advances in this potentially exciting discipline of TMJ diagnosis.

References

1. Katzberg RW: Temporomandibular joint imaging. Radiology 1989;*170*:297–307.
2. Kaplan PA, Helms CA: Current status of temporomandibular joint imaging for the diagnosis of internal derangements. AJR 1989;*152*:697–705.
3. Helms CA, Kaplan P: Diagnostic imaging of the temporomandibular joint: Recommendations for use of the various techniques. AJR 1990;*154*:319–322.
4. Manzione JV, Katzberg RW, Brodsky GL, Seltzer SE, Mellins HZ: Internal derangement of

the temporomandibular joint: Diagnosis by direct sagittal computed tomography. Radiology 1984;*150*:111–115.

5. Hüls A, Schulte W, Voigt K, Ehrlich-Treuenstätt V: Computed tomography of the temporomandibular joint; New diagnostic possibilities and initial clinical results. Electromedica 1983;*51*:14–19.

6. Christiansen EL, Thompson JR, Kopp S, Hasso AW, Hinshaw DB Jr: Radiographic signs of temporomandibular joint disease: An investigation utilizing x-ray computed tomography. Dentomaxillofac Radiol 1985;*14*:83–92.

7. Westesson P-L, Katzberg RW, Tallents RH, Sanchez-Woodworth RE, Svensson SA: CT and MRI of the temporomandibular joint: Comparison with autopsy specimens. AJR 1987;*148*:1165–1171.

8. Helms CA, Morrish RB, Kircos LT, Katzberg RW, Dolwick MF: Computed tomography of the meniscus of the temporomandibular joint: Preliminary observations. Radiology 1982;*145*:719–722.

9. Helms CA, Katzberg RW, Morrish R, Dolwick MF: Computed tomography of the temporomandibular joint meniscus. J Oral Maxillofac Surg 1983;*41*:512–517.

10. Helms CA, Vogler JB III, Morrish RB Jr: Diagnosis by computed tomography of temporomandibular joint meniscus displacement. J Prosthet Dent 1984;*51*:544–547.

11. Manco LG, Messing SG, Busino LJ, Fasulo CP, Sordill WC: Internal derangements of the temporomandibular joint evaluated with direct sagittal CT: A prospective study. Radiology 1985;*157*:407–412.

12. Christiansen EL, Thompson JR, Hasso AN, Hindshaw DB Jr, Moore RJ, Roberts D, Kopp S: CT number characteristics of malpositioned TMJ menisci: Diagnosis with CT number highlighting (blinkmode). Invest Radiol 1987;*22*:315–321.

13. Paz ME, Katzberg RW, Tallents RH, et al: CT assessment of TMJ meniscus density in internal derangements. Oral Surg Oral Med Oral Pathol 1988;*66*:519–524.

14. Hemmy DC, Tessier PL: CT of dry skulls with craniofacial deformities: Accuracy of three-dimensional reconstructions. Radiology 1985;*157*:113.

15. Silviera AM, Sommers EW, Katzberg RW, et al: Three-dimensional computerized tomographic scanning of craniofacial anomalies. J Craniomandib Pract 1988;*6*:217–223.

16. DeMarino DP, Steiner E, Poster RB, Katzberg RW, Hengerer AS, et al: Three-dimensional computerized tomography in maxillofacial trauma. Arch Otolaryngol Head Neck Surg 1986;*112*:146–150.

17. O'Mara RE, Charles ND: The osseous system. *In* Freeman LM, Johnson PM, eds: Clinical Scintillation Scanning. 2nd ed. New York, Grune and Stratton, 1975, pp 573–599.

18. Collier DB, Carrera GF, Messer EJ, Ryan DE, Gingrass D, Angell D, Palmer DW, Isitman AT, Hellman RS: Internal derangement of the temporomandibular joint: Detection by single-photon emission computed tomography. Radiology 1983;*149*:557–561.

19. Katzberg RW, O'Mara RE, Tallents RH, Weber DA: Radionuclide imaging and single photon emission computed tomography in suspected internal derangement of the temporomandibular joint. J Oral Maxillofac Surg 1984;*42*:782–787.

20. Watt DM: Temporomandibular joint sounds. J Dent 1980;*8*:119–127.

21. Oster C, Katzberg RW, Tallents RH, Morris TW, Bartholomew J, Miller TL, Hayakawa K: Characterization of temporomandibular joint sounds. A preliminary investigation with arthrographic correlation. Oral Surg 1984;*58*:10–16.

22. Eriksson L, Rohlin M, Westesson P-L: The correlation of temporomandibular joint sounds with joint morphology in fifty-five autopsy specimens. J Oral Maxillofac Surg 1985;*43*:194–200.

23. Heffez L, Blaustein D: Advances in sonography of the temporomandibular joint. Oral Surg Oral Med Oral Pathol 1986;*62*:486–495.

24. Thompson JR, Christiansen E, Sauser D, Hasso AN, Hindshaw DB Jr: Dislocation of the temporomandibular joint meniscus: Contrast arthrography vs. computed tomography. AJNR 1984;*5*:747–750.

25. Manzione JV, Seltzer SE, Katzberg RW, Hammerschlag SB, Chiango BF: Direct sagittal computed tomography of the temporomandibular joint. AJNR 1982;*3*:677–679.

26. Manzione JV, Katzberg RW, Manzione T: Internal derangements of the temporomandibular joint. I. Normal anatomy, physiology, and pathophysiology. Int J Periodont Restorative Dent 1984;*4*:9–16.

27. Christiansen EL, Thompson JR, Hasso AN, Hindshaw DB: Correlative thin section temporomandibular joint anatomy and computed tomography. RadioGraphics 1986;*6*:703–723.

28. Katzberg RW, Keith DA, Guralnick WC, Manzione JV, Ten Eick WR: Internal derangement and arthritis of the temporomandibular joint. Radiology 1983;*146*:107–112.

29. Westesson P-L, Rohlin M: Internal derangement related to osteoarthrosis in temporomandibular joint autopsy specimens. Oral Surg 1984;*57*:17–22.

30. Westesson P-L: Structural hard-tissue changes in temporomandibular joints with internal derangement. Oral Surg 1985;*59*:220–224.

31. MacAlister AD: A microscopic survey of the human temporomandibular joint. NZ Dent J 1954;*50*:161–172.

32. Bessette RW, Katzberg RW, Natiella JR, Rose MJ: Diagnosis and reconstruction of the human

temporomandibular joint after trauma or internal derangement. Plast Reconstr Surg 1985;75:192–203.

33. Bradley J, Lang H, Ledley R: Evaluation of calcium concentration in bones from CT scans. Radiology 1978;128:103–107.

34. Siegelman SS, Zerhouri EA, Leo FP, Nickolog EL, et al: CT of the solitary pulmonary nodule. In Donner MW, Herck FHW, eds: Radiology Today. Berlin, Springer-Verlag, 1981, pp 113–120.

35. Paz ME, Hartman L, Tallents RH, et al: Am J Orthod Dentofacial Orthop 1990;98:354–357.

36. Hansson T, Öberg T: En klinisk-bettfysiologisk undersökning av 67-åringar i Dalby. Tandläkartidningen 1971;63:650–655.

37. Helkimo M: Studies on function and dysfunction of the masticatory system. Thesis, University of Gothenburg, Sweden, 1974.

38. Hansson T, Nilner M: A study of the occurrence of symptoms of diseases of the temporomandibular joint musculature system and related structures. J Oral Rehabil 1975;2:313–324.

39. Solberg WK, Woo MW, Houston JB: Prevalence of mandibular dysfunction in young adults. J Am Dent Assoc 1979;98:25–34.

40. Ireland VE: The problem of "the clicking jaw." Proc R Soc Med 1951;44:363–372.

41. Boering G: Arthrosis deformans van het kaakegewricht. Thesis, Rijksuniversiteit te Groningen, 1966.

42. Laskin DM: Etiology of the pain-dysfunction syndrome. J Am Dent Assoc 1969;79:147–153.

43. Unsworth A, Dowson D, Wright V: "Cracking joints." A bioengineering study of cavitation in metacarpophalangeal joint. Ann Rheum Dis 1971;30:348–358.

44. Nanthaviroj S, Omnell K-A, Randow K, Öberg T: Clicking and temporary "locking" in the temporomandibular joint. A clinical, radiographical and electromyographical study. Dentomaxillofac Radiol 1976;5:33–38.

45. Isberg-Holm AM, Westesson P-L: Movement of disc and condyle in temporomandibular joints with and without clicking. A high-speed cinematographic and dissection study on autopsy specimens. Acta Odontol Scand 1982;40:167–179.

46. Isberg-Holm AM, Westesson P-L: Movement of disc and condyle in temporomandibular joints with clicking. An arthrographic and cineradiographic study on autopsy specimens. Acta Odontol Scand 1982;40:153–166.

47. Hutta JL, Morris TW, Katzberg RW, Tallents RH, Espeland MA: Separation of internal derangements of the temporomandibular joint using sound analysis. Oral Surg Oral Med Oral Pathol 1987;63:151–157.

48. Lysell L, Hansson T: Käkleder och käkledsmuskler (temporomandibular joints and masticatory muscles). In Lysell L, ed: Epidemiologic roentgendiagnostic study on teeth, jaws and temporomandibular joints in 67-year-old people in Dalby, Sweden. Thesis, University of Lund, Sweden, 1977.

49. Farrar WB: Diagnosis and treatment of anterior dislocation of the articular disc. NY J Dent 1971;41:348–351.

50. Farrar WB: Differentiation of temporomandibular joint dysfunction to simplify treatment. J Prosthet Dent 1972;28:629–636.

51. Farrar WB: Characteristics of the condylar path in internal derangements of the TMJ. J Prosthet Dent 1978;39:319–323.

52. Farrar WB, McCarty WL Jr: Inferior joint space arthrography and characteristics of condylar paths in internal derangements of the TMJ. J Prosthet Dent 1979;41:548–555.

53. Watt DM: Clinical applications of gnathosonics. J Prosthet Dent 1966;16:83–95.

54. Ekensten B: Phonograms of anomalies of the temporomandibular joint in motion. Odontol Tidskr 1952;60:235–242.

55. Ouellette PL: Temporomandibular joint sound prints: Electronic auscultation and sonographic and audiospectral analysis of the temporomandibular joint. J Am Dent Assoc 1974;89:623.

56. Widmalm SE, Westesson P-L, Brooks SL, et al: Temporomandibular joint sounds: Correlation to joint structure in fresh autopsy specimens. Am J Orthod Dentofac Orthop 1992;101:60–69.

Post-Treatmer

INDICATIONS FOR IMAGING AFTER TREATMENT

The primary goal of treatment of temporomandibular joint (TMJ) disorders is to eliminate pain and dysfunction. Secondary goals are to restore normal anatomy and prevent progression of disease. There is, however, no convincing documentation to confirm that treatment actually can prevent progression of disease. Preventive treatment is therefore not recommended. The majority of TMJ treatments are successful, so a clinical need for imaging after treatment is infrequent. If patients do not experience pain or dysfunction after treatment, in our opinion there is no need for post-treatment imaging unless it is for documentation of follow-up. If the results of treatment are going to be used in a systematic comparison with other treatment methods, imaging is mandatory.

The average success rate for conservative or nonsurgical treatment is estimated at around 80 per cent. The long-term success rate for surgical treatment with diskectomy has been reported at between 65 and 85 per cent.[1–6] Disk repositioning operation has been reported to have a success rate between 63 and 93 per cent.[7–10] The success with different forms of alloplastic implants was initially good,[11–13] but the long-term results are poor, and eventually all alloplastic disk replacement implants have to be removed.[14, 15]

Occasionally surgical and nonsurgical treatments do not result in symptom-free patients; in these patients, postoperative imaging can contribute significantly to treatment planning because of its accurate capability of evaluating the morphology of the joint and its surrounding structures. Patients who experience pain after treatment are puzzling, and it is frequently difficult with physical examination alone to determine the cause of residual or recurrent pain. One important question is whether the pain is caused by abnormalities within the joint or whether the muscles of mastication are the source of the post-treatment pain.

This chapter will review imaging after different forms of nonsurgical and surgical treatment and analyze findings relative to patient symptomatology. A basis for interpretation of postoperative imaging in the clinical situation will be presented.

PROTRUSIVE SPLINT THERAPY

Therapeutic Position

The principal idea of protrusive splint therapy is to reposition the mandible anteriorly and inferiorly so that a normal relationship between the disk and the condyle is established and maintained during jaw function (Fig. 7–1).[16–18] The mandibular position where the condyle-disk relationship is normal has been termed the therapeutic position.[19] In the early era of protrusive splint therapy, the therapeutic position was often established on clinical grounds. Thus, the patient was asked to open the jaw widely to reduce the displaced disk and then close in an anterior position. This position was such that the disk was not displaced. Then the patient was asked to slowly slide the teeth posteriorly and stop just before the closing click occurred. If the patient could open from this position without clicking or irregularity, it was thought that the disk was recaptured. This position was then used as the therapeutic position for the protrusive splint. The intention was to establish the therapeutic position as close as possible before the closing click.

Later studies found that this was not an optimal way of establishing the therapeutic position.[20] Thus an arthrogram study of patients in whom the therapeutic position was established clinically showed that only around 50 per cent had a normal condyle-disk relationship in the therapeutic position using clinical techniques alone.[20, 21] There are at least two reasons why the clinical method of establishing the therapeutic position did not work. First, arthrographic experience has later shown that the disk starts to displace anteriorly before the closing click appears. Thus a therapeutic position that is established close to the point where a closing click occurs may not represent a normal condyle-disk relationship even though clicking does not occur. Second, arthrographic studies of patients with reciprocal clicking have shown that 15 per cent of them actually have disk displacement without reduction.[22] This means that in spite of reciprocal clicking the diagnosis may be disk displacement without reduction.

Arthrographic studies after splint therapy are good examples of how imaging in association with treatment can be a powerful tool to understanding how treatment works. Failure to establish normal anatomy because of inaccurate mandibular registration technique could be one factor that influenced the relatively poor prognosis that has been reported by some investigators for protrusive splint therapy over the long term.[23] Based on these early observations,

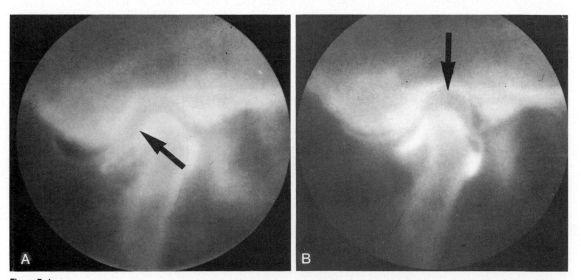

Figure 7–1
Therapeutic position. A, Dual-space double-contrast arthrotomogram at closed-mouth position, showing the anterior band of the disk (arrow) anterior to the condyle. B, After repositioning, the posterior band of the disk (arrow) is now in a normal relationship to the condyle.

it was suggested that the therapeutic position could be more accurately established with the aid of fluoroscopic arthrography.[20, 24, 25] It has been our clinical experience that the frequency of failure with protrusive splint therapy can be reduced significantly if the anatomy can be visualized with arthrography when the therapeutic position is established.[26] An example of anterior disk displacement with reduction and establishment of the therapeutic position with arthrographic control is shown in Figure 7–2. From a practical point of view, single-contrast arthrography is the standard method for establishing the therapeutic position. Magnetic resonance (MR) imaging, however, also can be used. With

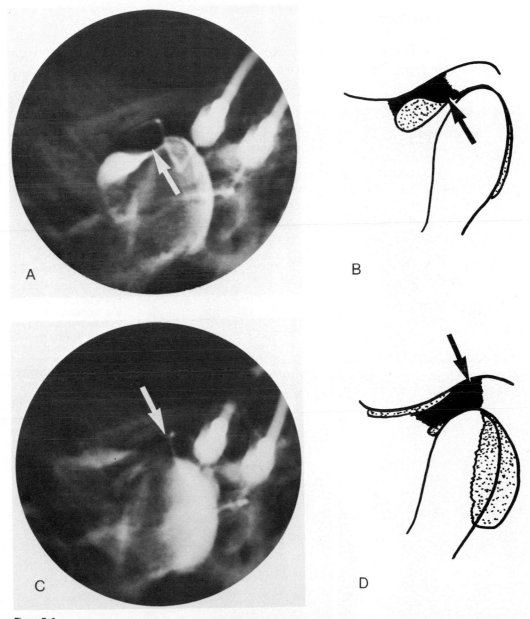

Figure 7–2
Disk repositioning with arthrographic guidance. A, Lower space single-contrast arthrogram and schematic drawing (B) showing the posterior band of the disk (arrow) anterior to the condyle. C, Lower and upper space single-contrast arthrogram and schematic drawing (D) after disk recapture. The disk is located with its posterior band (arrow) over the condyle.

this technique we produced a wax index that the patient takes into the scanner to put into the mouth when closing after opening wide. MR imaging is then used to confirm and possibly correct the therapeutic position. An example of how MR imaging was used to evaluate a therapeutic position is shown in Figure 7–3. The joint in Figure 7–3 shows anterior disk displacement with reduction, but there is also a medial component to the displacement. In the therapeutic position the anterior displacement is eliminated (Fig. 7–3*B*), but the medial displacement remains to a certain extent and makes the prognosis for repositioning splint therapy less favorable (Fig. 7–3*D*).[26] This is also an example of the value of the coronal plane of imaging that is possible with MR.

Long-Term Follow-Up

There is controversy with respect to long-term results of protrusive splint therapy.[27] In our experience, arthrographically guided splint therapy has a

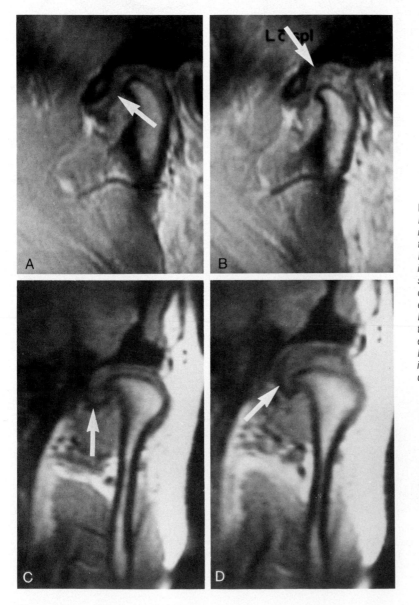

Figure 7–3
Disk displacement with splint. A, Sagittal magnetic resonance (MR) scan showing anterior disk displacement (arrow). B, Sagittal MR scan after reduction of disk position and insertion of an anterior repositioning splint, showing normal relationship between the condyle and disk. The posterior band of the disk is indicated by the arrow. C, Coronal MR scan showing medial displacement of the disk and widening of the medial recess of the lower joint space (arrow). D, Coronal MR scan with the anterior repositioning splint in place, showing persistence of slight medial disk displacement (arrow).

higher success rate than if this technique is based on a clinically determined therapeutic position. A study with post-treatment arthrography[28] showed that normal superior disk position remained in 82 per cent of patients treated with disk repositioning onlays followed by prosthodontics or orthodontics. In the patients with failure, medial displacement was more frequent than in those with successful long-term results.[28] The study suggested that medial and lateral disk displacement was more difficult to treat with protrusive splint therapy than anterior disk displacement. Other studies have reported a lower long-term success rate.[23, 29]

In our opinion, protrusive splint therapy, followed by permanent alteration of the dental occlusion to match the therapeutic position, is an effective method of eliminating symptoms related to disk displacement with reduction. The long-term results can be good.[28] Figure 7–4 shows images of a patient successfully treated with protrusive splint therapy, followed by orthodontic adjustment of the occlusion to the therapeutic position. A 6-year follow-up with MR imaging confirms the normal disk position. This illustrates that protrusive splint therapy with subsequent occlusal-orthodontic treatment can maintain the condyle-disk relationship for a long period of time. However, the treatment has a significant disadvantage in that it requires extensive dental treatment to maintain the therapeutic position. This can be done either with restorative dentistry or with orthodontics. The extensive amount and extent of dental treatment needed to maintain the therapeutic position permanently should be weighed relative to the severity of the symptomatology. Extensive treatment is probably not justified unless the symptoms are severe and other treatment methods have failed. We do not feel that there is justification for treating reciprocal clicking that is not associated with pain.

In our opinion the literature supports only treatment of patients with pain or severe mechanical dysfunction. The morphologic abnormality by itself rarely warrants intervention. However, documentation of an anatomic abnormality, even if nonsymptomatic, may be valuable as a baseline and to alert the patient that this abnormality might be a risk factor for future symptoms.

DISK REPOSITIONING SURGERY

Surgical Technique and Follow-Up Imaging Studies

The anteriorly displaced disk also can be anatomically corrected by surgical technique in the early stage of disease.[7] Disk repositioning surgery entails shortening of the posterior disk attachment and repositioning the displaced disk to a normal anatomic position. This surgical technique gained popularity in the late 1970s and early 1980s. Relatively few studies have been published on postsurgical imaging findings. An arthrographic study of ten patients evaluated the status of the joints after disk repositioning surgery utilizing arthrography.[30] Several of the studies in this investigation were inconclusive because of difficulty injecting contrast into the joint space. Some cases showed adhesions between the condyle and the disk, and some were documented to have normal function. The study concluded that arthrography was frequently nondiagnostic when performed after disk repositioning surgery. In a clinical follow-up of 33 patients 19 months after disk plication, Anderson and associates[9] reported a 79 per cent success rate with this surgical procedure, and Politis and colleagues[8] found a 63 per cent success rate with disk plication when associated with a high condylectomy.

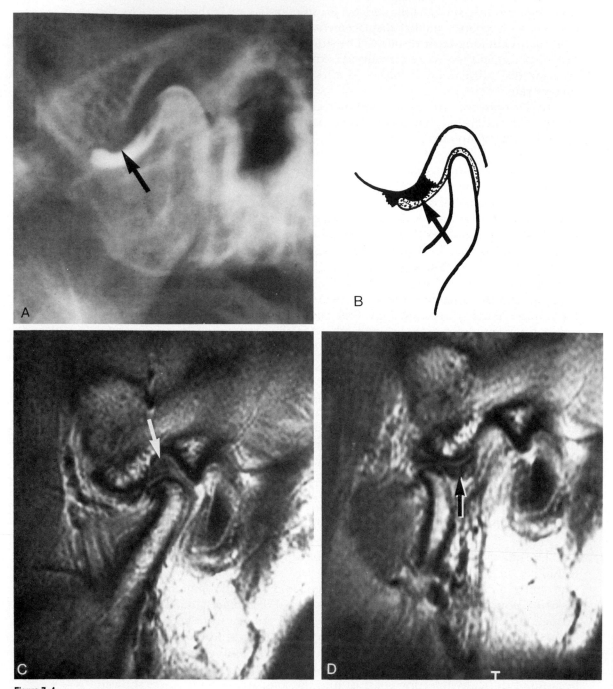

Figure 7–4
Six-year follow-up after protrusal splint therapy. A, Arthrogram showing anterior disk displacement (arrow). B, Schematic drawing showing the disk (arrow) anterior to the condyle. C, MR images at closed-mouth position 6 years after initiation of treatment, showing the disk (arrow) in normal superior position. D, MR image at 6-year follow-up obtained at maximal mouth opening, showing normal function of the disk (arrow).

The relationship between pain and disk position is not fully understood. There are conflicting opinions of how important repositioning the disk is to gain freedom from symptoms after operation. Conway and associates performed MR imaging after disk repositioning surgery of 25 joints and documented a strong correlation between good clinical results and normal superior disk position at follow-up.[31] In their study, those patients with poor clinical results showed MR evidence of disk displacement with no improvement, compared with preoperative images. Those patients with good or excellent clinical results had normal superior disk position at follow-up. The significance of disk position, however, is controversial, and MR imaging after arthroscopic surgery has shown persistent disk displacement in spite of clinical success.[32] These results have not prevented arthroscopic surgeons from trying to develop arthroscopic surgical techniques by which the disk position can be repositioned to restore normal anatomy.[33]

Our own limited experience indicates that the disk frequently is not repositioned all the way back into its normal position after disk repositioning surgery. Montgomery and coworkers showed disk displacement in 86 per cent of joints imaged an average of 2 years after surgery and concluded that disk repositioning surgery frequently failed to restore normal anatomy but still appeared to improve pain and dysfunction.[10] A joint with anterior disk displacement before surgery and correction of disk position after surgery is shown in Figure 7–5. The patient shown in Figure 7–6 shows improvement of disk position but not a complete restoration of normal anatomy. The patient was asymptomatic at follow-up. An example of failure to restore normal anatomy with disk repositioning surgery is shown in Figure 7–7. This follow-up MR examination 2 years after surgery shows the disk anterior to the condyle and significant remodeling of the upper part of the condylar head. The patient had pain and some limitation of opening.

Interpretation of Postsurgical Images

In the interpretation of postsurgical imaging after disk repositioning surgery, one should evaluate the position, configuration, and function of the disk. The osseous components should be evaluated for remodeling and arthrosis. Furthermore, the images should be evaluated for intra-articular adhesions and compared with the presurgical images. The criteria for interpretation of postoperative imaging in general are listed in Table 7–1.

Arthrography could be effective for studying postoperative intra-articular adhesions but may be technically difficult to perform. Peripheral adhesions, altered joint anatomy, and loss of distinct bony surfaces as anatomic landmarks may make joint puncture difficult. To be entirely normal, the joint spaces should have the same dimensions as before operation. If intra-articular adhesions are present, they usually are located in the periphery of the joint spaces; the contrast will appear irregular in outline, and the joint spaces may be significantly smaller than normal.[34] A joint with peripheral adhesions and disk perforation demonstrated with arthrography is shown in Figure 7–8. The observation of adhesions after operation is probably the most significant finding using arthrography.[34] Disk displacement with and without reduction, perforation, and deformation of the disk should be evaluated in the same way as in images before operation. Imaging after surgery should always be compared with the situation before treatment to determine whether there has been a progression of disease.

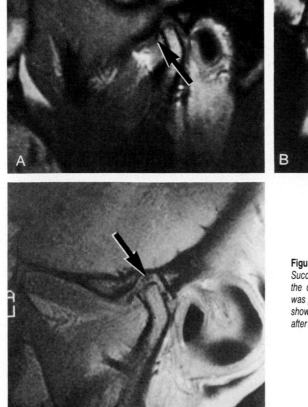

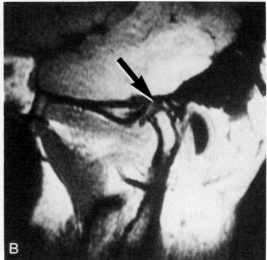

Figure 7–5
Successful surgical disk repositioning. A, Sagittal MR scan showing the disk (arrow) anteriorly displaced. Disk repositioning operation was performed. B, MR scan of the same joint 3 years after operation shows the normal position of the disk (arrow). C, MR scan 6 years after operation shows the normal position of the disk (arrow).

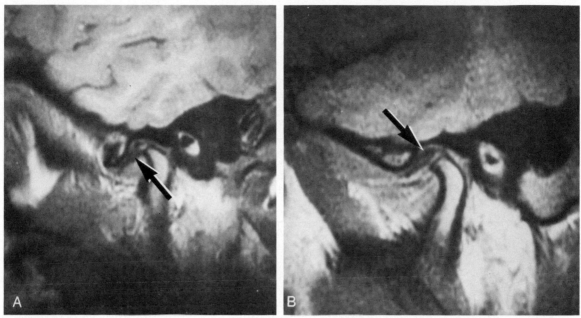

Figure 7–6
Improved disk position after disk repositioning operation. A, Sagittal MR scan showing anterior displacement of the disk (arrow). Disk repositioning operation was performed. B, Sagittal MR scan 1 year after surgery shows improved position of the disk (arrow). The disk-condyle relationship, however, is not totally normal.

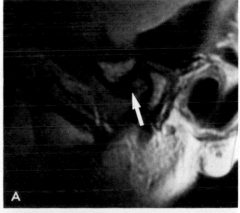

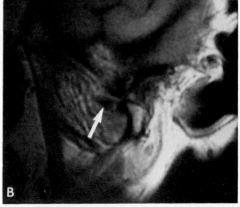

Figure 7–7
Failed disk repositioning surgery. A, Sagittal MR scan at closed-mouth position after disk repositioning operation shows the disk (arrow) remaining in an anterior position. The disk is also deformed. B, Sagittal open-mouth MR image showing the disk anterior to the condyle (arrow), also at the open-mouth position, suggesting disk displacement without reduction. There is also remodeling of the condyle.

Table 7–1
CRITERIA FOR INTERPRETATION OF POSTOPERATIVE IMAGES

Disk position	Normal disk position; disk displacement in anterior, medial, or lateral direction should be evaluated according to the same criteria as in preoperative imaging
Disk function	Normal function; disk displacement with or without reduction
Disk form	Normal or deformed according to the same criteria as used in preoperative imaging
Adhesions	Peripheral or central adhesions
Osseous changes	Normal, remodeling, or arthrosis

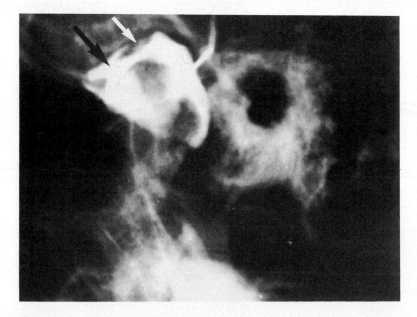

Figure 7–8
Perforation after disk repositioning operation. Arthrogram with contrast injection into the lower joint space shows perforation. The disk (white arrow) is in a relatively normal position over the condyle, but there is a perforation (black arrow) in the central part of the disk. There are also adhesions in the periphery of the joint, demonstrated as relatively small joint spaces, especially anteriorly.

Adhesions After Operation

Frequently after operation, scar tissue formation is seen in the lateral wall of the joint capsule (Figs. 7–9 and 7–10). This scar tissue is usually seen posterior and lateral to the joint. In a successful case, the scar tissue is seen on MR images as irregular areas of low signal intensity that do not extend into the joint space (Fig. 7–9). The scar tissue should be confined to the lateral capsule wall. Figure 7–10 shows an example of successful disk repositioning operation in which the disk is in a normal position but scar tissue is present in the lateral capsule wall. It has been our experience that as long as the scar tissue is only in the capsule, it does not impair joint function significantly.

Scar tissue that becomes extensive (Fig. 7–11) and extends into the joint space is frequently associated with residual pain and represents a partial fibrous ankylosis. Figure 7–11 shows failure of repositioning of the disk, complicated by extensive scar tissue in the lateral capsule wall extending into the lateral third of the joint space. Postoperative fibrous ankylosis is a possible complication of all TMJ surgery, but disk repositioning techniques are more prone to it. If there is clinical suspicion of fibrous ankylosis, MR imaging can be a powerful tool to evaluate the extent. Figure 7–12 shows a joint after disk repositioning surgery in which extensive fibrous tissue in the joint space extends to the medial capsule (Fig. 7–12B). It is essential that the imaging evaluation of this patient extend medially and laterally to depict all areas in the lateral capsule wall that

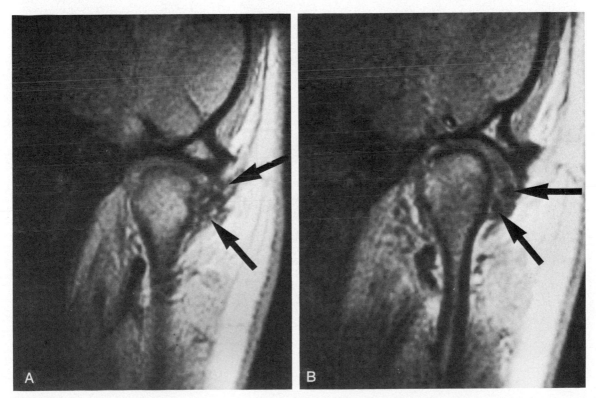

Figure 7–9
Scar tissue in the lateral part of the joint capsule after disk repositioning operation. A, Coronal MR scan showing an area of irregular low signal (arrows) lateral to the condyle. This is interpreted as fibrous scar tissue in the lateral capsule wall. B, Coronal MR scan of the same joint more anteriorly. Areas of low signal are seen in the lateral recess of the joint, indicating scar tissue. These do not extend into the joint space.

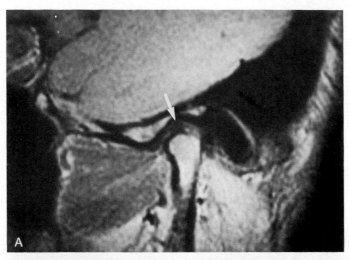

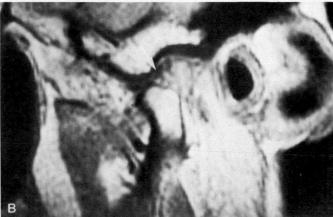

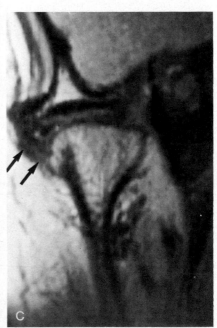

Figure 7–10

Successful disk repositioning. A, Sagittal MR image at the closed-mouth position, showing the disk (arrow) in normal location relative to the condyle after disk repositioning operation. B, On opening, the disk functions normally. The posterior band of the disk (arrow) is behind the condyle. C, A coronal MR image shows scar tissue (arrows) in the lateral capsule wall. The patient was asymptomatic at follow-up.

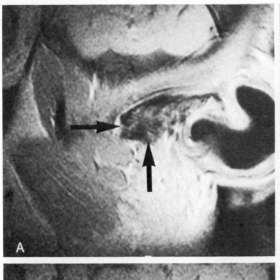

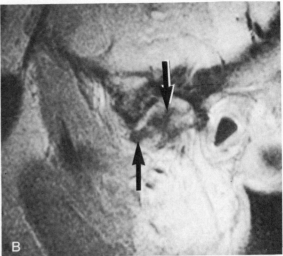

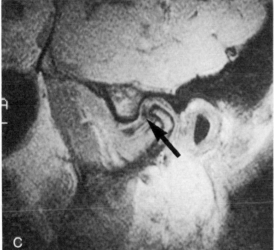

Figure 7–11

Extensive scar tissue in a patient with symptoms after disk repositioning operation. A, Sagittal MR image off the lateral aspect of the joint, showing an area of tissue with low signal intensity (arrows). B, Sagittal MR scan from the lateral third of the joint, showing that the tissue with low signal intensity extends into the joint space (arrows). C, Sagittal MR image from the central part of the joint, showing the disk (arrow) remaining in an anterior position. Both the anterior disk displacement and the scar tissue in the lateral part of the joint could be associated with the patient's persistent pain symptoms.

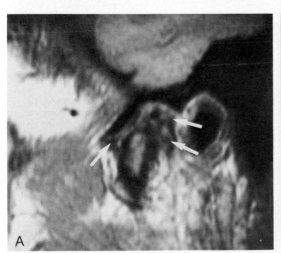

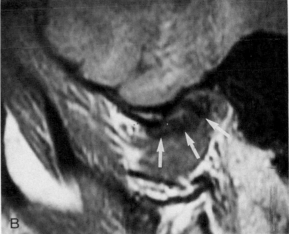

Figure 7–12

Fibrous ankylosis. A, Sagittal MR scan from the lateral part of the joint after disk repositioning operation in a patient with persistent pain. The scan shows multiple bandlike areas of low signal (arrows) that are suggestive of fibrous ankylosis. B, Sagittal MR image medial to the joint, showing an irregular area of low signal intensity (arrows) in the medial capsule wall. This is suggestive of fibrous ankylosis extending into the medial wall of the joint.

might be involved with fibrous ankylosis. A massive fibrous ankylosis following TMJ surgery is shown in Figure 7–13.

Plain Film and Tomograms

Imaging evaluation after disk repositioning surgery should also involve the osseous components of the joint. This could be done with plain film, tomography, or computed tomography. In the successful disk repositioning case there should be no significant progression of the osseous changes. Significant arthrosis that develops after disk repositioning surgery is an indication that the disk repositioning operation has not been successful.

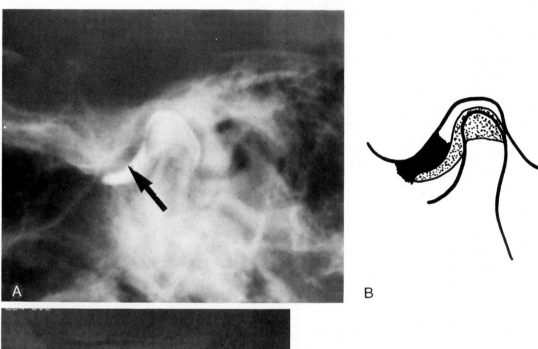

Figure 7–13

Extensive fibrous ankylosis after disk repositioning operation. A, Presurgical single-contrast lower compartment arthrogram showing anterior disk displacement. The enlarged anterior recess of the lower joint space indicates disk displacement (arrow). B, Schematic drawing of the arthrogram in A. C, Magnetic resonance scan 2 years after surgery shows a massive fibrous ankylosis from the low neck of the condyle to the base of the skull. The area of fibrous tissue is indicated by arrows.

Imaging Strategy

Screening of symptomatic postsurgical joints can be done with plain film, tomography, or panoramic radiography. This can be especially valuable if previous films are available for comparison. If there is a clinical suspicion of abnormalities within the joint, the next imaging technique performed should be MR to assess soft tissue of the joint. CT imaging should not be used as a primary imaging modality after disk repositioning surgery, but could be valuable if osseous ankylosis is present. For fibrous ankylosis, which is more common, MR imaging is clearly superior to CT.

DISKECTOMY

Persistent Joint Space

More information is available concerning findings of diagnostic imaging after diskectomy than after disk repositioning. The first observation reported was during the late 1940s when it was demonstrated that the joint space between the condyle and the glenoid fossa frequently remained after diskectomy. This has been a consistent observation over the years. Despite the disk being removed and the articular soft tissue cover on the condyle and in the glenoid fossa amounting to less than a millimeter, the joint space seems to remain after diskectomy (Fig. 7–14). Follow-up studies with arthrography after diskectomy have shown that this persistent joint space is maintained by a thickened soft tissue cover in the glenoid fossa and to some degree also on the mandibular condyle.[35] Figure 7–15 shows a joint in which a thick articular soft tissue cover developed after diskectomy. This soft tissue cover appears to maintain the joint space—that is, the radiolucent distance between the mandibular condyle and the glenoid fossa. An arthrogram of this joint before surgery showed no significant thickness of the soft tissue layer in the glenoid fossa (Fig. 7–15A), whereas a tomogram 21 months after operation (Fig. 7–15B) and an arthrogram

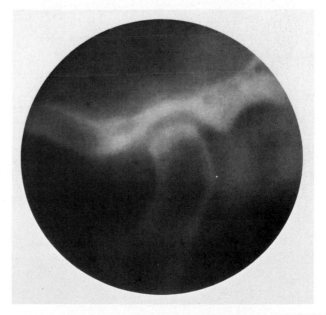

Figure 7–14
Minimal changes 29 years after diskectomy. Sagittal tomogram of a joint treated with diskectomy 29 years earlier. Only minimal remodeling changes on the temporal joint component are seen. A joint space remains between the condyle and the glenoid fossa.

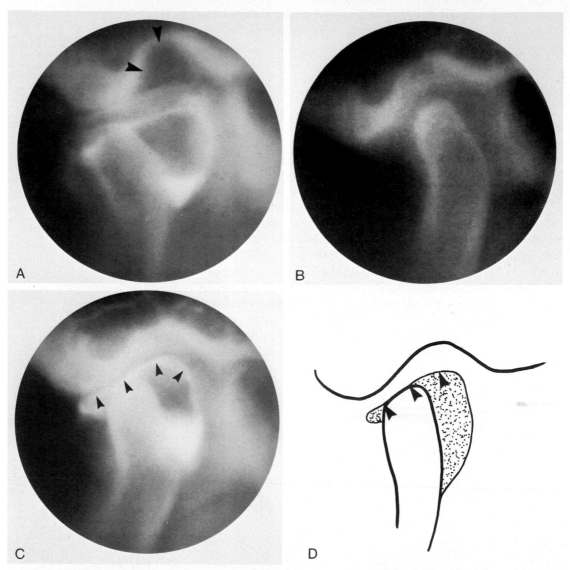

Figure 7–15

Thickening of articular soft tissue cover after diskectomy. A, Dual-space double-contrast arthrotomogram showing no significant thickness of the articular soft tissue cover in the glenoid fossa (arrowheads). B, Tomogram 21 months after diskectomy, showing the condyle separated from the glenoid fossa by a radiolucent distance. C, Double-contrast arthrotomogram 21 months after diskectomy, showing thickening of the articular soft tissue cover (arrowheads) along the glenoid fossa and articular tubercle. D, Schematic drawing of the arthrotomogram shown in C.

(Fig. 7–15C and D) showed a substantial thickening of this layer. It is our opinion that the thickened soft tissue cover in the glenoid fossa accounts for the persistence of the joint space frequently seen after diskectomy. If the disk is perforated or thin when removed, only a thin articular soft tissue cover will be seen after operation (Fig. 7–16). Apparently the thickened soft tissue cover is a response to fill the empty space after the disk has been removed and not an active process by which the new cartilage pushes the condyle anteriorly and inferiorly.

Condylar Position and Bone Remodeling

The position of the condyle frequently changes after diskectomy. If the condyle is located posteriorly in the glenoid fossa before operation (Fig. 7–17), it is frequently in a more central position at follow-up (Fig. 7–17D).[36] The reason for this change of position is not clearly understood but it seems reasonable to assume that the anteriorly displaced disk presses the condyle posteriorly. When the disk is eliminated, the mandible shifts slightly forward.

Remodeling of the bone after diskectomy was studied by Agerberg and Lundberg.[37] They showed that the outline of the osseous contours of the condyle and temporal component frequently are indistinct in the first 2 years after diskectomy. Follow-up studies of larger materials have shown that different degrees of remodeling consistently follow diskectomy, with, however, a wide variation of the degree. Mild remodeling (Fig. 7–18) has been seen in up to 30 years after diskectomy. However, extensive remodeling with osteophytosis and flattening of the articular eminence also has been seen in long-term follow-up after diskectomy (Fig. 7–19). There appears to be no clear association between osseous changes in the form of remodeling and clinical symptoms.[4] Thus, in

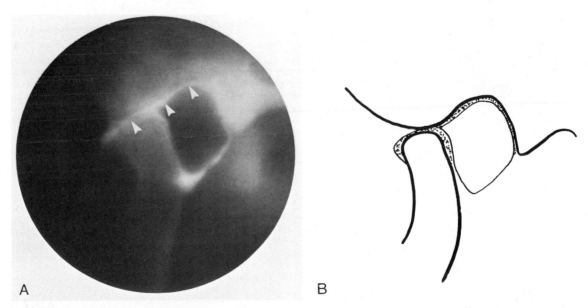

A   B

Figure 7–16
Thin articular soft tissue cover after diskectomy. A, Double-contrast arthrotomogram after diskectomy, showing a thin, articular soft tissue cover (arrowheads) along the temporal joint component in this joint that had a perforation of the removed disk. B, Schematic drawing of the double-contrast arthrotomogram shown in A.

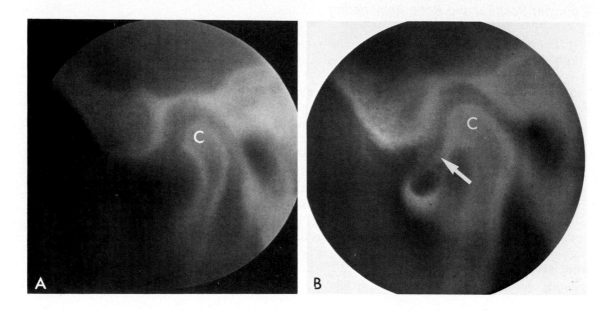

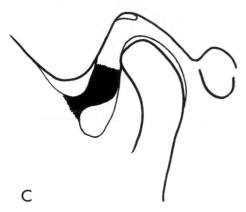

Figure 7–17
Condylar and soft tissue changes after diskectomy. A, Sagittal tomogram before diskectomy, showing the condyle (C) posterior in the glenoid fossa. There are no osseous changes. B, Dual-space double-contrast arthrotomogram, showing the disk (arrow) anterior to the condyle. C, Schematic drawing of the dual-space double-contrast arthrotomogram shown in B.

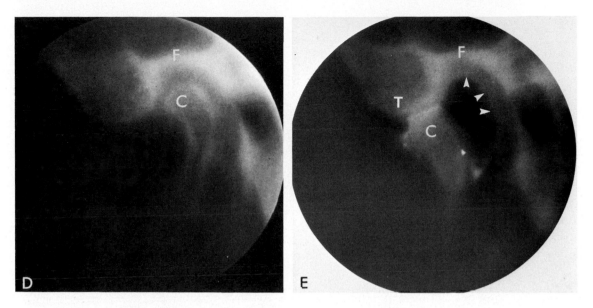

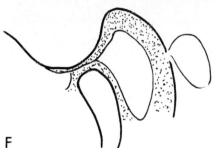

Figure 7–17 Continued

D, *Sagittal tomogram 18 months after diskectomy, showing the condyle (C) in a central position in the glenoid fossa (F). E, Double-contrast arthrotomogram showing thickening of the articular soft tissue cover in the glenoid fossa (arrowheads). The arthrotomogram was obtained at mouth opening, and the condyle (C) is articulating against the posterior slope of the articular tubercle (T). The most pronounced thickening of the articular soft tissue cover is in the glenoid fossa (F). F, Schematic drawing of the double-contrast arthrotomogram shown in E.*

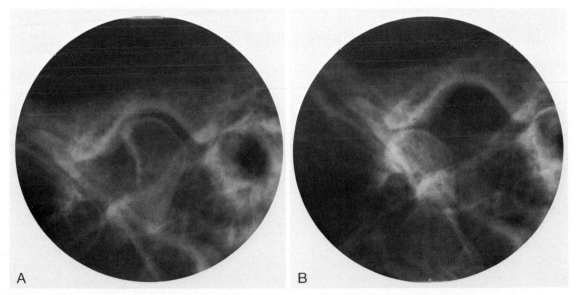

Figure 7–18

Thirty-year follow-up with mild narrowing of joint space in a patient without symptoms. A, Transcranial image of the closed-mouth position 30 years after diskectomy, showing mild narrowing of the joint space and mild osteophytosis on the condyle. B, Open-mouth transcranial image showing narrowing of the joint space but good range of motion.

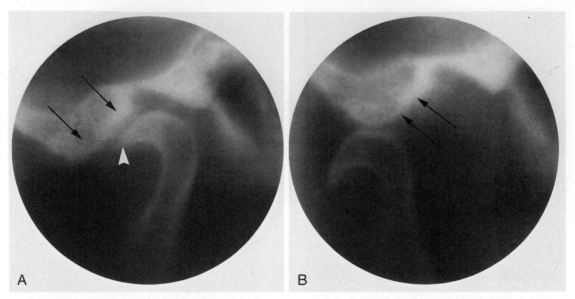

Figure 7–19
Extensive osseous changes 30 years after diskectomy in a patient without symptoms. A, Closed-mouth tomogram showing a large osteophyte on the condyle (arrowhead) and progressive remodeling of the articular eminence (arrows). B, Open-mouth image showing good range of motion but loss of distance between the condyle and the articular eminence. Again, progressive remodeling of the posterior slope of the articular eminence (arrows) is well visualized.

spite of extensive osseous changes as shown in Figures 7–19, 7–20, and 7–21, the patient might be clinically asymptomatic at follow-up. Figure 7–20 is an example of relatively extensive remodeling in an asymptomatic patient 2 years after diskectomy. The osseous changes include sclerosis of both condyle and temporal component, osteophytosis of the condyle, and flattening of the condyle and articular eminence.

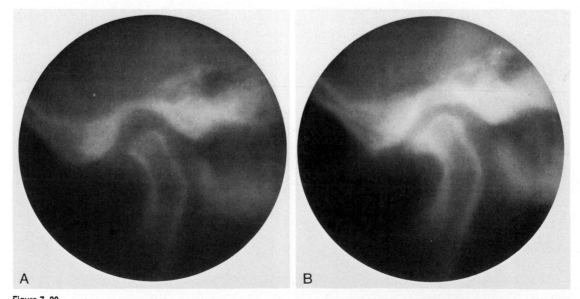

Figure 7–20
Extensive remodeling 2 years after diskectomy. A, Sagittal tomogram before diskectomy, showing mild remodeling of the condyle. B, Sagittal tomogram of the same joint 2.5 years after diskectomy, showing osteophytosis and sclerosis of the condyle and significant sclerosis in the fossa and articular eminence. Note that a radiolucent distance remains between the condyle and temporal joint component.

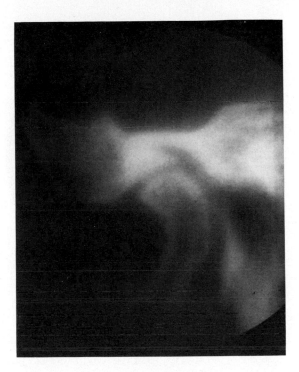

Figure 7–21
Characteristic remodeling after diskectomy; 5-year follow-up. Characteristic progressive remodeling in the glenoid fossa and along the posterior slope of the articular eminence after diskectomy. Also the remodeling of the condyle is characteristic. This change is a reflection of the altered function when the disk has been removed.

After diskectomy, the condyle characteristically demonstrates flattening superiorly and anterior osteophyte formation (Fig. 7–21). The temporal component also will be flattened, and the joint will change its function from a rotational and translational joint to a sliding or translational joint.[38] These osseous changes characteristically are seen after diskectomy in both symptomatic and asymptomatic patients and should not necessarily be regarded as arthrosis. This means that plain film and tomography are valuable for follow-up of osseous changes but correlate poorly to clinical symptomatology after diskectomy. Therefore we recommend soft tissue imaging in symptomatic patients to acquire accurate information about the status of the soft tissues.

Soft Tissue Changes

Arthrography can be employed after diskectomy to assess soft tissue changes.[35] The arthrographic images have proved useful in assessing the mechanisms responsible for persistence of the radiolucent distance between the condyle and glenoid fossa, as described above. Experience with clinical arthrography has shown that the size of the joint compartment is a significant element in the evaluation of patients after diskectomy.[34] The larger the joint space, the better. A narrow joint space that tightly surrounds the condyle with an irregular periphery (Fig. 7–22) is indicative of peripheral adhesions and could be associated with persistent or recurrent pain and limitation of opening. However, even though arthrography is excellent for evaluating the size of the joint compartment, it is more difficult to perform than other imaging modalities, such as MR. It would appear to be easy to inject the TMJ after the disk has been removed, since the joint space should be larger. However, this is not the case, since peripheral and central adhesions can make injection more difficult. Furthermore, the bony surface of the condyle is not as distinct with thickening of the soft tissue cover, and the anatomic landmarks are altered.

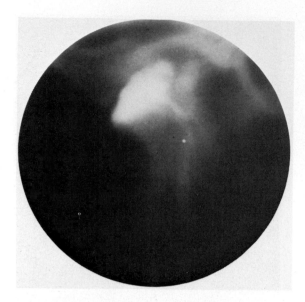

Figure 7–22
Narrowing of joint space after diskectomy due to peripheral adhesions. Contrast was injected into the joint space and shows narrowing anteriorly and posteriorly. The joint space is smaller than normal. The upper and posterior outlines of the joint space are irregular, suggestive of peripheral adhesions. The arthrotomogram was obtained at mouth opening.

MR Imaging

MR imaging is an alternative technique to evaluate soft tissue changes after diskectomy.[39] Studies have shown that MR imaging is useful in differentiating painful from nonpainful joints.[40] An example of an MR image before and after diskectomy in a patient with no residual pain is shown in Figure 7–23. There should be a good range of motion and no evidence of areas of low signal between the condyle and temporal component within the joint space in a successful diskectomy joint (Fig. 7–24). Coronal imaging in combination with sagittal imaging is valuable for assessment of the tissue condition in the lateral part of the joint (Fig. 7–25). In a follow-up study of 28 consecutive patients

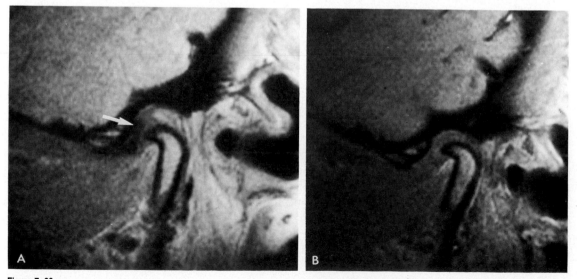

Figure 7–23
Successful diskectomy. A, Sagittal MR scan before diskectomy, showing remodeling of the condyle and the disk (arrow) slightly anterior. B, MR scan of the same joint 2 months after diskectomy, showing maintenance of joint space, but the disk is absent.

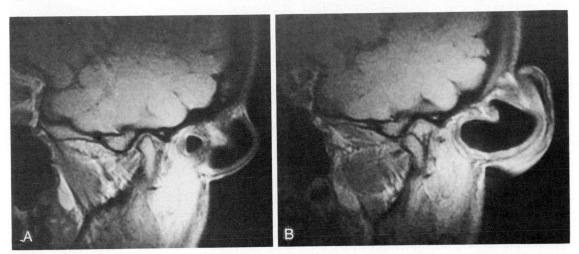

Figure 7–24
Successful diskectomy. A, Sagittal MR scan after diskectomy. The disk is absent. The joint space is present, with tissue of relatively high signal. B, On opening, the condyle translates almost to the apex of the articular eminence. The distance between the condyle and temporal component is smaller on opening than at closed-mouth position.

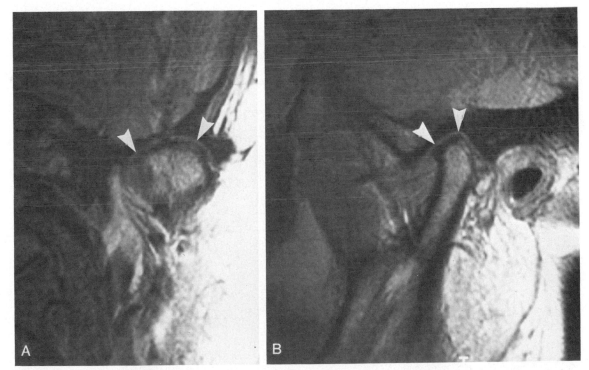

Figure 7–25
Coronal and sagittal images of successful diskectomy. A, Coronal MR image after diskectomy, showing persistent joint space with intermediate signal (arrowheads). B, Sagittal image showing persistent joint space (arrowheads).

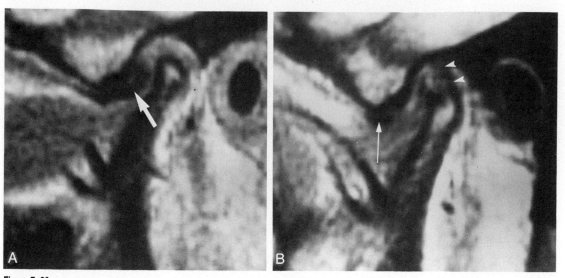

Figure 7–26

Failed diskectomy. A, MR image before diskectomy shows the disk (arrow) anterior to the condyle. B, MR image 12 months after diskectomy shows areas of low signal (arrowheads) in the joint space between the condyle and the glenoid fossa. Small remnants of disk (arrow) are seen inferior to the articular eminence. The postoperative pain symptoms were probably related to the fibrous tissue between the condyle and glenoid fossa. The small remnants of the disk were insignificant, because this is seen in both asymptomatic and symptomatic individuals. MR images were obtained on a 0.3 Tesla magnet.

who had unilateral diskectomy without disk replacement implant, a correlation was identified between MR findings of fibrous tissue in the joint space at follow-up (Fig. 7–26) and pain and limitation of opening at follow-up.[40] Patients who experienced no pain at follow-up generally had an area of relatively high signal in the joint space (Fig. 7–27). The area of low signal in the joint space at follow-up (Fig. 7–26) was probably representative of fibrous tissue and could indicate a partial fibrous ankylosis.

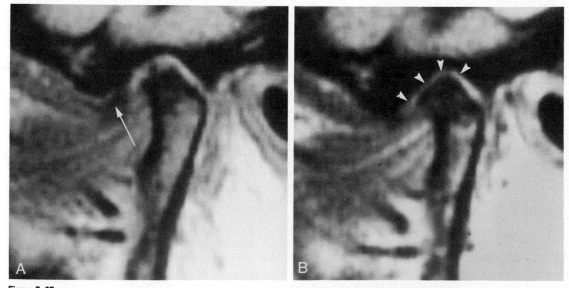

Figure 7–27

Successful diskectomy. A, MR image before diskectomy showing the disk (arrow) anteriorly displaced. B, MR image 17 months after diskectomy, showing an area of high signal (arrowheads) in the joint space between the glenoid fossa and mandibular condyle. This is characteristic of a postoperative image of a successful diskectomy. MR images were obtained on a 0.3 Tesla magnet.

The same study evaluated other features in postoperative MR ima␣ as the vertical dimension of the joint space, signal changes from ␣ marrow of the condyle (Fig. 7–28), fibrous tissue confined to the ␣ capsule, signal void from minuscule metal particles, and remnant␣ anteriorly. This study could not identify any statistically significan␣ with these features and patient symptomatology at follow-up.[40] The on␣ imaging finding at follow-up that was significantly associated with residual pain and dysfunction was areas of low signal intensity in the joint space suggestive of partial fibrous ankylosis (Fig. 7–26).

Imaging Strategy

Based on our experience with plain film, arthrography, CT, and MR, we recommend MR as the primary imaging modality for follow-up of patients experiencing pain or dysfunction after diskectomy (Table 7–2). Plain film, tomography, or panoramic radiography may be used as a routine follow-up after diskectomy if there is a clinical need to document the remodeling of the bone that will occur.

SILICONE IMPLANT

Surgeons have used various forms of silicone implants in many areas of the human body for reconstruction and to prevent postoperative ankylosis.[41–48] The first mention of silicone implants used in the TMJ came at the end of 1960.[49, 50] Initially a high success rate was reported when the removed disk was replaced by a sheet of medical-grade silicone material (Silastic, Dow Corning Corporation, Midland, Michigan) (Fig. 7–29).[51, 52] However, the long-term results and the orthopedic experience with Silastic as a temporary or permanent

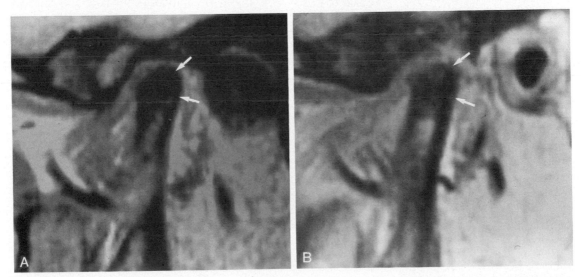

Figure 7–28
Stable area of dark signal in condyle. A, Sagittal MR image before diskectomy, showing an area of dark signal in the condyle (arrows). B, MR image 15 months after diskectomy shows the area of low signal essentially unchanged (arrows). There is some remodeling, with a diffuse outline of the condyle and glenoid fossa. This is characteristic during the first 1 to 2 years after diskectomy. The patient was asymptomatic at follow-up. MR images were obtained on a 0.3 Tesla magnet.

7–2

GGESTIONS FOR IMAGING FOLLOWING TEMPOROMANDIBULAR JOINT SURGERY

Surgical Technique	Asymptomatic Patients	Symptomatic Patients
Diskectomy without implant	Plain film, tomography, or panoramic radiography 12 months after operation as a baseline for future follow-up of osseous morphology	MR scan at the time patient returns with symptoms
Diskectomy with temporary silicone implant	Plain film, tomography, or panoramic radiography 12 and 24 months after operation. If conditions are stable at 24 months, no further imaging in asymptomatic patients. If conditions are not stable, further imaging as clinically needed but no less than every 12 months	MR scan at the time the patient returns with symptoms
Diskectomy with Proplast-Teflon or silicone implants; implant in place	MR and/or CT every 6 months as long as the implant is in place	MR and/or CT every 6 months as long as the implant is in place
Diskectomy with Proplast-Teflon or silicone implant that has been removed	CT, MR, or tomography at 12 and 24 months after removal of the implant. Imaging should continue every 12 months until stable conditions have developed	MR scan at the time the patient presents with symptoms

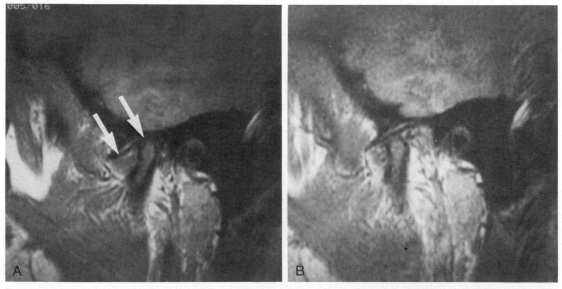

Figure 7–29
Silastic in good position. A, MR image in the closed-mouth position, showing Silastic (arrows) in good position 2 years after surgery. There is no surrounding widening or enlargement of the joint capsule. B, Open-mouth MR image, showing the condyle to translate anterior inferiorly along the inferior surface of the implant.

implant in a functional area such as the TMJ was not discussed at this early stage. Fragmentation or fracture of the implant does occur, and the particles from the implant are distributed into the surrounding soft tissues. Numerous articles in the medical literature report the disadvantage of silicone due to foreign body reaction against the fragmented silicon.[53-64] Fragmentation appears to be a problem that is difficult to avoid when natural surfaces are sliding against an artificial material.

Imaging Following Silicone Implant

Imaging following silicone implant in the TMJ, both long-term[65] and short-term,[66] has revealed a variety of remodeling changes similar to those seen in diskectomy without an implant. As long as the remodeling changes are confined to flattening, sclerosis, and osteophytosis, they should not be alarming. However, several studies[65, 66] have shown that erosive changes of the bone following silicone implant are frequent (Fig. 7–30). These can be seen radiographically as osteolysis of the most superior part of the condyle (Fig. 7–30) or as rounded, punched-out erosions in the condyle (Fig. 7–31) or temporal joint component

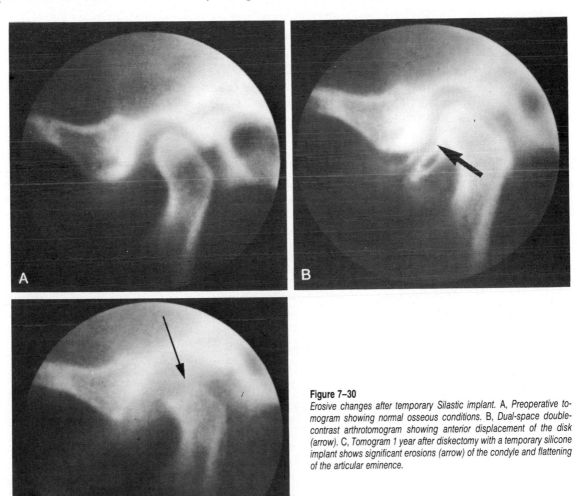

Figure 7–30
Erosive changes after temporary Silastic implant. A, Preoperative tomogram showing normal osseous conditions. B, Dual-space double-contrast arthrotomogram showing anterior displacement of the disk (arrow). C, Tomogram 1 year after diskectomy with a temporary silicone implant shows significant erosions (arrow) of the condyle and flattening of the articular eminence.

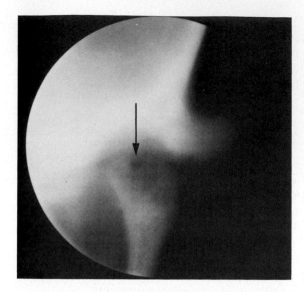

Figure 7–31
Erosion in condyle 5 years after diskectomy. Coronal tomogram showing punched-out erosion (arrow) in the center of the mandibular condyle 5 years after diskectomy with a temporary silicone implant.

(Fig. 7–32). Erosions are rarely seen in nonoperated joints or postsurgically in joints operated without an implant. If an erosion (Figs. 7–30, 7–31, and 7–32) is seen after operation, it is highly likely to be associated with the placement of a temporary or permanent implant. A removed condyle with such erosion has shown particulated silicone material and cyst formation in the condyle head (Fig. 7–33).

Two types of silicone implant have been used in the TMJ. One is reinforced with Dacron (Fig. 7–34), and the other is nonreinforced high-performance silicone material (Fig. 7–35). The Dacron-reinforced material has a tendency to fracture during function (Fig. 7–34). The fractures occur along the mesh of Dacron fibers, and the separated material becomes particulated and dispersed in the periarticular soft tissue.[66, 67] The high-performance nonreinforced silicone material does not have the same tendency for fracture, but the material does not stand the functional load of articulating against natural surfaces (Fig. 7–35). Thus wear facets have been observed after functioning in the TMJ for only a few months.

MR imaging of TMJ with silicone implants is excellent in demonstrating displacement of the implants and capsular enlargement secondary to granulation tissue around the implant[68] (Fig. 7–36). A joint with severe arthrosis, a displaced silicone implant, and capsular enlargement is shown in Figure 7–37.

Clinical Results of Temporary Silicone Implant

A recent 5-year follow-up on diskectomy with and without a temporary silicone implant failed to show any positive effect on clinical symptomatology.[65] Instead, the results showed a higher frequency of poor results in patients treated with an implant compared with those treated without a temporary silicone implant (Table 7–3). Silicone implants also have a tendency to create cysts in the mandibular condyle (see Fig. 7–33; Fig. 7–38). In advanced cases

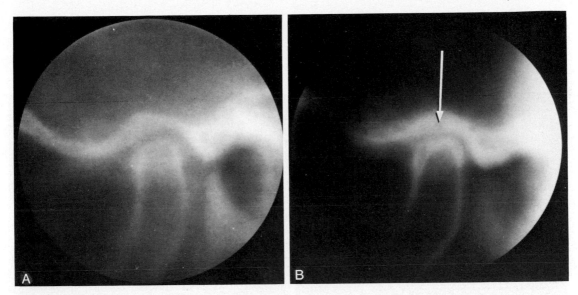

Figure 7-32
Erosions in the glenoid fossa 5 years after diskectomy. A, Tomogram before diskectomy, showing remodeling of the condyle and the temporal component. B, Tomogram 5 years after diskectomy with a temporary silicone implant, showing lytic lesions in the remodeled bone of the glenoid fossa (arrow).

the cyst formation in the condyle may be associated with bony ankylosis and erosions of the glenoid fossa toward the middle cranial fossa (Fig. 7–38). There are contradictory opinions about the value of silicone implants in the TMJ,[69-72] but we see no justification at this time for the use of temporary silicone implants in primary diskectomy cases. The situation might be different in surgery of joints with fibrous ankylosis or in operations of previously operated joints. These conditions must await further studies.

Imaging Strategy

For imaging of patients with silicone implants, we recommend MR imaging as the primary modality to assess the position and integrity of the implant and the surrounding soft and hard tissues. In cases with extensive osseous involvement, CT scan can provide additional information about cyst formation, erosions, and bony ankylosis. Imaging studies should be obtained to serve as a baseline for follow-up both when the implant is removed immediately and when removal is postponed.

Follow-up imaging studies after the implant has been removed are probably best done with thin-section direct coronal CT scan. After removal of the implant there is probably no need to image more often than once per year. In many cases with mild changes, a longer interval can be elected. It has been our experience that mild and moderate changes usually do not progress significantly after the implant has been removed. Advanced osseous changes have shown a more variable pattern. Little experience is available on follow-up imaging after removal of silicone implants, but coronal thin-section CT scan on a yearly basis for the first couple of years until stable conditions have developed is suggested. A suggestion for imaging of joints reconstructed with silicone is shown in Table 7–2.

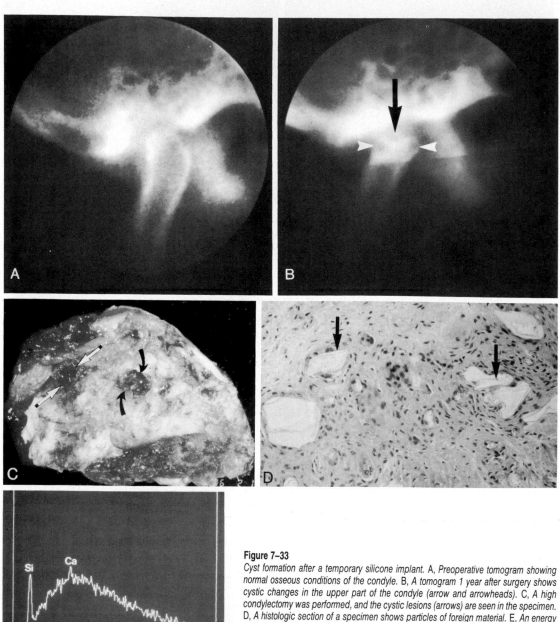

Figure 7–33

Cyst formation after a temporary silicone implant. A, Preoperative tomogram showing normal osseous conditions of the condyle. B, A tomogram 1 year after surgery shows cystic changes in the upper part of the condyle (arrow and arrowheads). C, A high condylectomy was performed, and the cystic lesions (arrows) are seen in the specimen. D, A histologic section of a specimen shows particles of foreign material. E, An energy and dispersive x-ray microanalyzer of the tissue shows a marked peak corresponding to silicone.

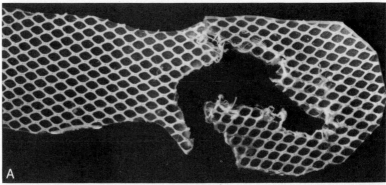

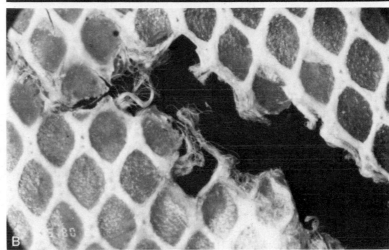

Figure 7–34
Dacron-reinforced silicone implants. A, This implant was removed after 4 months; extensive fracture and loss of material are revealed. B, Close-up view showing the fracture lines along the Dacron reinforcement.

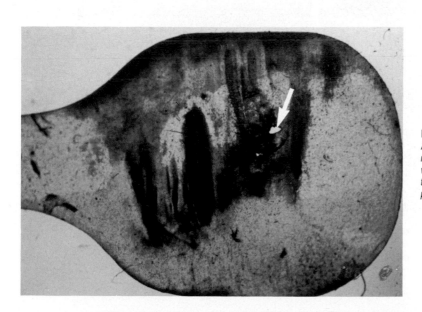

Figure 7–35
A high performance silicone implant removed after 4 months shows a significant wear facet from the condyle moving against the undersurface of the implant. A small perforation (arrow) is also seen.

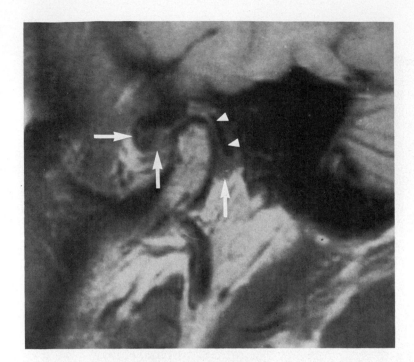

Figure 7–36
Fractured and displaced silicone implant. An MR image of a TMJ with implant (arrowheads) being displaced posterior to the condyle. There is enlargement of the joint capsule (arrows), suggestive of granulation tissue around the implant.

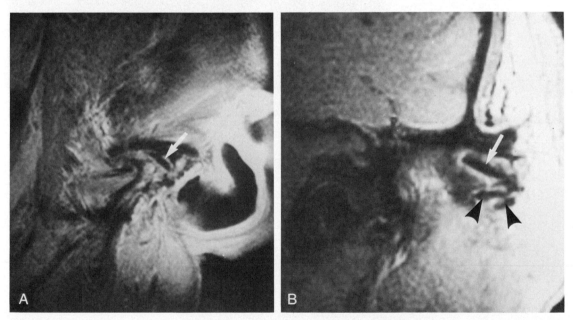

Figure 7–37
Displaced fractured silicone implant with arthrosis. A, Sagittal MR image showing the implant (arrow) posterior and superior to the condyle. The condyle demonstrates advanced arthrosis. B, A coronal image shows the implant (arrow) laterally displaced. Surrounding the implant are small areas of low signal that are interpreted as implant particles in the periarticular soft tissue (arrowheads).

Table 7–3
RESULTS OF DISKECTOMY WITH AND WITHOUT TEMPORARY SILICONE IMPLANT AT 5-YEAR FOLLOW-UP (N = 43 PATIENTS)

	No Implant (N = 21 Patients)	Temporary Silicone (N = 22 Patients)
Good	18	12
Acceptable	3	5
Failures	0	5

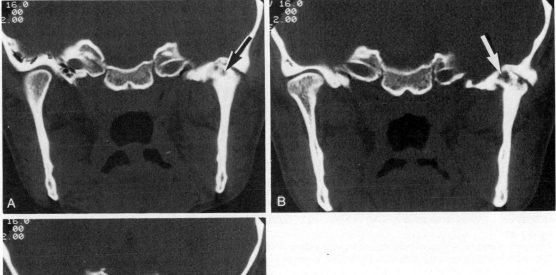

Figure 7–38
Bony ankylosis and subchondral cysts following silicone implant. A, Coronal CT scan shows subchondral cysts in the left TMJ (arrow). B, More anteriorly, there are more extensive cyst formation (arrow) and evidence of bony ankylosis between the medial part of the condyle and the glenoid fossa. C, Further anteriorly, destructive changes of the articular eminence (arrowheads) are seen.

PROPLAST-TEFLON IMPLANTS

Another type of implant used in the TMJ is Proplast-Teflon. Proplast is a porous form of Teflon (polytetrafluoroethylene) and has been fused with carbon (Proplast 1), aluminum oxide (Proplast 2), or synthetic hydroxy apatite (Proplast HA). The Proplast portion of the implant is placed against the temporal bone; it is designed to encourage growth of the soft and hard tissue into the upper surface of the implant to stabilize it (Fig. 7–39). The idea was that bony ingrowth to the superior surface should stabilize the implant, and the smooth undersurface should serve as a functional articulating surface against the condyle. The patient shown in Figure 7–39 has bilateral Proplast-Teflon implants in good position. On the right side there is ossification suggestive of bony ingrowth into the superior part of the implant. However, arthrotic changes of the condyle with a small cyst are seen. On the left side, the implant is in good position, but there appears to be a defect in the implant (Fig. 7–39). This illustrates a generic problem with this type of implant material, namely insufficient resistance to wear from articulating against a natural surface such as the condyle. The degree of wear is probably greater in cases with arthrotic changes of the condyle, as well as in patients with parafunction.

The Proplast-Teflon implant has been used in more than 20,000 joints since 1983,[14] and the initial success rate was in the 90 per cent range.[73] Other

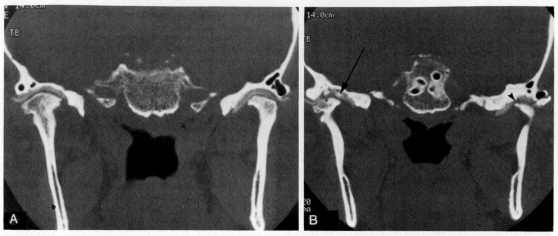

Figure 7–39
Proplast-Teflon implants. A, Proplast-Teflon implants in good position in the left and right TMJ. Arthrotic changes of the left and right condyles are seen. B, More anteriorly, bony ingrowth into the implant in the right joint (long arrow) is noted. On the left side is a small defect in the implant (arrowhead).

studies have also shown positive results with a similar success rate.[74] However, the failures are expected to occur later since they are related to wear of the material. The long-term prognosis is poor; Ryan reported failure at between 70 and 84 per cent.[14] The long-term results are doubtful,[15] and it seems reasonable to assume that eventually all implants have to be removed. The problems with alloplastic implants in the TMJ are inadequate wear characteristics,[75] tissue reaction to the particulated material—known in the orthopedic community as early as 1963,[76, 77] and difficulty achieving adequate stabilization of the implant against both the temporal bone and the mandible.

Imaging Following Proplast-Teflon Implant

Assessment of Proplast-Teflon implants can be done with CT or MR imaging. CT provides an excellent depiction of the implant itself (Figs. 7–39 and 7–40) and the osseous structures. CT is also excellent for demonstrating displacement of the implant (Fig. 7–41) and erosion of the bone. The sagittal image (Fig. 7–41A) shows an erosion of the articular eminence that penetrates almost into the middle cranial fossa. The erosive changes can be so extensive that the dura is exposed.[15] Erosive changes are indications for removal of the implant. Erosions can be seen both on sagittal (Fig. 7–41) and coronal projections (Fig. 7–42), but the coronal projection is more easily obtained in a routine clinical practice. The coronal imaging plane is therefore recommended instead of the direct sagittal for routine use. Axial CT images are less desirable, because this projection does not provide as much information about the roof of the glenoid fossa as does the coronal.

MR imaging has also been applied to patients with Proplast-Teflon implants. This technique shows the implant as a low signal structure in the joint space between the condyle and temporal joint component (Fig. 7–43). A patient who has had a Proplast-Teflon implant for 5 years with no significant clinical symptoms is shown in Figure 7–43. The implant is in a good location, but there is enlargement of the joint capsule posteriorly, suggestive of soft tissue granulation around the implant. This is in accordance with the medical literature,

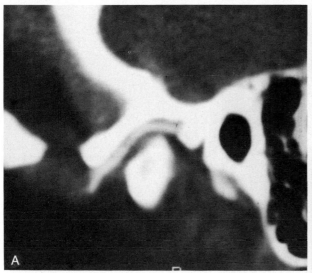

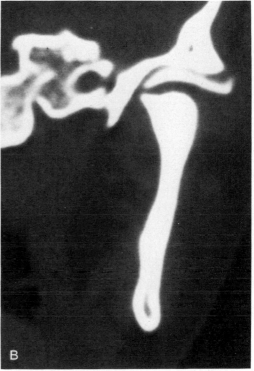

Figure 7–40
A, A sagittal CT scan showing a Proplast implant in good position. B, A coronal image of the same patient also shows the implant in good position.

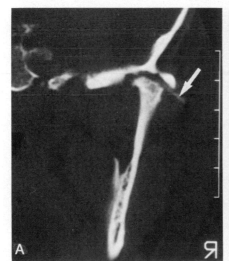

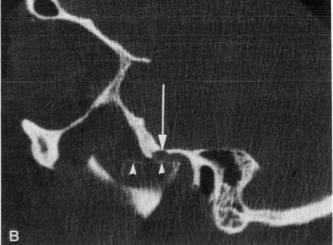

Figure 7–41
Displacement of Proplast-Teflon implant. A, Coronal CT scan showing displacement of the implant (arrow) laterally. B, Sagittal image of the same joint showing the implant (arrowheads) displaced anteriorly. There is a large erosion of the articular eminence (arrow).

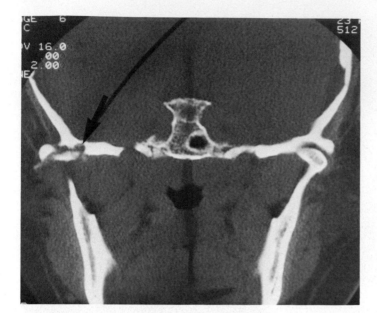

Figure 7–42
Erosion with Proplast-Teflon implant. Coronal CT scan showing erosion (arrow) approaching the middle fossa on the right side.

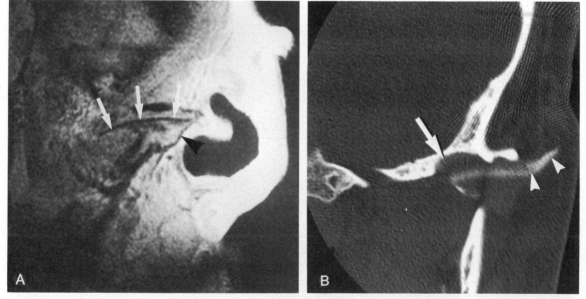

Figure 7–43
Sagittal MR image showing a Proplast-Teflon implant (arrows) that has been in place for 5 years. Arthrotic changes of the condyle and widening of the joint capsule posteriorly (arrowhead) are clearly seen. The patient was asymptomatic at follow-up. B, CT 1 year later shows displacement of the implant laterally (arrowheads) and erosion of the medial part of the articular tubercle (arrow) in the patient depicted in A. The patient continued to be asymptomatic but could palpate the implant under the skin.

which indicates that significant changes can be seen also in patients who are clinically asymptomatic.[78] However, foreign body reaction with granulation tissue around the implant is frequently seen (Fig. 7–44). MR imaging has been of great value to assess the extent of granulation tissue surrounding the implant, displacement and perforation of the implant (Fig. 7–45), and also the spread of dispersed particulate material in the periarticular soft tissue (Fig. 7–46)[79–82] around the joint with the implant.

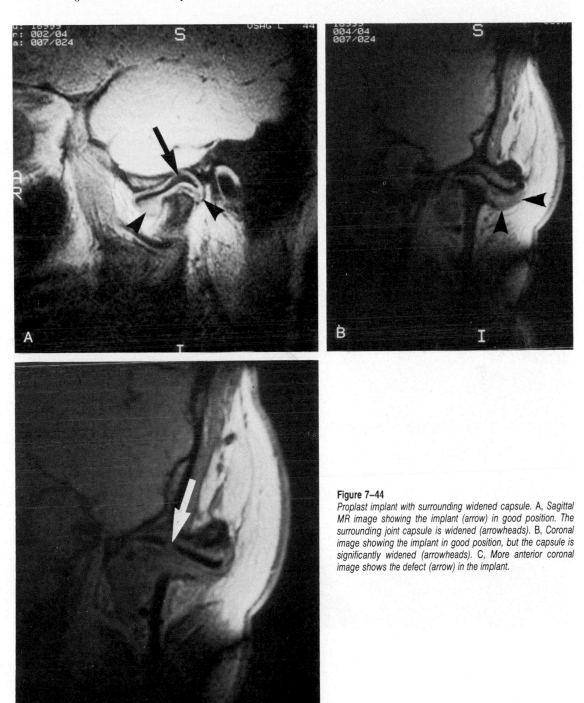

Figure 7–44
Proplast implant with surrounding widened capsule. A, Sagittal MR image showing the implant (arrow) in good position. The surrounding joint capsule is widened (arrowheads). B, Coronal image showing the implant in good position, but the capsule is significantly widened (arrowheads). C, More anterior coronal image shows the defect (arrow) in the implant.

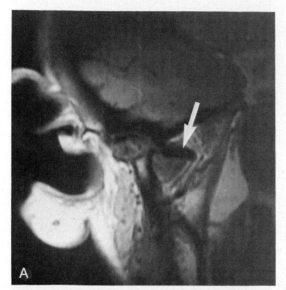

Figure 7–45
Proplast-Teflon implant displacement and dispersement of material within the capsule. A, Sagittal MR image showing a Proplast-Teflon implant (arrow) fractured and displaced. One part of the implant is anterior to the articular eminence and another part is behind the mandibular condyle. The joint capsule is expanded, and there are areas of low signal within the capsule that probably represent particulated material. B, A coronal image shows the expansion of the capsule (arrowheads). C, A coronal image further anterior shows lateral displacement of the implant and the defect of the implant (arrows).

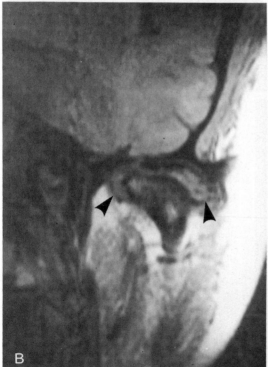

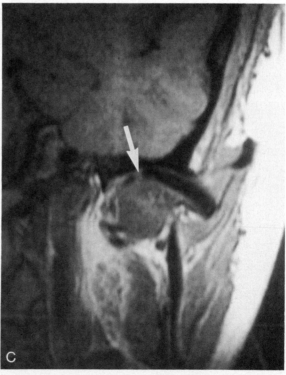

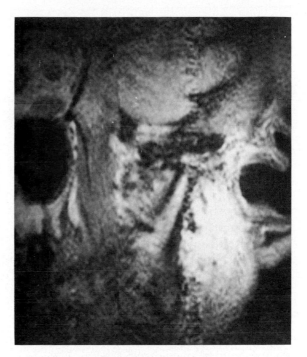

Figure 7–46
Fragmentation of Proplast-Teflon implant. Sagittal MR scan showing extensive arthrotic changes of both the condyle and the temporal joint component. Surrounding the joint are multiple areas of low signal suggestive of dispersed fragments of foreign material in the periarticular tissue.

T2-weighted MR images have a capacity to show the inflammatory nature of the granulation tissue around the implant. In Figure 7–47, a joint with a Proplast-Teflon implant is shown in good position. By CT criteria this would have been relatively unremarkable, with arthrotic changes of the condyle and possibly on the temporal component. MR imaging, however, shows enlargement of the capsule suggestive of granulation tissue surrounding the implant. The T2-weighted image shown in Figure 7–47 shows high signal of the tissue between the implant and the temporal joint component, suggestive of the

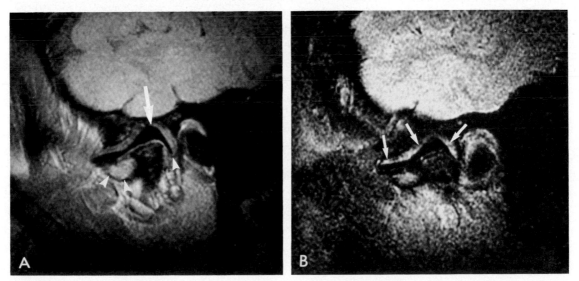

Figure 7–47
Proplast-Teflon implant with granulation tissue. A, Sagittal MR image showing the Proplast-Teflon implant (arrow). The joint capsule is expanded (arrowheads). B, A T2-weighted image shows a high signal of tissue between the implant and the temporal joint component (arrows) suggestive of granulation tissue.

inflammatory nature of this tissue. This is probably a further indication of the active process in the joint. More advanced changes occur with these implants when small particles from the implants are dispersed into the periarticular tissue (Fig. 7–46). Then a diffuse inflammatory reaction around the joint will develop. This is frequently associated with swelling and pain but may also be asymptomatic. Erosions into the middle cranial fossa do occur with Proplast-Teflon implant, and these are best evaluated with thin-section coronal CT scans.

Imaging Strategy

What strategy should be employed when imaging patients with Proplast-Teflon implants? We recommend plane film as an initial screening modality.[83] The second imaging choice is MR imaging. This shows the implant, possible defects in the implant, and the extent of granulation tissue in the periarticular tissue. To evaluate the integrity of the roof of the glenoid fossa and the articular eminence with respect to the possibility of erosions and perforations into the middle cranial fossa, thin-section CT scan is frequently necessary. This can be done with both direct sagittal and direct coronal CT scans, but the direct coronal scan is more easily obtained in a routine clinical practice and is therefore recommended over direct sagittal scan.

Follow-up imaging after removal of the Proplast-Teflon implant is not well documented. Thin-section coronal CT scan is probably optimal for the first few years until stable conditions have developed. A suggestion for imaging protocol of joints with Proplast-Teflon implant is described in Table 7–2.

DERMAL GRAFT

Because of the problem with alloplastic implants, there has been a trend in TMJ surgery to find alternative disk replacement material. One is the autogenous dermal graft.[84–86] Surgical procedures using autogenous dermal graft began in the early 20th century and involved bone, joints, and gastrointestinal tract.[87, 88] In 1957 to 1962, Georgiade and coworkers published articles on the use of dermal grafts in the TMJ.[84, 89] They suggested that the disk is necessary to prevent development of arthrosis,[90] and in order not to leave the condyle directly against the temporal component they suggested that some material has to be used to replace the disk. Instead of using alloplastic material with its inherent disadvantage, clinicians have attempted to use dermal graft. Other surgeons have attempted to use autogenous cartilage from the external ear,[91] a pedicled temporalis/pericranial flap,[92] and a temporalis muscle flap.[93, 94] Imaging evaluation of joints with ear cartilage or temporalis flap is probably similar to that of joints with dermal grafts. In all these situations we recommend baseline postoperative MR imaging for future evaluation of the joint.

COMPLICATIONS OF TEMPOROMANDIBULAR JOINT SURGERY

Unsuccessful TMJ surgery can lead to bony ankylosis. This can be evaluated with plain film, tomography, or computed tomography (Fig. 7–48). Computed

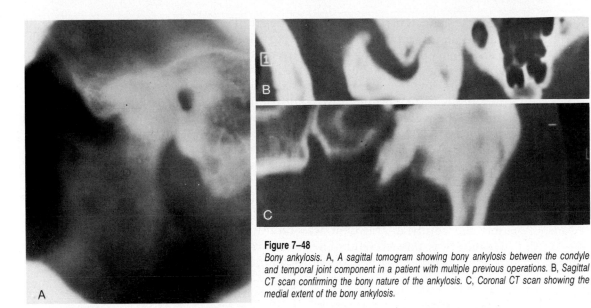

Figure 7–48
Bony ankylosis. A, A sagittal tomogram showing bony ankylosis between the condyle and temporal joint component in a patient with multiple previous operations. B, Sagittal CT scan confirming the bony nature of the ankylosis. C, Coronal CT scan showing the medial extent of the bony ankylosis.

tomography is preferred over regular plain film tomography because of higher soft and hard tissue resolution. Direct coronal imaging is of significant value for the assessment of the medial part of the joint. Both direct sagittal and direct coronal imaging can be performed, but the coronal plane of imaging is usually more practical. For planning of operation for ankylosis of the TMJ, extensive ankylosis in the medial part of the joint has to be evaluated preoperatively to provide information about how deep it extends and its relationship to the vital structures medial to the joint.

Another sequela of TMJ surgery may be small metallic fragments in the osseous and soft tissue structures of the joint. This is not a complication of the surgery, but when postoperative MR imaging is performed (Fig. 7–49), the

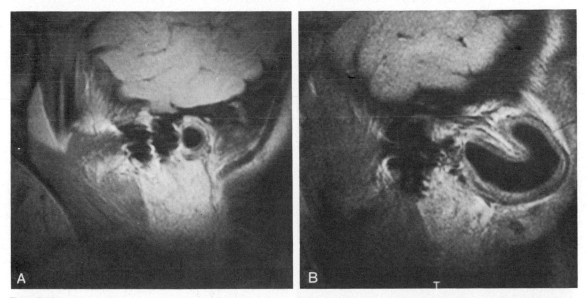

Figure 7–49
Metal artifact. A, MR image of a patient with metal wires in the articular eminence. The irregular areas of signal void bordered by areas of higher signal are indicative of metal artifacts. B, Metal artifacts from a prior operation in which metallic instruments were used. The metallic fragments were not seen on plain films or tomograms.

metallic artifacts can deteriorate the image. The metallic fragments are probably the result of minuscule metallic particles left from scraping with metallic instruments on the bony surface, from drilling, or from wires used to fixate an implant (Fig. 7–49). The fragments are usually so small that they are not seen with plain images or even with CT scanning. They are seen in both painful and nonpainful postoperative joints[40] and are probably of no clinical significance. Their greater significance is the prevention of diagnostic MR images in some cases.

If the metallic particles are located outside the joint, MR imaging of the joint proper usually can be successful. Metallic screws or other fixation devices outside the joint are no contraindication to MR imaging.

Failure of healing of a high condylar fracture in spite of attempts with fixation is shown in Figure 7–50. The patient sustained a high condylar fracture, and the condylar fragment was repositioned and fixated with a metal pin. Healing was unsuccessful. The metal fixation pin moved out of the condylar fragment, which became ankylosed in the glenoid fossa.

TOTAL JOINT REPLACEMENT

Total replacement of the TMJ has been attempted for many years.[95, 96] There continue to be problems with stabilization of both the glenoid and condyle parts of the prosthesis. A custom-made implant based on a model of the bone generated from CT scanning is presently under development. This is still in the experimental stage, and further research will show whether adequate stabilization, function, and long-term results can be achieved.

Imaging of the joint with total replacement is somewhat limited because of the large metallic component. Attempts have been made to use MR imaging, but the signal void artifacts from the metal condyle have been so extensive that conclusive images usually cannot be obtained. CT imaging cannot be optimally performed because of extensive metallic artifacts. Conventional tomography is frequently the only imaging technique that routinely produces diagnostic images (Fig. 7–51). In conventional tomography it is essential to evaluate evidence of

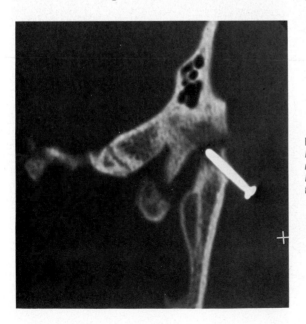

Figure 7–50
Pseudarthrosis. Coronal CT scan showing a metallic pin located only in a ramus fragment. The condylar fragment ankylosed with the glenoid fossa. Lytic changes in the bone around the metallic pin are seen. A fragment of the condyle is displaced medially and inferiorly.

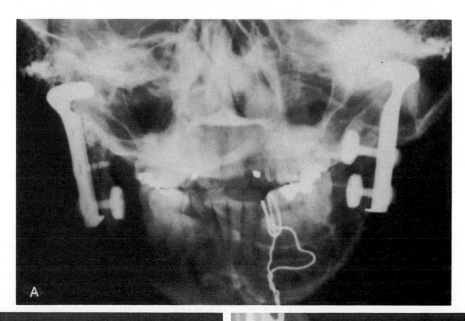

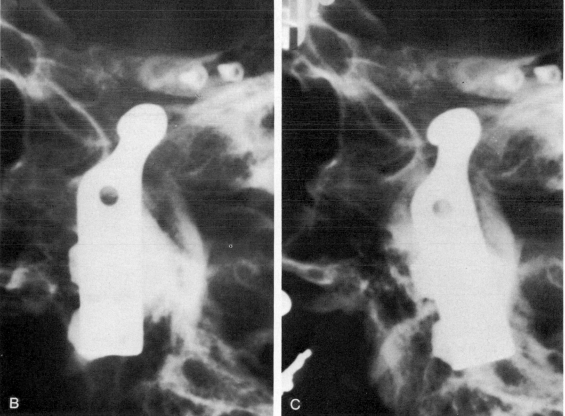

Figure 7–51
Bilateral total joints. A, AP plain film showing bilateral total joint replacement. The condylar fragments are attached to the ramus of the mandible. A Proplast-Teflon fossa implant is attached to the articular eminence and the zygomatic arch with screws. B, Closed-mouth view showing the implant in place. C, Open-mouth view showing rotation and translation of the implant.

loosening or displacement of the implants. The interphase between the implant and the bone should be carefully studied.

COSTOCHONDRAL GRAFTS

Early work in the area of costochondral graft to the TMJ was done by Blackwood, Meikle, Poswillo, and Laskin and their associates.[97–100] Indications for reconstruction with costochondral graft include ankylosis, aplasia, hypoplasia, extensive infectious disease, osteoarthrosis, rheumatoid arthritis, and other conditions in which there is significant condylar resorption, such as neoplastic disease. In young individuals, costochondral grafts do have a potential for growth, and in some cases gross asymmetries of the mandible can be avoided by their use.[101–104] More recently, since Proplast is no longer available and total joint replacement is used less frequently, costochondral grafts have enjoyed increased popularity for reconstruction of the postsurgical adult TMJ.

Imaging of the costochondral graft can be done with plain films, conventional tomography, and computed tomography. However, these techniques all have the disadvantage of not showing the nonmineralized parts of the implant that articulate against the temporal component. Figure 7–52 shows a patient with healed bilateral costochondral grafts close to the ramus of the mandible on both left and right sides. The nonmineralized superior parts of the implant are not visualized with CT. With CT scanning a three-dimensional image can be produced (Fig. 7–53). This is an excellent technique for evaluation of the positional relationship between the facial skeleton, mandible, and costochondral graft.

A superior way to image costochondral grafts is MR imaging, because the nonmineralized parts of the costochondral graft can also be visualized. Figure 7–54 is an example of a patient with a costochondral graft placed several years ago who is now free of symptoms. The patient was imaged because of symptoms on the opposite side. Another example of MR imaging of a costochondral graft approximately 1 year after operation is shown in Figure 7–55. The patient continued to experience pain in the operated joint. The T2-weighted MR image shows joint effusion in the joint space, which suggests the presence of inflammatory changes. There was a good range of motion. The implants were secured to the mandible with metallic wires, as seen in the illustration but these

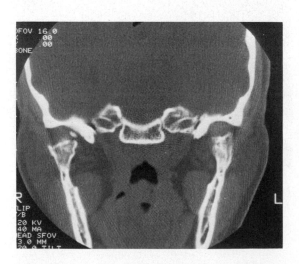

Figure 7–52
Costochondral graft. A coronal CT scan shows bilateral costochondral grafts that are well healed to the ramus of the mandible on both left and right sides. The osseous parts of the rib grafts are visualized. The cartilaginous parts by which the implant is articulating against the glenoid fossa are not visualized on this CT scan.

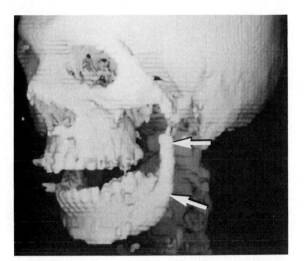

Figure 7–53
Three-dimensional CT scan of a patient operated on with a costochondral graft for hemifacial microsomia. The rib graft (arrows) is seen to substitute for the mandibular ramus. There is anterior open bite. The cartilaginous part of the costochondral graft is not visualized on this scan.

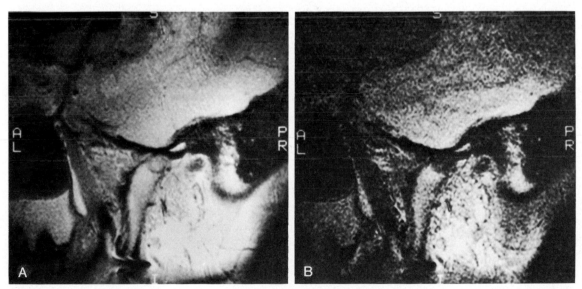

Figure 7–54
Costochondral graft. A, Sagittal MR scan showing a costochondral graft in a patient with hemifacial microsomia. The rib graft is well visualized. The articular eminence is underdeveloped, which is characteristic for the hemifacial microsomia. The temporal bone and the mastoid air cells are also underdeveloped. B, A T2-weighted image of the same joint shows no area of high signal that could suggest joint effusion.

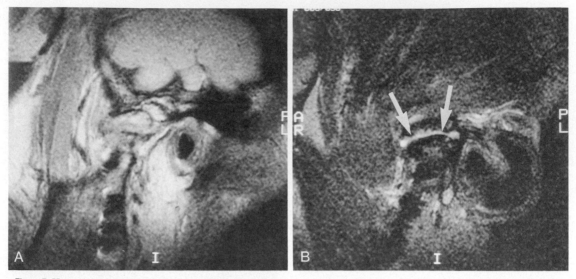

Figure 7–55
Painful costochondral graft. A, Sagittal MR scan showing the ramus of the mandible with multiple areas of artifact from wires that are holding a rib graft in place. The rib graft is visualized. B, In the lateral aspect of the joint is an area of high signal along the top surface of the rib graft (arrows) that suggests some inflammatory reaction.

were located inferiorly enough that they did not interfere with the image of the joint.

Imaging Strategy

MR imaging is the preferred method for imaging of costochondral grafts. If there is a specific question with regard to the osseous status of the implant or the glenoid fossa, thin-section coronal CT scan is recommended.

CONCLUSION

Postsurgical imaging of patients who continue to experience pain or dysfunction after surgery or conservative treatment may be of significant value for assessment of joint morphology. In general, MR imaging is the procedure of choice if there is no metallic implant in the joint region. CT scan may be necessary to evaluate the integrity of the roof of the glenoid fossa when perforation of the glenoid fossa into the middle cranial fossa is suspected. In cases with a large metallic implant, conventional tomography is the imaging modality of choice.

References

1. Boman K: Temporomandibular joint arthrosis and its treatment by extirpation of the disc. Acta Chir Scand (Suppl 118) 1947;*95*:1–225.
2. Silver CM: Long-term results of meniscectomy of the temporomandibular joint. Cranio 1984;*3*:47–57.
3. Hall HD: Meniscectomy for damaged disks of the temporomandibular joint. South Med J 1985;*78*:569–572.

4. Eriksson L, Westesson P-L: Long-term evaluation of meniscectomy of the temporomandibular joint. J Oral Maxillofac Surg 1985;*43:*263–269.
5. Tolvanen M, Oikarinen VJ, Wolf J: A 30-year follow-up study of temporomandibular joint meniscectomies: A report on five patients. Br J Oral Maxillofac Surg 1988;*26:*311–316.
6. Wilkes CH: Surgical treatment of internal derangements of the temporomandibular joint. A long-term study. Arch Otolaryngol Head Neck Surg 1991;*117:*64–72.
7. McCarty WL Jr, Farrar WB: Surgery for internal derangements of the temporomandibular joint. J Prosthet Dent 1979;*42:*191–196.
8. Politis C, Stoelinga PJ, Gerritsen GW, Heyboer A: Long-term results of surgical intervention on the temporomandibular joint. Cranio 1989;*7:*319–330.
9. Anderson DM, Sinclair PM, McBride KM: A clinical evaluation of temporomandibular joint disk plication surgery. Am J Orthod Dentofac Orthop 1991;*100:*156–162.
10. Montgomery MT, Gordon SM, Van Sickels JE, Harms SE: Changes in signs and symptoms following temporomandibular joint disc repositioning surgery. J Oral Maxillofac Surg 1992;*50:*320–328.
11. Gallagher DM, Wolford LM: Comparison of Silastic and Proplast implants in the temporomandibular joint after condylectomy for osteoarthritis. J Oral Surg 1982;*40:*627–730.
12. Carter JB: Meniscectomy in the management of chronic internal derangements of the TMJ. Abstracts of the Scientific Sessions, Annual Meeting of the American Association of Oral and Maxillofacial Surgeons, 1983.
13. Kiersch TA: The use of Proplast implants for meniscectomy and disk repair in the temporomandibular joint. Abstracts of the Clinical Congress of the American Academy of Oral and Maxillofacial Surgeons, 1984.
14. Ryan DE: Alloplastic implants in the temporomandibular joint. Oral Maxillofac Surg Clin North Am 1989;*1:*427–441.
15. Spagnoli D, Kent JN: Multicenter evaluation of temporomandibular joint Proplast-Teflon disk implant. Oral Surg Oral Med Oral Pathol 1992;*74:*411–421.
16. Farrar WB: Diagnosis and treatment of anterior dislocation of the articular disc. NY J Dent 1971;*41:*348–351.
17. Farrar WB: Differentiation of temporomandibular joint dysfunction to simplify treatment. J Prosthet Dent 1972;*28:*629–636.
18. Farrar WB: Characteristics of the condylar path in internal derangement of the TMJ. J Prosthet Dent 1978;*39:*319–323.
19. Lundh H, Westesson P-L, Kopp S, Tillström B: Anterior repositioning splint in the treatment of temporomandibular joints with reciprocal clicking. Comparison with a flat occlusal splint and an untreated control group. Oral Surg Oral Med Oral Pathol 1985;*60:*131–136.
20. Manzione JV, Tallents R, Katzberg RW, Oster C, Miller TL: Arthrographically guided splint therapy for recapturing the temporomandibular joint meniscus. Oral Surg Oral Med Oral Pathol 1984;*57:*235–240.
21. Tallents RH, Katzberg RW, Miller TL, Manzione J, Macher DJ, Roberts C: Arthrographically assisted splint therapy: Painful clicking with a nonreducing meniscus. Oral Surg Oral Med Oral Pathol 1986;*61:*2–4.
22. Miller TL, Katzberg RW, Tallents RH, Bessette RW, Hayakawa K: Temporomandibular joint clicking with nonreducing anterior displacement of the meniscus. Radiology 1985;*154:*121–124.
23. Moloney F, Howard JA: Internal derangements of the temporomandibular joint. III. Anterior repositioning splint therapy. Aust Dent J 1986;*31:*30–39.
24. Tallents RH, Katzberg RW, Miller TL, Manzione JV, Oster C: Arthrographically assisted splint therapy. J Prosthet Dent 1985;*53:*235–238.
25. Tallents RH, Katzberg RW, Miller TL, Manzione JV, Oster C: Evaluation of arthrographically assisted splint therapy in treatment of TMJ disk displacement. J Prosthet Dent 1985;*53:*836–838.
26. Lundh H, Westesson P-L: Temporomandibular joint displacement: Arthrographic and tomographic followup after six months of treatment with disc repositioning onlays. Oral Surg Oral Med Oral Pathol 1988;*66:*271–278.
27. Clark GT: A critical evaluation of orthopedic interocclusal appliance therapy: Design, theory, and overall effectiveness. J Am Dent Assoc 1984;*108:*359–364.
28. Lundh H, Westesson P-L: Long-term follow-up after occlusal treatment to correct an abnormal temporomandibular joint disk position. Oral Surg Oral Med Oral Pathol 1989;*67:*2–10.
29. Le Bell Y, Kirveskari P: Treatment of reciprocal clicking of the temporomandibular joint using a mandibular repositioning splint and occlusal adjustment. Proc Finn Dent Soc 1985;*81:*251–255.
30. Bronstein SL: Post surgical TMJ arthrography. J Craniomandib Pract 1984;*2:*165–171.
31. Conway WF, Hayes CW, Campbell RL, Laskin DM, Swanson KS: Temporomandibular joint after meniscoplasty: Appearance at MR imaging. Radiology 1991;*180:*749–753.
32. Moses JJ, Sartoris D, Glass R, Tanaka T, Poker I: The effect of arthroscopic surgical lysis and lavage of the superior joint space on TMJ disc position and mobility. J Oral Maxillofac Surg 1989;*47:*674–678.

33. McCain JP, Podrasky EA, Zabiegalski NA: Arthroscopic disc repositioning and suturing: A preliminary report. J Oral Maxillofac Surg 1992;*50:*568–579.

34. Kaplan PA, Reiskin AB, Tu HK: Temporomandibular joint arthrography following surgical treatment of internal derangement. Radiology 1987;*163:*217–220.

35. Westesson P-L, Eriksson L: Diskectomy of the temporomandibular joint: A double-contrast arthrotomographic follow-up study. Oral Surg Oral Med Oral Pathol 1985;*59:*435–440.

36. Eriksson L, Westesson P-L: Diskectomy in the treatment of anterior disk displacement of the temporomandibular joint. A clinical and radiological one-year follow-up study. J Prosthet Dent 1986;*55:*106–116.

37. Agerberg G, Lundberg M: Changes in the temporomandibular joint after surgical treatment. A radiologic followup study. Oral Surg Oral Med Oral Pathol 1971;*32:*865–875.

38. Steinhardt G: Zur Entstehung und konservativen Behandlung der Kiefergelenkstörungen (insbesondere der Bewegungsstörungen und des Gelenkknackens). Osterr Z Stomatol 1957;*54:*69–76.

39. Vogl T, Kellermann O, Randzio J, Kniha H, Requardt H, Tiling R, Lissner J: Results of magnetic resonance tomography of the temporomandibular joint using optimized surface coils. Rofo: Fortschr Gebiete Rontgenstr Nuklearmed 1988;*149:*502–507.

40. Hansson L-G, Eriksson L, Westesson P-L: Temporomandibular joint: Magnetic resonance evaluation after diskectomy. Oral Surg Oral Med Oral Pathol 1992;*74:*801–810.

41. Silagi J, Schow C: Temporomandibular joint arthroplasty: Review of literature and report of case. J Oral Surg 1970;*28:*920–926.

42. Wukelich S, Marshall J, Walden R, et al: Use of a Silastic testicular implant in reconstruction of the temporomandibular joint of a 5-year old child. Oral Surg Oral Med Oral Pathol 1971;*32:*4–9.

43. Palmer D, Perdersen GW: Arthroplasty for bilateral temporomandibular joint ankylosis: Report of case. J Oral Surg 1972;*30:*816–820.

44. Estabrooks LN, Murnane TW, Doku HC: The role of condylotomy with interpositional silicone rubber in temporomandibular joint ankylosis. Oral Surg Oral Med Oral Pathol 1972;*34:*2–6.

45. Hartwell SW Jr, Hall MD: Mandibular condylectomy with silicone rubber replacement. Plast Reconstr Surg 1974;*53:*440–444.

46. Lewin RW, Wright JA: Silastic ulnar head prosthesis for use in surgery of the temporomandibular joint. J Oral Surg 1978;*36:*906–914.

47. Alpert B: Silastic tubing for interpositional arthroplasty. J Oral Surg 1978;*36:*153.

48. DeChamplain RW, Gallagher CS Jr, Marchall ET Jr: Autopolymerizing Silastic for interpositional arthroplasty. J Oral Maxillofac Surg 1988;*46:*522–525.

49. Hansen WC, Dezhazo BW: Silastic reconstruction of temporomandibular joint meniscus. Plast Reconstr Surg 1969;*43:*388–391.

50. Henny FA: Surgical treatment of the painful temporomandibular joint. J Am Dent Assoc 1969;*79:*171–177.

51. Sanders B: Surgical treatment of the TMJ. Abstracts of the Clinical Congress of the American Association of Oral and Maxillofacial Surgeons, 1981.

52. Ryan DE: Meniscectomy with Silastic implants. Abstracts of the Clinical Congress of the American Association of Oral and Maxillofacial Surgeons, 1984.

53. Aptekar RG, Davie JM, Cattell HS: Foreign body reaction to silicone rubber: Complication of a finger joint implant. Clin Orthop 1974;*98:*231–232.

54. Worsing RA Jr, Engber WD, Lange TA: Reactive synovitis from particulate Silastic. J Bone Joint Surg 1982;*64A:*581–585.

55. Rosenthal DJ, Rosenberg AE, Schiller AL, Smith RJ: Destructive arthritis due to silicone: A foreign-body reaction. Radiology 1983;*149:*69–72.

56. Eiken O, Lindström C, Jonsson K: Silicone carpal implants: Risk or benefit? Scand J Plast Reconstr Surg 1985;*19:*295–304.

57. Martini AK, Rohe K: Synovitis of the wrist joint following silicone replacement of the carpal bones. Handchir Mikrochir Plast Chir 1988;*20:*295–300.

58. Shergy WJ, Urbaniak JR, Polisson RP: Silicone synovitis: Clinical, radiologic, and histologic features. South Med J 1989;*82:*1156–1158.

59. Verhaar J, Vermeulen A, Bulstra S, Walenkamp G: Bone reaction to silicone metatarsophalangeal joint hemiprosthesis. Clin Orthop 1989;*245:*228–232.

60. Christie AJ, Pierret G, Levitan J: Silicone synovitis. Semin Arthritis Rheum 1989;*19:*166–171.

61. Sennwald G: Silastic implant and synovitis. Schweiz Med Wochenschr 1989;*119:*1010–1012.

62. Perlman MD, Schor AD, Gold ML: Implant failure with particulate silicone synovitis (detritic synovitis). J Foot Surg 1990;*29:*584–588.

63. Wanivenhaus A, Lintner F, Wurnig C, Missaghi-Schinzi M: Long-term reaction of the osseous bed around silicone implants. Arch Orthop Trauma Surg 1991;*110:*146–150.

64. Trepman E, Ewald FC: Early failure of silicone radial head implants in the rheumatoid elbow. A complication of silicone radial head implant arthroplasty. J Arthroplasty 1991;*6:*59–65.

65. Eriksson L, Westesson P-L: Temporomandibular joint diskectomy: No positive effect of temporary silicone implant in a five-year follow-up. Oral Surg Oral Med Oral Pathol 1992;*74:*259–272.

66. Westesson P-L, Eriksson L, Lindström C: Destructive lesions of the mandibular condyle following diskectomy with temporary silicone implant. Oral Surg Oral Med Oral Pathol 1987;*63:*143–150.

67. Dolwick MF, Aufemorte TB: Silicone-induced foreign body reaction and lymphadenopathy after temporomandibular joint arthropathy. Oral Surg Oral Med Oral Pathol 1985;*59:*449–452.

68. Kneeland JB, Carrera GF, Ryan DL, Jesmanowicz A, Froncisz W, Hyde JS: MR imaging of a fractured temporomandibular disk prosthesis. J Comput Assist Tomogr 1987;*11:*199–200.

69. Hartman LC, Bessette RW, Baier RE, Meyer AE, Wirth J: Silicone rubber temporomandibular joint (TMJ) meniscal replacements: Post implant histopathologic and material evaluation. J Biomed Mater Res 1988;*22:*475–484.

70. Tucker MR, Burkes EF Jr: Temporary Silastic implantation following discectomy in the primate temporomandibular joint. J Oral Maxillofac Surg 1989;*12:*1290–1295.

71. Grundlach KKH: Long-term results following surgical treatment of internal derangement of the temporomandibular joint. J Craniomaxillofac Surg 1990;*18:*206–209.

72. Bosanquet AG, Ishimaru J-I, Goss AN: The effect of Silastic replacement following discectomy in sheep temporomandibular joints. J Oral Maxillofac Surg 1991;*49:*1204–1209.

73. Kiersch TA: The use of Proplast-Teflon implants for meniscectomy and disk repair in the use temporomandibular joint (abstract). Presented at the 63rd annual AAOMS Clinical Congress on Reconstructive Biomaterials: Current Assessment and Temporomandibular Joint: Surgical Update. San Diego, California, January 1984.

74. Estabrooks LN, Fairbanks CE, Collett RJ, Miller L: A retrospective evaluation of 301 TMJ Proplast-Teflon implants. Oral Surg Oral Med Oral Pathol 1990;*70:*381–386.

75. Fontenot MG, Kent JN: In vitro wear performance of Proplast TMJ disc implants. J Oral Maxillofac Surg 1992;*50:*133–139.

76. Scales JT, Stinson NB: Tissue reaction to polytetrafluoroethylene. Lancet 1964;*7323:*169.

77. Charnley J: Tissue reaction to polytetrafluoroethylene. Lancet 1963;*7322:*1379.

78. Heffez L, Mafee MF, Rosenberg H, Langer B: CT evaluation of TMJ disc replacement with a Proplast-Teflon laminate. J Oral Maxillofac Surg 1987;*45:*657–665.

79. Lagrotteria L, Skipino R, Granston AS, Felgenhauer D: Patients with lymphadenopathy following temporomandibular joint arthroplasty with Proplast. Cranio 1986;*4:*172–178.

80. Kneeland JB, Ryan DE, Carerra G, Jesmanowicz A, Froncisz W, Hyde JS: Failed temporomandibular joint prosthesis: MR imaging. Radiology 1987;*165:*179–181.

81. Schellhas KP, Wilkes CH, El Deeb M, Lagrotteria LB, Omlie MR: Permanent Proplast temporomandibular joint implants. MR imaging of destructive complications. AJR 1988;*151:*731–735.

82. Katzberg RW, Laskin DM: Radiographic and clinical significance of temporomandibular joint alloplastic disk implants. AJR 1988;*151:*736–737.

83. Kaplan PA, Ruskin G, Tu HK, Knibbe MA: Erosive arthritis of the temporomandibular joint caused by Teflon-Proplast implants: Plain film features. AJR 1988;*151:*337–339.

84. Georgiade N, Altany F, Pickrell K: Experimental and clinical evaluation of autogenous dermal grafts used in the treatment of TMJ ankylosis. Plast Reconst Surg 1957;*19:*321–336.

85. Zetz MR, Irby WB: Repair of the adult temporomandibular joint meniscus with an autogenous dermal graft. J Oral Maxillofac Surg 1984;*42:*167–171.

86. Meyer RA: The autogenous dermal graft in temporomandibular joint disc surgery. J Oral Maxillofac Surg 1988;*16:*948–954.

87. Loewe O: Ueber Hautimplantation an stelle der freien Faszienplastik. Münch Med Wochensch 1913;*60:*1320–1328.

88. Rehn E, Miyauchi Y: Das cutane und subcutane Bindegewebe in veränderter Funktion. Arch Klin Chir 1914;*105:*1–15.

89. Georgiade N: The surgical correction of temporomandibular joint dysfunction by means of autogenous dermal grafts. Plast Reconstr Surg 1962;*30:*68–73.

90. Ioannides C, Freihofer HP: Replacement of the damaged interarticular disc of the TMJ. J Craniomaxillofac Surg 1988;*16:*273–278.

91. Witsenburg B, Freihofer HPM: Replacement of the pathological temporomandibular articular disc using autogenous cartilage of the external ear. Int J Oral Surg 1984;*13:*401–405.

92. Feinberg SE, Larsen PE: The use of a pedicled temporalis muscle–pericranial flap for replacement of the temporomandibular joint disc: Preliminary report. J Oral Maxillofac Surg 1989;*47:*142–146.

93. Albert TW, Merrill RG: Temporal myofascial flap for reconstruction of the temporomandibular joint. Oral Maxillofac Surg Clin North Am 1989;*1:*341–349.

94. Brusati R, Raffaini M, Sesenna E, Bozzetti A: The temporalis muscle flap in temporomandibular joint surgery. J Craniomaxillofac Surg 1990;*18:*352–358.

95. Kent JN, Misiek DJ, Akin RK, Hinds EC, Homsy CA: Temporomandibular joint condylar prosthesis: A ten-year report. J Oral Maxillofac Surg 1983;*41:*245–254.

96. Kent JN, Block MS, Homsy CA, Prewitt JM III, Reid R: Experience with a polymer glenoid fossa prosthesis for partial or total temporomandibular joint reconstruction. J Oral Maxillofac Surg 1986;*44:*520–533.

97. Laskin DM, Sarnat G, Bain J: Respiration and anaerobic glucolysis of transplanted cartilage. Proc Soc Exp Biol Med 1952;*79:*474–482.

98. Blackwood HJJ: Growth of the mandibular condyle of the rat studied with tritiated thymidine. Arch Oral Biol 1966;*2:*394–398.

99. Meikle MC: In vivo transplantation of the mandibular joint of the rat: An autoradiographic investigation into cellular changes at the condyle. Arch Oral Biol 1973;*18:*1011–1020.

100. Poswillo D: Experimental reconstruction of the mandibular joint. Int J Oral Surg 1974;*3:*400–411.

101. Politis C, Fossion E, Bossuyt M: The use of costochondral grafts in arthroplasty of the temporomandibular joint. J Craniomaxillofac Surg 1987;*15:*345–354.

102. Daniels S, Ellis E III, Carlson DS: Histologic analysis of costochondral and sternoclavicular grafts in the TMJ of the juvenile monkey. J Oral Maxillofac Surg 1987;*45:*675–682.

103. Obeid G, Guttenberg SA, Connole PW: Costochondral grafting and condylar replacement and mandibular reconstruction. J Oral Maxillofac Surg 1988;*48:*177–188.

104. MacIntosh RB: Costochondral and dermal grafts in temporomandibular joint reconstruction. Oral Maxillofac Surg Clin North Amer 1989;*1:*363–397.

PART THREE

Imaging Miscellaneous Conditions

CHAPTER EIGHT

Tore A. Larheim

Rheumatoid Arthritis and Related Joint Diseases

GENERAL DISEASE CHARACTERISTICS

Rheumatoid arthritis and related joint diseases consist of a number of inflammatory disorders that are characterized by prominent inflammation of the synovial membrane. Rheumatoid arthritis (RA) is the most frequent, but other well-known diseases are the seronegative spondyloarthropathies, e.g., ankylosing spondylitis and psoriatic arthropathy. RA occurs in 4.5 per cent of people over the age of 55 years in the United States.[1] Because of the chronic nature of the disease, the prevalence increases with age. An average age at onset of 40 years (SD 14 years) is compatible with what would be expected, based on current knowledge of RA.[2] Women are affected two to three times more often than men. Most frequently, the joint involvement is symmetric with afflictions of small joints, in particular the metacarpophalangeal joints, proximal interphalangeal joints, wrists, and metatarsophalangeal joints.[3, 4]

Affected joints are usually swollen, and joint motion is limited. The main clinical symtoms are morning stiffness and joint pain; however, great variations are seen in the clinical picture. A fluctuating, but progressive, disease course is typical, with exacerbations and remissions. Some patients will be completely disabled.[2] Disease activity and impairment of joint mobility usually will have a great impact on patients' health status and quality of life.

PATHOLOGIC AND IMAGING ABNORMALITIES

Edema and cellular accumulation result in a macroscopically evident thickened synovial membrane, with synovial villous formation and joint effusion. These changes in peripheral joints are accompanied by characteristic radiographic abnormalities:[5, 6] fusiform soft tissue swelling, peri-articular osteoporosis, uniform loss of interosseous space because of cartilage reduction and destruction, and marginal erosion of bone, which relates to the location of the aggressive inflammatory synovial tissue, or pannus, in peripheral portions of the joint where bone does not possess protecting cartilage. Though these four radiographic abnormalities are considered classic early manifestations of RA, they may not all be evident on the initial radiographic examination. In more advanced stages of the disease, bone destruction may occur with lytic defects in cortical bone, corresponding to intraosseous extension of inflamed synovium. In long-standing RA, secondary osteoarthrosis may be observed, and the end-stage may become intra-articular fibrous ankylosis or, occasionally, bony ankylosis.

A recent review of the roles of radiography and other imaging techniques in evaluation of arthritis concluded that conventional radiography is still the mainstay of all examinations in arthritic patients.[7] However, in this era of advancing imaging technology, magnetic resonance imaging (MRI), computed tomography (CT), ultrasound, nuclear medicine imaging, and arthrography are all being used to study patients with arthritis.

A challenge in diagnostic imaging has been the assessment of disease activity, which in clinical practice is determined by physical examination findings. One feature common to most forms of arthritis is increased regional blood flow. This may be evident on flow images of technetium-99m phosphate or diphosphonate bone study.[7] Because of destructive and productive changes in adjacent bones, static images from bone scintigraphy will also reveal increased uptake of radionuclide in periarticular regions. Though very nonspecific, the increase in periarticular uptake of bone-scanning radionuclides may precede conventional radiographic findings in arthritis.[8, 9] Most recently, gadopentetate-enhanced MRI has been used to evaluate activity of disease in RA. The use of gadopentetate dimeglumine as an MR contrast agent allows the identification of an active synovial proliferative disease and allows the synovial membrane to be distinguished from joint effusion in RA.[10–12]

Juvenile rheumatoid arthritis (JRA) affects patients below 16 years of age. Although the histologic picture is similar to that of RA in adults, JRA differs in many respects.[13] Some of the illustrations in this chapter are of adults with JRA; TMJ abnormalities in such patients are sometimes quite similar to those found in patients with adult onset of chronic arthritis.

INVOLVEMENT OF THE TEMPOROMANDIBULAR JOINT

Villous synovitis, the major pathologic abnormality found also in the temporomandibular joint (TMJ), may lead to formation of synovial granulomatous tissue, pannus, growing into fibrocartilage and bone,[6] paralleling findings in other joints involved by chronic arthritic diseases. Evidence of arthritic disease in the TMJ has been demonstrated in surgical procedures,[14, 15] in autopsy specimens,[16] and by the different imaging modalities discussed in the following sections.

TMJ involvement has been known since the term *rheumatoid arthritis* was introduced more than a century ago,[17] and a frequency of 68 per cent in a series of 293 patients was reported as early as 1898.[18] Though the frequency of clinical TMJ affection has varied considerably, most studies indicate that at least 50 per cent of the patients with RA will exhibit symptoms or signs of TMJ involvement during the disease course.[17] The TMJ may also be involved in the seronegative spondyloarthropathies, though fewer studies than on RA are available. Pain, stiffness/tiredness, sounds (crepitus), tenderness on palpation, and limited mouth opening are the most frequent symptoms or signs of TMJ involvement in chronic arthritic diseases. Joint swelling is occasionally reported by patients, but it is seldom observed at clinical examination. Disturbances of the dental occlusion associated with arthritic TMJ involvement are loss of occlusal support, occlusal interferences, and, most characteristically, anterior bite opening. Discrepancies between subjective symptoms and radiographic abnormalities may be found; symptomatic joints may show little or no bone abnormality,[19] whereas silent joints may show mutilating abnormalities.[20]

PLAIN RADIOGRAPHY, TOMOGRAPHY, AND COMPUTED TOMOGRAPHY

Bone destruction or deformation, a result of the inflammatory process, until recently has been the only abnormality of importance in the radiographic assessment of TMJ involvement. Although similar in appearance, bony TMJ abnormalities have been associated with different arthritic diseases. Besides RA, the most important are ankylosing spondylitis and psoriatic arthropathy.[17] The frequency of TMJ abnormalities varies in the different diseases but seems to be highest in RA; most comprehensive studies indicate figures in the range of 50 to 80 per cent.[17] Bony TMJ abnormalities may be depicted with plain film as well as panoramic radiography, but such methods are inferior to tomography concerning minor cortical erosions.[19, 21]

In a series of patients with RA, including some with ankylosing spondylitis and psoriatic arthropathy, any of the radiographic methods evaluated (panoramic, transcranial, or transpharyngeal) demonstrated about 80 per cent of the abnormal TMJs, as revealed by oblique sagittal hypocycloidal tomography.[19] If other radiographic methods are negative or uncertain in such patients, tomographic examination, preferably with hypocycloidal motion, is recommended for better visualization of the bony structures. With tomography, bone destruction may characteristically be found as "punched-out" destructions at various locations throughout the joint (Figs. 8–1, 8–2, and 8–3).

A recent study of patients with chronic arthritic disease indicated computed tomography to be superior to hypocycloidal tomography for depicting subtle bony abnormalities,[22] although agreement between CT and tomography was high concerning the total number of abnormal TMJs. Of 30 joints examined in 15 adults, 21 were found to be abnormal using CT and 20 were abnormal on tomography. The bony details were better demonstrated by the multiplanar CT imaging, particularly in the most lateral and medial parts of the joint, owing to superior contrast and spatial resolution (Fig. 8–3). In two joints in

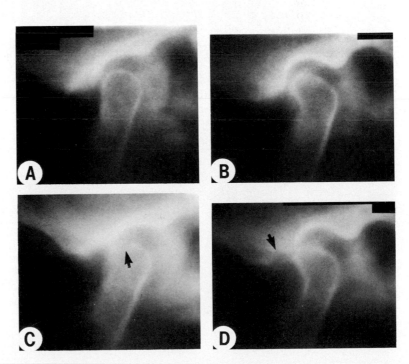

Figure 8–1
Hypocycloidal (oblique sagittal) tomography of a 60-year-old woman with rheumatoid arthritis. A and B, Initial studies show normal condyle and temporal bone. C and D, One-year follow-up studies show cortical erosion in the condyle and eminence (arrows). (B and D from Larheim TA: Imaging of the temporomandibular joint in rheumatic disease. In Westesson P-L, Katzberg R, eds: Imaging of the Temporomandibular Joint. Baltimore, Williams & Wilkins, 1991, pp 133–153.)

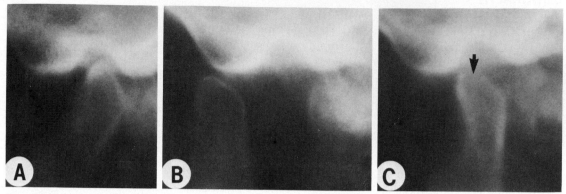

Figure 8–2

Hypocycloidal (oblique sagittal) tomography of a 34-year-old woman with psoriatic arthropathy. A, Closed-, and B, open-mouth tomograms show normal bone and condylar translation. C, A 7-month follow-up study (with a severely impaired ability to open the mouth) shows cortical erosion on the posterosuperior aspect of the condyle (arrow) and severely impaired translation. (From Larheim TA, Smith H-J, Aspestrand F: Rheumatic disease of temporomandibular joint with development of anterior disk displacement as revealed by magnetic resonance imaging. A case report. Oral Surg Oral Med Oral Pathol 1991;71:246–249.)

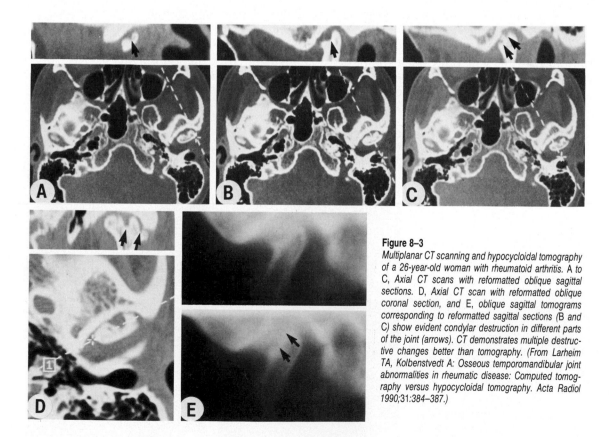

Figure 8–3

Multiplanar CT scanning and hypocycloidal tomography of a 26-year-old woman with rheumatoid arthritis. A to C, Axial CT scans with reformatted oblique sagittal sections. D, Axial CT scan with reformatted oblique coronal section, and E, oblique sagittal tomograms corresponding to reformatted sagittal sections (B and C) show evident condylar destruction in different parts of the joint (arrows). CT demonstrates multiple destructive changes better than tomography. (From Larheim TA, Kolbenstvedt A: Osseous temporomandibular joint abnormalities in rheumatic disease: Computed tomography versus hypocycloidal tomography. Acta Radiol 1990;31:384–387.)

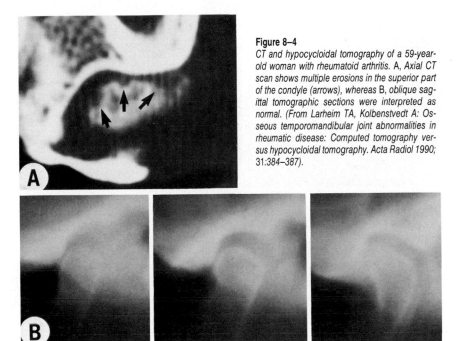

Figure 8–4
CT and hypocycloidal tomography of a 59-year-old woman with rheumatoid arthritis. A, Axial CT scan shows multiple erosions in the superior part of the condyle (arrows), whereas B, oblique sagittal tomographic sections were interpreted as normal. (From Larheim TA, Kolbenstvedt A: Osseous temporomandibular joint abnormalities in rheumatic disease: Computed tomography versus hypocycloidal tomography. Acta Radiol 1990; 31:384–387).

which CT showed minor erosions in the most superior parts of the condyle, tomography was normal in one and uncertain in the other (Fig. 8–4). In my experience, CT is particularly valuable in the assessment of bony ankylosis.

Longitudinal examinations are essential to show progression of abnormalities in arthritic patients (see Figs. 8–1, 8–2, and 8–5). With hypocycloidal tomography it is possible to demonstrate development or progression of small cortical erosions during a period as short as 3 months (Fig. 8–5). In joints with high disease activity, severe bone destruction may develop (Fig. 8–6). Although unilateral abnormalities may occur, bilateral TMJ abnormalities are most frequently seen.[17, 19]

In postoperative imaging of arthritic patients, plain film and tomographic methods are valuable to show TMJ remodeling and reparative changes, which are seen in arthritic joints after synovectomy and diskectomy (Figs. 8–7 and 8–8).

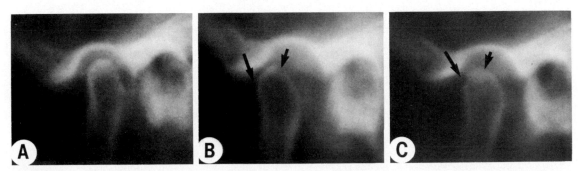

Figure 8–5
Hypocycloidal (oblique sagittal) tomography of a 31-year-old woman with rheumatoid arthritis. A, Initial study shows normal bone. B, A 3-month follow-up study shows small condylar cortical erosions (arrows). C, A 6-month follow-up study shows progression of the condylar erosions (arrows). Bone erosions were confirmed at operation. (From Larheim TA: Imaging of the temporomandibular joint in rheumatic disease. In Westesson P-L, Katzberg R, eds: Imaging of the Temporomandibular Joint. Baltimore, Williams & Wilkins, 1991, pp 133–153.)

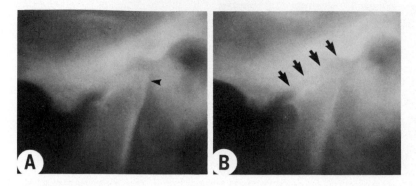

Figure 8–6

Hypocycloidal tomography (oblique sagittal sections) of a 64-year-old woman with rheumatoid arthritis (same joint as shown in Figure 8–1). A shows a severely deformed condyle with apposition of bone posteriorly (arrowhead), and B shows obvious bone apposition that has created a new fossa/eminence (arrows). Advanced bone abnormalities were confirmed at operation. (B from Larheim TA, Smith H-J, Aspestrand F: Temporomandibular joint abnormalities associated with rheumatic disease: Comparison between MR imaging and arthrotomography. Radiology 1992;183:221–226.)

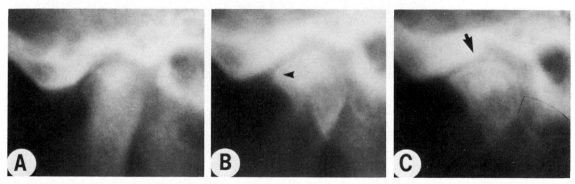

Figure 8–7

Hypocycloidal (oblique sagittal) tomography of a 28-year-old woman with juvenile rheumatoid arthritis (same joint as shown in Figure 8–15). A, Initial section shows normal bone. B and C, Three-year postoperative sections; after diskectomy (normally positioned disk with perforation in the central thin part) and synovectomy with removal of synovial proliferation, condylar remodeling (arrowhead) and flattening/apposition of bone in the eminence/fossa (arrow) are seen.

Figure 8–8

Transcranial radiography (A, B, D, and E) and hypocycloidal (oblique sagittal) tomography (C and F) of a 38-year-old woman with psoriatic arthropathy (same joint as shown in Figure 8–20). A, B, and C, Preoperative studies (B at maximally opened mouth) show severely impaired condylar translation and condylar destruction (arrow). D and E, Postoperative 1-year (E at maximally opened mouth) and F, 3-year studies; after diskectomy (anteriorly displaced disk) and synovectomy with removal of synovial proliferation/pannus formation in the condylar destruction, excellent condylar translation, and condylar remodeling and evident bone apposition (arrowheads) in the fossa are seen. C, Condyle.

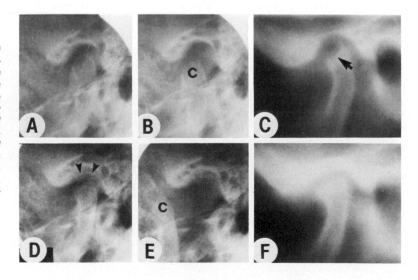

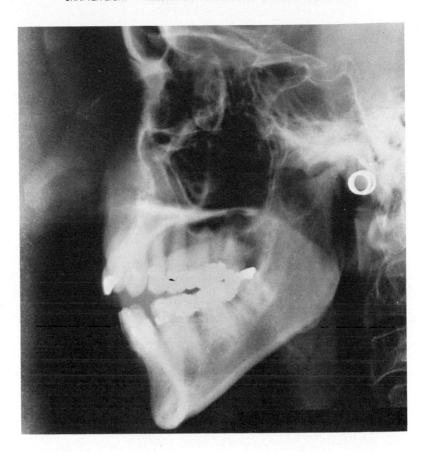

Figure 8–9
Lateral cephalogram of a 52-year-old man with rheumatoid arthritis shows severe anterior open bite with contact only on the second molars caused by complete destruction of both condyles. (From Larheim TA, Storhaug K, Tveito L: Temporomandibular joint involvement and dental occlusion in a group of adults with rheumatoid arthritis. Acta Odontol Scand 1983;41:301–309.)

Collapse of the mandibular condyles may lead to a posterior rotation of the mandible with anterior bite opening as a result (Fig. 8–9). This complication is not frequent and is seen in patients with bilateral and severe TMJ involvement.[17, 20, 23] Severe destructive changes may be accompanied by evident remodeling and reparative changes even in older patients (see Fig. 8–6), though productive and reparative bone changes seem to be more dominating in patients with childhood onset of arthritis[13] (Fig. 8–10). The two patients illustrated in Figures 8–6 and 8–10A did not show any evidence of anterior bite opening and mandibular rotation, probably because of the severe TMJ remodeling.

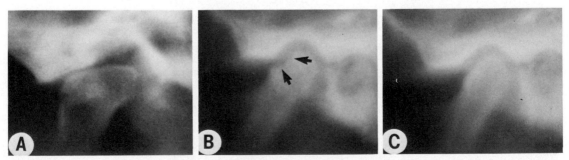

Figure 8–10
Hypocycloidal (oblique sagittal) tomography of patients with juvenile rheumatoid arthritis. A shows a severely deformed TMJ with extensive remodeling of the condyle and fossa/eminence. (This is the contralateral joint of the 28-year-old woman shown in Figure 8–7.) B, The initial study of an 18-year-old patient shows condylar destruction (arrows). C, A 3-year follow-up study of the patient in B shows an apparently normal condyle, indicating bony healing. At follow-up study, the patient was in general disease remission and had not received specific TMJ treatment.

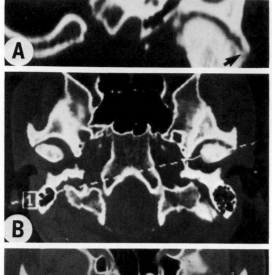

Figure 8–11
CT of a 25-year-old woman with ankylosing spondylitis. A, Reformatted oblique coronal section, and B and C, axial scans show severe bone abnormalities, with bony fusion in the most lateral part of the joint (arrows). Bony ankylosis was confirmed at operation. (From Larheim TA, Kolbenstvedt A: Osseous temporomandibular joint abnormalities in rheumatic disease. Computed tomography versus hypocycloidal tomography. Acta Radiol 1990;31:383–387.)

Another serious, though infrequent, complication of arthritic TMJ involvement is development of osseous ankylosis. This abnormality, which needs surgical treatment, seems to be best depicted with CT (Figs. 8–11 and 8–12). In both cases of osseous TMJ ankylosis in the patient series previously mentioned,[22] we had to supplement our TMJ studies with CT. Bony fusion was demonstrated only with CT in one case and more clearly with CT than hypocycloidal tomography in the other. It is interesting that both patients had ankylosing spondylitis, which is generally considered to be more bone productive than RA.[6]

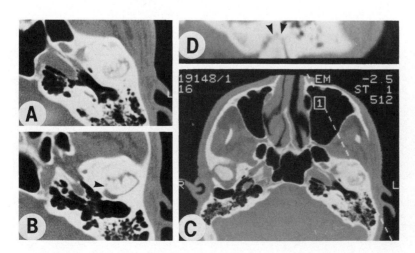

Figure 8–12
CT of a 32-year-old man with ankylosing spondylitis. A to C, Axial scans, and D, oblique sagittal reformatted image show bony fusion in different parts of the joint (arrowheads), confirmed at operation. (From Larheim TA, Bjørnland T, Smith H-J, et al: Imaging temporomandibular joint abnormalities in rheumatic disease: Comparison with surgical observations. Oral Surg Oral Med Oral Pathol 1992;73:494–501.)

Figure 8–13
Arthrotomography and MRI (oblique sagittal sections) of a 30-year-old woman with juvenile rheumatoid arthritis. A, Tomogram shows a flattened condyle with subcortical sclerosis (arrow). B, T1-weighted image shows a flattened condyle with subcortical decreased signal intensity (arrowhead) (corresponding to sclerosis on the tomogram) and an apparently normal disk. Due to the normal disk position, the degenerative changes are interpreted as secondary to chronic arthritis. (From Larheim TA, Smith H-J, Aspestrand F: Rheumatic disease of the temporomandibular joint: MR imaging and tomographic manifestations. Radiology 1990;175:527–531.)

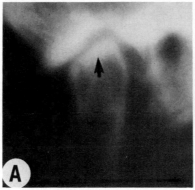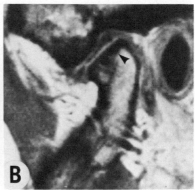

In summary, osseous TMJ abnormalities in patients with chronic arthritic disease show a great range of variation. Destructive changes may vary from minor cortical erosion to severe and complete condylar destruction; bony reaction may be evident and occasionally may lead to osseous ankylosis. Follow-up studies are of great value for observing progression of bone destruction, which may be rapid and severe in chronic TMJ arthritis. However, even reparative changes may be seen. Though punched-out destructions at variable sites throughout the joint or completely destroyed condyles (sometimes accompanied by anterior open bite) may be considered rather characteristic of arthritic TMJ involvement, the radiographic abnormalities, particularly when accompanied by productive changes, may be similar to those of degenerative TMJ disease. Examination of the soft tissue may then be necessary to verify the TMJ diagnosis (Fig. 8–13). Recent studies have shown that soft tissue abnormalities caused by chronic arthritic disease may be indicated by arthrotomography or magnetic resonance imaging.[24, 25]

Table 8–1 indicates the relative merits of the different imaging modalities for the assessment of cortical bone abnormalities in the TMJ in patients with chronic arthritic diseases.

ARTHROTOMOGRAPHY

Arthrotomographic TMJ studies in arthritic patients have demonstrated that abnormalities in the soft tissue are frequent in joints with bone abnormalities.[24] Irregularity in the outline of contrast medium and small joint compartment(s) is an indirect sign of synovial proliferation/pannus formation (Fig. 8–14).

Perforation between joint compartments, as revealed by contrast medium flowing from the lower to the upper compartment, has been found in 40 per cent of TMJs involved by chronic arthritis.[24] In contrast to internal TMJ

Table 8–1
VALUE OF TMJ IMAGING MODALITIES FOR CORTICAL BONE CHANGES IN ARTHRITIS

Plain Film or Panoramic Radiography	MRI	Tomography (Hypocycloidal)	CT
+	+ +	+ + +	+ + + +

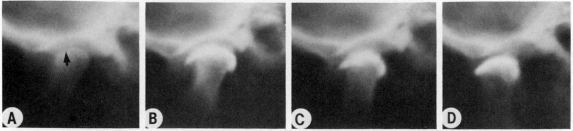

Figure 8–14
Hypocycloidal tomography and arthrotomography (oblique sagittal sections) of a 20-year-old woman with rheumatoid arthritis. A, Tomogram shows condylar flattening with erosion (arrow). B, C, and D, Corresponding arthrotomograms at closed (B), half open (C), and maximally open mouth (D), show contrast medium in the lower compartment with irregularity in the outline and a small anterior recess, indicative of synovial proliferation/pannus formation. Note the abnormal configuration of the posterior recess at the mouth opening despite no (or minimal) filling in the anterior recess, suggesting normal disk position. (From Larheim TA, Björnland T: Arthrographic findings in the temporomandibular joint in patients with rheumatic disease. J Oral Maxillofac Surg 1989;47:780–784.)

derangement, perforation may be found in arthritic joints showing normal bone and in the central thin part of a normally positioned disk (Fig. 8–15).

The arthrotomographic characteristics of arthritic involvement versus internal derangement are demonstrated in Figure 8–16, showing a patient with RA who was re-examined with TMJ arthrotomography after a period of 3.5 years.

MAGNETIC RESONANCE IMAGING

MRI has recently demonstrated its potential to assess soft tissue abnormalities associated with arthritic TMJ involvement.[25] Soft tissue abnormalities as evaluated with this imaging modality may show a great range of variation: flattening, fragmentation, heterogeneity, or poor delineation of the disk (Figs. 8–17 and 8–18). In severe rheumatic disease the disk may be completely destroyed (Fig. 8–19). These findings are indirect signs of synovial proliferation/pannus formation, which seems to be difficult to visualize directly by unenhanced MRI in a small joint like the TMJ.[25] MRI, however, may show other signs of inflammation, such as joint effusion and condylar marrow edema.

Disk Position

Both arthrotomographic and MRI studies have shown that the position of the disk most frequently is normal in TMJs involved by chronic arthritis (see

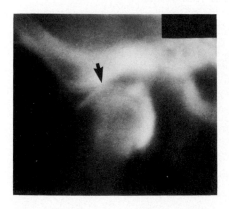

Figure 8–15
Arthrotomogram (oblique sagittal) of a 28-year-old woman with juvenile rheumatoid arthritis (same joint as shown in Figure 8–7) shows contrast medium in both compartments (filling through perforation, preoperatively judged to be in the central thin part of the disk, arrow), small joint compartments (0.45 ml injected), some irregularity in outline of the contrast medium, normal disk position, and normal bone (cf. Figure 8–7A). Surgical therapy showed synovial proliferation consistent with rheumatic involvement, the disk in normal position, perforation in the central thin part of the disk, and normal bone. (From Björnland T, Larheim TA, Haanaes HR: Surgical treatment of temporomandibular joints in patients with chronic arthritic disease: Pre-operative findings and one-year follow-up. J Craniomandib Pract 1992;10:205–210.)

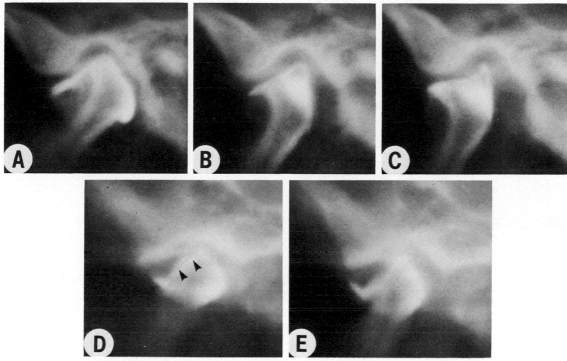

Figure 8–16

Arthrotomography (oblique sagittal) of a woman (23 years old at initial examination) with rheumatoid arthritis. A, B, and C, Initial studies show contrast medium (0.6 ml injected) in the lower compartment at closed (A), half open (B), and maximally open mouth (C) consistent with anterior disk displacement with reduction. D and E, Follow-up studies 3.5 years later show a small lower compartment (0.3 ml injected) with irregularities in outline (arrowheads), indicating rheumatic involvement, and an enlarged anterior recess at E, indicating anterior disk displacement without reduction. (Tomography showed cortical erosions both in the condyle and eminence.) Synovial proliferation/pannus formation consistent with rheumatic involvement and cortical erosions were found at operation (the disk position, however, was interpreted as normal). (D and E from Larheim TA, Smith H-J, Aspestrand F: Temporomandibular joint abnormalities associated with rheumatic disease: Comparison between MR imaging and arthrotomography. Radiology 1992;183:221–226.)

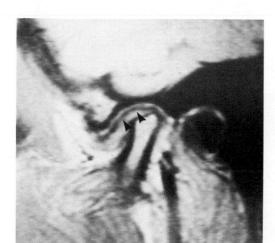

Figure 8–17

Proton density-weighted (oblique sagittal) MR image of a 20-year-old woman with juvenile arthritis shows an abnormal disk (arrowheads), flattened with uniform thickness, and a deformed condyle. (From Larheim TA, Smith H-J, Aspestrand F: Rheumatic disease of the temporomandibular joint: MR imaging and tomographic manifestations. Radiology 1990;175:527–531.)

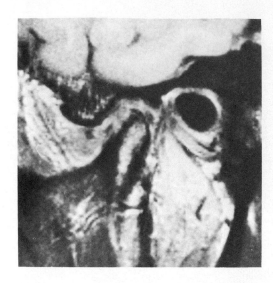

Figure 8–18
T1-weighted (oblique sagittal) MR image of a 28-year-old man with psoriatic arthropathy shows a fragmented disk and condylar destruction. (From Larheim TA, Smith H-J, Aspestrand F: Rheumatic disease of the temporomandibular joint: MR imaging and tomographic manifestations. Radiology 1990;175:527–531.)

Figs. 8–13 through 8–15), though anterior disk position may occur (Figs. 8–16 and 8–20).[24, 25] In a recent surgical TMJ study on patients with chronic arthritic diseases, the occurrence of either normal or anterior disk position in joints involved by arthritis was confirmed.[15] In some joints a completely destroyed disk, as indicated by MRI, was surgically verified. In TMJs involved by chronic arthritis, even a posterior position of the disk has been reported (Fig. 8–21). However, the disk position in arthritic joints may be difficult to decide, even with MRI.

The rather high proportion of anterior disk displacement in joints involved by arthritic disease is an interesting observation. This may be coincidental, but a recent case study suggests that there may be a causal relationship between the two conditions.[26] Another aspect to be further studied is whether anterior disk displacement in a TMJ involved by chronic arthritis may complicate the condition for the patient and have implications for the treatment decision.[15]

Magnetic Resonance Imaging Versus Arthrotomography

As noted, both arthrotomography and MRI have the potential to depict soft tissue and bone abnormalities associated with arthritic TMJ involvement. In recent comparative imaging studies, correlating with surgical observations,[27, 28] these imaging modalities frequently demonstrated soft tissue as well

Figure 8–19
MRI and hypocloidal tomography (oblique sagittal sections) of a 25-year-old woman with ankylosing spondylitis. A, T1-weighted MR image shows the disk completely destroyed, replaced by soft tissue (showing no increased signals on T2-weighted images), and severe bone destruction. Fibrous pannus without any disk structure and bone destruction were found at operation. B, Tomogram shows severe bone destruction (arrow) and condylar sclerosis corresponding to reduced signal intensity on the MR image.

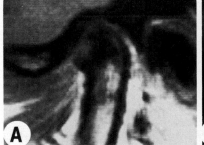
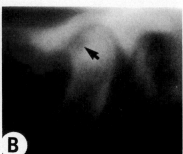

(From Larheim TA, Bjørnland T, Smith H-J, et al: Imaging temporomandibular joint abnormalities in patients with rheumatic disease: Comparison with surgical observations. Oral Surg Oral Med Oral Pathol 1992;73:494–501.)

Figure 8–20

Arthrotomography (oblique sagittal) of a 38-year-old woman with psoriatic arthropathy (same joint as shown in Figure 8–8). A, Closed, and B, open mouth show an enlarged anterior recess consistent with anterior disk displacement without reduction, irregularity in outline of the contrast medium, and gaps between the contrast medium and bone (arrowheads), consistent with synovial proliferation/pannus formation. Bone destruction, anterior disk displacement, and synovial proliferation/pannus formation were confirmed at operation. (From Larheim TA,

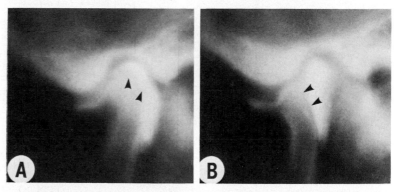

Bjørnland T: Arthrographic findings in the temporomandibular joint in patients with rheumatic disease. J Oral Maxillofac Surg 1989;47:780–784.)

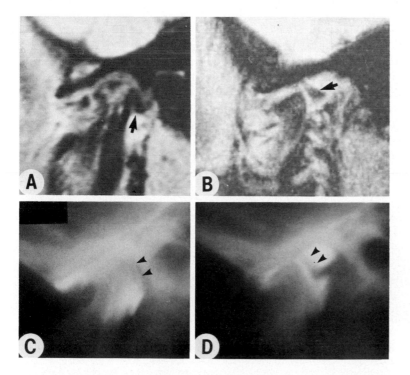

Figure 8–21

MRI and arthrotomography (oblique sagittal sections) of a 17-year-old woman with juvenile rheumatoid arthritis. A, Proton density-weighted MR image at closed mouth, and B, FLASH (fast low angle shot) image at open mouth show larger disk fragment (arrows) posterior and adherent to the abnormally flat condyle. C and D, Corresponding arthrotomograms at closed (C) and open mouth (D) show contrast medium in small (0.45 ml injected) lower and upper compartments (filling of upper compartment through perforation), and an adherent disk in posterior position (arrowheads) on the abnormally flat condyle. (From Larheim TA, Smith H-J, Aspestrand F: Temporomandibular joint abnormalities associated with rheumatic disease: Comparison between MR imaging and arthrotomography. Radiology 1992;183:221–226.)

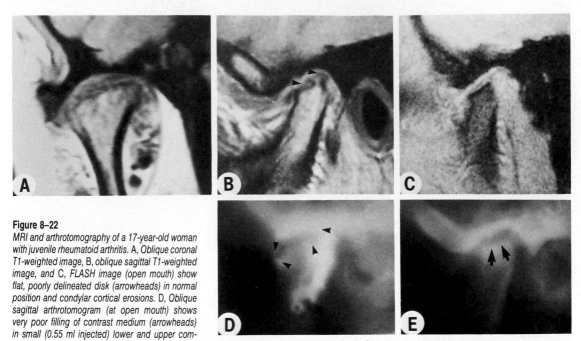

Figure 8–22
MRI and arthrotomography of a 17-year-old woman with juvenile rheumatoid arthritis. A, Oblique coronal T1-weighted image, B, oblique sagittal T1-weighted image, and C, FLASH image (open mouth) show flat, poorly delineated disk (arrowheads) in normal position and condylar cortical erosions. D, Oblique sagittal arthrotomogram (at open mouth) shows very poor filling of contrast medium (arrowheads) in small (0.55 ml injected) lower and upper compartments (filling of upper compartment through perforation), with some irregularities in outline and disk in normal position. E, Oblique sagittal tomogram shows condylar cortical erosions (arrows). Synovial proliferation/pannus formation consistent with rheumatic involvement, a normally positioned disk with perforation in the posterior attachment, and condylar erosions were found at operation. (From Larheim TA, Smith H-J, Aspestrand F: Temporomandibular joint abnormalities associated with rheumatic disease: Comparison between MR imaging and arthrotomography. Radiology 1992;183:221–226.)

as bone abnormalities in joints with evident arthritic involvement (Fig. 8–22). Whereas arthrotomography in such joints showed irregularly outlined joint spaces and small joint compartments, MRI showed abnormal disks. These complementary findings are indirect signs of synovial proliferations. Occasionally, arthrotomography depicted irregularities in the articular space not shown by MRI (Fig. 8–23). In joints with evident arthritic involvement, both hypocycloidal tomography and MRI frequently showed cortical bone erosions (Figs. 8–22 and 8–23).

In TMJs with more severe arthritic involvement, MRI was found to be superior to arthrotomography. As the only examination method, it can directly visualize a completely destroyed disk. If condylar translation is severely impaired

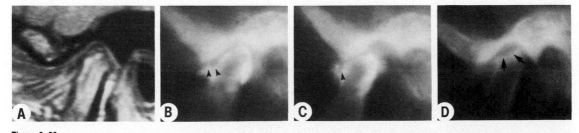

Figure 8–23
MRI and arthrotomography (oblique sagittal sections) of a 17-year-old woman with juvenile rheumatoid arthritis. A, T1-weighted MR image shows abnormally thin anterior band of the disk, normal disk position, and condylar erosion. B and C, Corresponding hypocycloidal arthrotomograms at closed (B) and open mouth (C) show contrast medium in small (0.4 ml injected) lower compartment, with irregularities in outline (arrowheads) indicating rheumatic involvement, and an apparently enlarged anterior recess indicating an anterior disk position. D, Corresponding hypocycloidal tomogram (closed mouth) shows condylar erosion (arrows). Synovial proliferation/pannus formation consistent with rheumatic involvement, normal disk position, and bone erosions were found at operation. (From Larheim TA, Smith H-J, Aspestrand F: Temporomandibular joint abnormalities associated with rheumatic disease: Comparison between MR imaging and arthrotomography. Radiology 1992;183:221–226.)

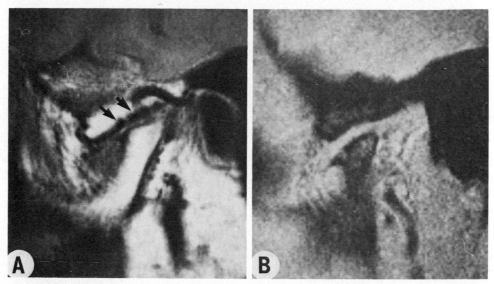

Figure 8–24
MRI (oblique sagittal sections) of a 64-year-old woman with rheumatoid arthritis (same joint as shown in Figures 8–1 and 8–6). A, T1-weighted image shows interosseous space with no evidence of disk (replacement by soft tissue showing no increased signal on T2-weighted images); a deformed, flat condyle; and a flat, entirely new fossa/eminence (arrows). B, FLASH (fast low angle shot) image at open mouth shows severely impaired condylar translation. Arthrography was not successful despite the evident interosseous space as assessed from tomography; see Figure 8–6. Fibrous ankylosis with no evidence of disk structure and a deformed condyle were found at operation. (A from Larheim TA, Smith H-J, Aspestrand F: Temporomandibular joint abnormalities associated with rheumatic disease: Comparison between MR imaging and arthrotomography. Radiology 1992;183:221–226.)

and the disk is replaced by a soft tissue that does not show increased signal on T2-weighted images, the condition most likely represents fibrous ankylosis (Figs. 8–19 and 8–24). The initial radiographic examination made of the joint shown in Figure 8–24 is shown in Figure 8–25, indicating development of a fibrous condition (surgically confirmed) within a period of 7.5 years. In TMJs showing such advanced arthritic abnormalities, arthrotomographic examination may be impossible to perform, despite an evident interosseous space as revealed by tomography (see Fig. 8–6). An autopsy study earlier indicated that fibrous ankylosis may be an end-stage of arthritic TMJ involvement,[16] in accordance with the general view on rheumatoid arthritis.[6] This also was confirmed in a recent surgical TMJ study of patients with chronic arthritis.[15]

In early involvement of the TMJ with arthritic disease, i.e., in cases with normal bone or small or uncertain cortical erosions, arthrotomographic examination may be more valuable than MRI. Arthrotomographic signs of arthritic TMJ involvement—small joint compartments, irregularity in outline of contrast medium, and disk perforation, not shown with MRI—have been demonstrated

Figure 8–25
A and B, Transcranial (oblique sagittal) radiography of a 57-year-old woman with rheumatoid arthritis (same joint as shown in Figures 8–1, 8–6, and 8–24). This initial examination was made 7.5 years prior to the imaging and surgical confirmation of a fibrous joint condition as shown in Figure 8–24 and indicates normal bone and excellent condylar translation at open mouth (B). The patient was initially referred for TMJ pain that was considered clinically to be caused by myalgia. C, Condyle.

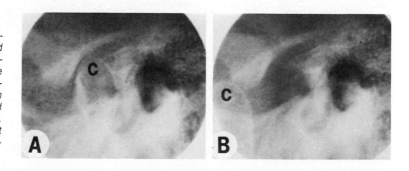

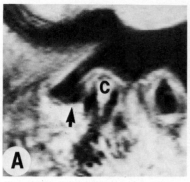

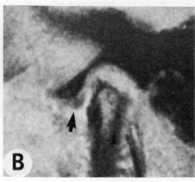

Figure 8–26

MRI (oblique sagittal sections) of a 26-year-old woman with rheumatoid arthritis (same joint as shown in Figure 8–16). A, Proton density-weighted image at closed mouth, and B, FLASH image at open mouth show internal derangement; anterior disk displacement without reduction (arrows); and normal bone. C, Condyle. Soft tissue abnormalities indicative of rheumatic involvement were demonstrated only by arthrotomography (see Figure 8–16D and E) and confirmed by the findings of synovial proliferation at operation.

(From Larheim TA, Smith H-J, Aspestrand F: Temporomandibular joint abnormalities associated with rheumatic disease: Comparison between MR imaging and arthrotomography. Radiology 1992;183:221–226.)

in joints with normal bone (see Fig. 8–15). Such arthrotomographic signs of chronic arthritis also have been demonstrated in joints with MRI interpretation of internal derangement (Figs. 8–16, 8–26, and 8–27). The assessment of joint compartment reduction as revealed by arthrotomographic follow-up studies (Fig. 8–27), strongly indicating arthritic development, is another advantage of arthrotomography over MRI. That thickened synovium indirectly seen by arthrotomography could not be directly depicted with MRI should perhaps be an expected finding. It has been shown that fibrous adhesions in internal TMJ derangement are not seen with MRI, although they may be indicated by arthrotomography[29, 30] or directly seen with arthroscopy.[31]

Arthroscopic examination probably will be of great value also for early detection of arthritic TMJ involvement, as recently demonstrated in a comprehensive study on knee joints involved by RA.[32]

Arthrotomographic interpretation may be false-positive concerning synovial proliferations, however. In 2 of 12 joints with similar arthrotomographic interpretation in patients with chronic arthritic disease, surgical therapy showed fibrous adhesions (and internal derangement).[28] Severe adhesions between disk and bone could explain the irregularly outlined joint space and poor filling,

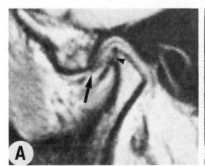

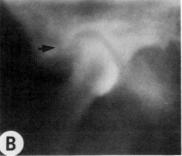

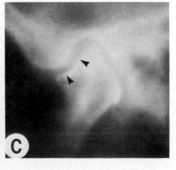

Figure 8–27

MRI and arthrotomography (oblique sagittal sections) of a 26-year-old woman with rheumatoid arthritis. A, T1-weighted MR image shows the disk in anterior position (arrow) and minor condylar cortical erosions (arrowhead). B, Arthrotomogram at the same time shows very poor and somewhat irregular filling of the anterior recess in the small (0.3 ml of contrast medium injected) lower compartment and erosion in the eminence (arrow). (Tomography showed minor condylar erosions.) C, Arthrotomogram made 3 years earlier of the same joint indicates the anterior disk position (arrowheads) but otherwise smooth and satisfactory filling of the lower compartment (0.6 ml of contrast medium injected) and normal bone in the eminence. (Tomography showed a normal condyle.) Note the similarity between A and C. MRI at the same time as C showed a similar appearance to A. Synovial proliferation/pannus formation consistent with rheumatic involvement, the disk in an anterior position, and resorption in the eminence and condyle were found at operation. (From Larheim TA, Bjørnland T, Smith H-J, et al: Imaging temporomandibular joint abnormalities in patients with rheumatic disease: Comparison with surgical observations. Oral Surg Oral Med Oral Pathol 1992;73:494–501.)

simulating arthritic involvement. The occurrence of fibrous adhesions in inter-nal TMJ derangement is a well-documented feature.[29-31] Arthrotomographic differentiation between joints showing anterior disk displacement, with and without arthritic involvement, may thus be difficult or impossible. The most important arthrotomographic sign seems to be the smaller joint compartments in arthritic joints.[28]

In the aforementioned comparative imaging studies of arthritic TMJs,[27, 28] the power of MRI probably has been underestimated. Oblique sagittal sections routinely have been used and oblique coronal sections only occasionally. More important, all MRI studies have been unenhanced. Contrast-enhanced MRI has proved to be of more value than unenhanced MRI in depicting synovial proliferations in the knee,[11-13] and our studies indicate its usefulness for depicting synovial proliferation also in the TMJ[33] (Fig. 8–28).

Perforation between compartments in TMJs with arthritic involvement is most reliably assessed with arthrographic examination,[28] in agreement with the general view that arthrography is the "gold standard" for imaging such pathology.[34] In arthritic joints with large perforations and disk fragmentations (see Fig. 8–21), however, good agreement between arthrotomography and MRI may be found.[27]

Disk position in joints involved by arthritic disease is reliably assessed with either dual-space arthrotomography or MRI (see Figs. 8–21 and 8–22),[27, 28] in accordance with studies on internal TMJ derangement.[34] However, in arthritic joints without perforations, MRI was found to be more reliable than lower space arthrotomography.[27, 28] By arthrotomography the disk may be incorrectly assessed as anterior due to irregular contrast filling of the anterior recess, also at impaired mouth opening (see Fig. 8–23). Or it may be incorrectly assessed as normal due to poor contrast filling of the anterior recess (Fig. 8–27). Thus, the assessment of disk position by lower space arthrography seems to be more difficult in arthritic joints than in joints with internal derangement, also because of the severely impaired condylar translation that frequently occurs in joints with chronic arthritis. It has been stressed that evaluation of the disk position by lower space arthrography should be based not only on the morphology of

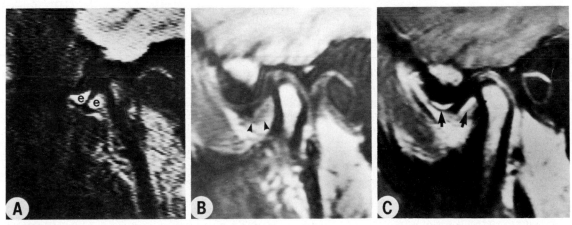

Figure 8–28
MRI (oblique sagittal sections) of a 34-year-old woman with rheumatoid arthritis, before (A and B) and after (C) intravenous contrast injection. A, Unenhanced T2-weighted image shows large effusion (e) in the anterior recess of both the upper and lower compartment. B, Unenhanced T1-weighted image shows an anteriorly displaced disk and a fluid-filled, bulging joint cavity of intermediate signal intensity (arrowheads). C, Contrast enhanced T1-weighted image shows a layer of enhancement on both sides of the disk (arrows). The effusion in the lower compartment is still intermediate gray. Synovial proliferation along the disk surface and normal bone was surgically confirmed. (From Smith H-J, Larheim TA, Aspestrand F: Rheumatic and non-rheumatic disease in the temporomandibular joint: Gadolinium-enhanced MR imaging. Radiology 1992;185:229–234.)

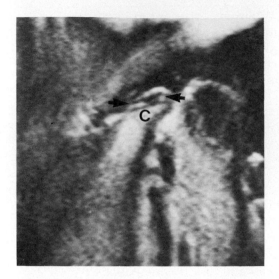

Figure 8–29
T2-weighted (oblique sagittal) MR image of a 64-year-old woman with rheumatoid arthritis (same joint as shown in Figure 8–4) shows an abnormal disk (arrows) (thin, no visible anterior band), joint effusion, and a deformed (flat) condyle (C). The disk position was assessed as normal in relation to the fossa/eminence. Synovial proliferation/pannus formation consistent with rheumatic involvement, the disk in normal position, and a deformed condyle were found at operation. (From Larheim TA, Bjørnland T, Smith H-J, et al: Imaging temporomandibular joint abnormalities in patients with rheumatic disease: Comparison with surgical observations. Oral Surg Oral Med Oral Pathol 1992;73:494–501.)

the anterior recess but also on functional (videofluoroscopic) analysis.[35, 36] In joints involved by chronic arthritis, the disk position may be difficult to determine even with MRI, due to abnormal disk morphology (see Fig. 8–17) or abnormal condylar morphology (Fig. 8–29). In cases with evident condylar destruction or deformation, the disk position should be considered in relation to the fossa and eminence.

In summary, soft tissue abnormalities in patients with chronic arthritic disease may vary considerably. In cases of severe arthritic involvement when arthrography is difficult or impossible to perform, MRI may directly depict disk destruction with soft tissue replacement, in addition to bone abnormalities. In these patients, MRI seems to be the procedure of choice for both diagnostic purposes and preoperative evaluation, although when osseous ankylosis is suspected, CT is preferred. In early arthritic involvement, MRI without contrast enhancement seems to be of limited value because of its inability to show synovial proliferation. Arthrotomography may indicate the presence of early chronic arthritis by showing irregularity in the outline of contrast medium, small joint compartments, and disk perforation, changes not shown by MRI. The procedure of choice in early arthritic TMJ involvement cannot be settled until the value of contrast-enhanced MRI has been clarified.

Table 8–2 summarizes the arthrotomographic and nonenhanced MRI signs indicative of chronic arthritic TMJ disease.

Table 8–2
ARTHROTOMOGRAPHIC AND NONENHANCED MRI SIGNS INDICATIVE OF CHRONIC ARTHRITIC TMJ DISEASE

Disease Characteristics	Arthrotomography	MRI
Irregularly outlined and small joint compartment	+	−
Perforation of normally positioned disk	+	−
Disk abnormality/destruction*	+	+
Fibrous ankylosis	−	+
Bone marrow abnormalities	−	+
Joint effusion	−	+

*In less advanced TMJ involvement, arthrotomography may be superior to nonenhanced MRI, whereas in more advanced TMJ involvement, MRI seems to be the superior method.

Magnetic Resonance Imaging Versus Hypocycloidal Tomography and Computed Tomography

The majority of the most characteristic bony abnormalities, i.e., the cortical erosions, will be depicted with hypocycloidal tomography, CT, or even MRI. In a series of patients with chronic arthritic diseases, multisection tomography— used as the routine method for assessing bony TMJ abnormalities—was false-negative concerning minor cortical erosions in 2 of 22 TMJs.[28] Possibly these could have been depicted with CT, which previously has proved to show bony details better than tomography. Cortical bone erosions also may be found with MRI, and a rather high agreement between hypocycloidal tomography and MRI concerning such erosions has been found.[25] However, MRI was recently found to be somewhat less accurate than hypocycloidal tomography concerning minor cortical erosions;[28] of 14 TMJs examined with both imaging modalities, MRI was false-negative in two and false-positive in one, compared with tomography and surgical observations. This is in agreement with two autopsy studies comparing MRI and cryosectional anatomy.[35, 36] In one of these studies MRI could give a false impression of bone erosion,[37] and in the other MRI was found to be inferior to CT for depicting cortical bone abnormalities.[38]

Magnetic resonance imaging is definitely superior, compared with hypocycloidal tomography and CT, in demonstrating other signs of inflammation, such as joint effusion and condylar marrow edema (Figs. 8–29, 8–30, and 8–31). Such inflammatory signs have been demonstrated both in TMJs with chronic arthritic diseases[25, 26] and in joints with internal derangement.[39] This capability of MRI makes it convenient to show exacerbation and subsidence of inflammation through increased and reduced signal intensity in the joint space and the condylar marrow, by longitudinal examinations[26] (Fig. 8–31).

Further, it has been demonstrated that MRI may show more severe arthritic TMJ involvement than is demonstrated by tomography,[25, 26] as indicated by the altered signal intensity within the condylar marrow (see Figs. 8–5 and 8–32). Similar signal intensity alterations also have been demonstrated in internal TMJ derangement.[40] Reduced signal intensity within the condylar marrow may also be reversible (Figs. 8–22, 8–31, and 8–33), if not representing sclerotic changes as shown with tomography (see Figs. 8–13 and 8–19).

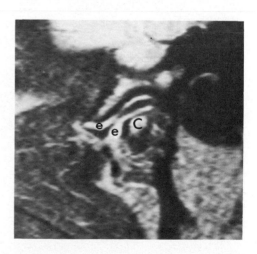

Figure 8–30
T2-weighted (oblique sagittal) MR image of a 14-year-old girl with juvenile rheumatoid arthritis shows normal disk position, deformed (flat) condyle (C), and increased signal intensity in both compartments consistent with joint effusion (e), as well as increased signal intensity in the condylar marrow, probably due to inflammatory edema. (From Larheim TA, Smith H-J, Aspestrand F: Rheumatic disease of the temporomandibular joint: MR imaging and tomographic manifestations. Radiology 1990;175:527–531.)

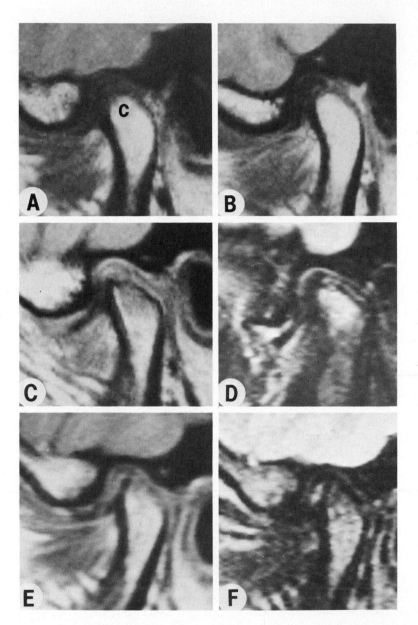

Figure 8–31
MRI (oblique sagittal) of a symptomatic (A and C to F) and an asymptomatic (B) joint in a 34-year-old woman with psoriatic arthropathy. A, Initial T1-weighted image of symptomatic right TMJ suggests a somewhat flat and poorly delineated disk in normal position and possibly slight cortical thinning in the superior part of the condyle (C). B, T1-weighted image of asymptomatic and presumably normal left TMJ for comparison. C, T1-weighted image 7 months later shows cortical destruction in the posterosuperior part of the condyle and reduced signal intensity in the marrow. D, Corresponding T2-weighted image shows increased signal in the lower and upper compartment consistent with joint effusion, and increased signal in the condylar marrow consistent with inflammatory edema. E, T1-weighted image 8 months later (i.e., 15 months after initial examination shown in A) shows almost normal signal intensity in the condylar marrow and, apparently, a partially destroyed disk with a more heterogeneous structure than on previous examinations. F, Corresponding T2-weighted image shows a slightly reduced signal intensity in the condylar marrow and minimal joint effusion. (From Larheim TA, Smith H-J, Aspestrand F: Rheumatic disease of temporomandibular joint with development of anterior disk displacement as revealed by magnetic resonance imaging. A case report. Oral Surg Oral Med Oral Pathol 1991; 71:246–249.)

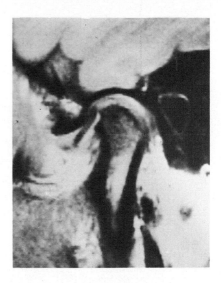

Figure 8–32
MRI (oblique sagittal, T1-weighted) of a 31-year-old woman with rheumatoid arthritis shows an anteriorly displaced and flat ("discoid") disk, condylar cortical erosions, and decreased signal intensity in the condylar marrow. Compare with the corresponding tomogram of the same joint (Figure 8–5C), which shows erosions but no abnormalities within the condylar marrow, corresponding to the extensive area of reduced signal intensity on the MR image, which represents rather extensive arthritic involvement. (From Larheim TA, Smith H-J, Aspestrand F: Rheumatic disease of the temporomandibular joint: MR imaging and tomographic manifestations. Radiology 1990;175:527–531.)

IMAGING STRATEGY

An imaging strategy for patients with chronic arthritic diseases and TMJ symptoms is presented in Table 8–3. Initial TMJ imaging should focus on bone abnormalities, since cortical destruction frequently is associated with rheumatic TMJ involvement in such patients. Plain film or panoramic examinations usually will show moderate or advanced bone destruction. Thus, in patients with severe TMJ involvement, such methods may be sufficient for radiographic diagnosis. For the assessment of minor cortical erosions, tomography or CT is necessary and should be performed if the initial examinations are negative or uncertain or if more detailed information is needed concerning the bony abnormalities, as for preoperative planning. If osseous ankylosis is suspected, CT is the method of choice.

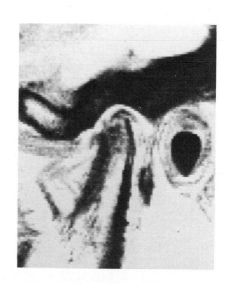

Figure 8–33
MRI (oblique sagittal, T1-weighted) of a 17-year-old woman with juvenile rheumatoid arthritis shows condylar cortical erosions and reduced signal intensity in the condylar marrow, indicating rather extensive arthritic involvement. The corresponding MR image of the same joint made half a year later (Figure 8–22B) shows almost normal signal intensity in the condylar marrow, indicating subsidence of inflammatory involvement. (From Larheim TA: Imaging of the temporomandibular joint in juvenile rheumatoid arthritis. In Westesson P-L, Katzberg R, eds: Imaging of the Temporomandibular Joint. Baltimore, Williams & Wilkins, 1991, pp 155–172.)

Table 8–3
IMAGING STRATEGY IN PATIENTS WITH CHRONIC ARTHRITIC DISEASE AND TMJ SYMPTOMS

1. Bone imaging:	2. Soft tissue imaging:
Plain film or panoramic radiography	MRI*
Tomography	Arthrotomography
CT	

*Gadolinium-enhanced imaging may depict the proliferating synovium.

For examination of the soft tissue, MRI is the first choice, if available. Disk displacement as a differential diagnosis may then be ruled out, and abnormal or completely destroyed disk (fibrous ankylosis) may be assessed. Additionally, the presence of joint effusion and condylar marrow edema indicative of disease activity may be evaluated. MRI is also valuable for assessment of bone. For depicting the proliferating synovium, gadolinium-enhanced imaging is necessary. Arthrotomographic examination should be performed if MRI is not available or is nondiagnostic, since disk perforation and small compartments indicative of synovial proliferation may be assessed only with arthrotomography. In cases scheduled for operative treatment, both soft tissue and bone imaging should be performed; soft tissue as well as bone abnormalities are frequently present in TMJs involved by chronic arthritic disease.

FUTURE PERSPECTIVES

A challenge in future imaging research of the TMJ in patients with chronic arthritic diseases probably will be the visualization of the synovial proliferation, which is a keypoint in distinguishing chronic arthritic diseases from other TMJ disorders. The capability of advanced imaging technology to detect active inflammatory changes within the joint probably will be utilized in longitudinal studies to monitor or perhaps even alter treatment. The disk displacement in chronic arthritic TMJs, whether or not incidental, and its significance for patient management, also should be a subject for future research in this field.

Acknowledgment

I thank Hans-Jørgen Smith, MD, PhD, for reviewing the text and illustrations of this chapter.

References

1. McDuffie FC: Morbidity impact of rheumatoid arthritis in society. Am J Med 1985;*78*:1–5.
2. Sherrer YS, Block DA, Mitchell DM, Young DY, Fries FJ: The development of disability in rheumatoid arthritis. Arthritis Rheum 1986;*29*:494–500.
3. Harris ED Jr: The clinical features of rheumatoid arthritis. *In* Kelley WN, Harris ED, Ruddy S, Sledge CB, eds: Textbook of Rheumatology. 3rd ed. Philadelphia, WB Saunders, 1989, pp 943–981.
4. Larsen A, Dale K: Standardized radiological evaluation of rheumatoid arthritis in therapeutic trials. *In* Dumonde DC, Jasani MK, eds: The Recognition of Anti-rheumatic Drugs. Lancaster, MTP Press, 1978, pp 285–292.
5. Larsen A, Dale E, Eek M: Radiographic evaluation of rheumatoid arthritis and related conditions by standard reference films. Acta Radiol [Diagn] (Stockh) 1977;*18*:481–491.
6. Resnick D: Common disorders of synovium-lined joints: Pathogenesis, imaging abnormalities, and complications. AJR 1988;*151*:1079–1093.

7. Kaye JJ: Arthritis: Roles of radiography and other imaging techniques in evaluation. Radiology 1990;*177*:601–608.
8. McCarty DJ, Polcyn RE, Collins PA: [99m]Technetium scintiphotography in arthritis. II. Its nonspecificity and clinical and roentgenographic correlations in rheumatoid arthritis. Arthritis Rheum 1970;*13*:21–32.
9. Weissberg DL, Resnick D, Taylor A, Becker M, Alazaraki N: Rheumatoid arthritis and its variants: Analysis of scintiphotographic, radiographic, and clinical examinations. AJR 1978;*131*:665–673.
10. Reiser MF, Bongartz GP, Erlemann R, et al: Gadolinium-DTPA in rheumatoid arthritis and related diseases: First results with dynamic magnetic resonance imaging. Skeletal Radiol 1989;*18*:591–597.
11. König H, Sieper J, Wolf K-J: Rheumatoid arthritis: Evaluation of hypervascular and fibrous pannus with dynamic MR imaging enhanced with Gd-DTPA. Radiology 1990;*176*:473–477.
12. Kursunoglu-Brahme S, Riccio T, Weisman MH, et al: Rheumatoid knee: Role of gadopentetate-enhanced MR imaging. Radiology 1990;*176*:831–835.
13. Larheim TA: Imaging of the temporomandibular joint in juvenile rheumatoid arthritis. *In* Westesson P-L, Katzberg R, eds: Imaging of the Temporomandibular Joint. Baltimore, Williams & Wilkins, 1991, pp 155–172.
14. Haanæs HR, Larheim TA, Nickerson JW, Pahle JA: Discectomy and synovectomy of the temporomandibular joint in the treatment of rheumatoid arthritis: Case report with three-year follow-up study. J Oral Maxillofac Surg 1986;*44*:905–910.
15. Bjørnland T, Larheim TA, Haanæs HR: Surgical treatment of temporomandibular joints in patients with chronic arthritic disease: Preoperative findings and one-year follow-up. J Craniomandib Pract 1992;*10*:205–210.
16. Blackwood HJJ: Arthritis of the mandibular joint. Br Dent J 1963;*115*:317–326.
17. Larheim TA: Imaging of the temporomandibular joint in rheumatic disease. *In* Westesson P-L, Katzberg R, eds: Imaging of the Temporomandibular Joint. Baltimore, Williams & Wilkins, 1991, pp. 133–153.
18. Chalmers IM, Blair GS: Rheumatoid arthritis of the temporomandibular joint. Q J Med 1973;*166*:369–386.
19. Larheim TA, Johannessen S, Tveito L: Abnormalities of the temporomandibular joint in adults with rheumatic disease. A comparison of panoramic, transcranial and transpharyngeal radiography with tomography. Dentomaxillofac Radiol 1988;*17*:109–113.
20. Åkermann S, Kopp S, Nilner M, Petersson A, Rohlin M: Relationship between clinical and radiologic findings of the temporomandibular joint in rheumatoid arthritis. Oral Surg Oral Med Oral Pathol 1988;*66*:639–643.
21. Petersson A, Rohlin M: Rheumatoid arthritis of the temporomandibular joint. Evaluation of three different radiographic techniques by assessment of observer performance. Dentomaxillofac Radiol 1988;*17*:115–120.
22. Larheim TA, Kolbenstvedt A: Osseous temporomandibular joint abnormalities in rheumatic disease. Computed tomography versus hypocycloidal tomography. Acta Radiol 1990;*31*:383–387.
23. Larheim TA, Storhaug K, Tveito L: Temporomandibular joint involvement and dental occlusion in a group of adults with rheumatoid arthritis. Acta Odontol Scand 1983;*41*:301–309.
24. Larheim TA, Bjørnland T: Arthrographic findings in the temporomandibular joint in patients with rheumatic disease. J Oral Maxillofac Surg 1989;*47*:780–784.
25. Larheim TA, Smith H-J, Aspestrand F: Rheumatic disease of the temporomandibular joint: MR imaging and tomographic manifestations. Radiology 1990;*175*:527–531.
26. Larheim TA, Smith H-J, Aspestrand F: Rheumatic disease of temporomandibular joint with development of anterior disk displacement as revealed by magnetic resonance imaging. A case report. Oral Surg Oral Med Oral Pathol 1991;*71*:246–249.
27. Larheim TA, Smith H-J, Aspestrand F: Temporomandibular joint abnormalities associated with rheumatic disease: Comparison between MR imaging and arthrotomography. Radiology 1992;*183*:221–226.
28. Larheim TA, Bjørnland T, Smith H-J, Aspestrand F, Kolbenstvedt A: Imaging temporomandibular joint abnormalities in patients with rheumatic disease: Comparison with surgical observations. Oral Surg Oral Med Oral Pathol 1992;*73*:494–501.
29. Donlon WC, Moon KL: Comparison of magnetic resonance imaging, arthrotomography and clinical and surgical findings in temporomandibular joint internal derangements. Oral Surg Oral Med Oral Pathol 1987;*64*:2–5.
30. Schellhas KP, Wilkes CH, Omlie MR, et al: The diagnosis of temporomandibular joint disease: two-compartment arthrography and MR. AJNR 1988;*9*:579–588.
31. Rao VM, Farole A, Karasick D: Temporomandibular joint dysfunction: Correlation of MR imaging, arthrography, and arthroscopy. Radiology 1990;*174*:663–667.
32. Paus AC, Pahle AJ: Arthroscopic evaluation of the synovial lining before and after open synovectomy of the knee joint in patients with chronic inflammatory joint diseases. Scand J Rheumatol 1990;*19*:193–201.

33. Smith H-J, Larheim TA, Aspestrand F: Rheumatic and nonrheumatic disease in the temporomandibular joint: Gadolinium-enhanced MR imaging. Radiology 1992;*185*:229–234.
34. Katzberg RW: Temporomandibular joint imaging. Radiology 1989;*170*:297–307.
35. Kaplan PA, Tu HK, Sleder PR, Lydiatt DD, Laney TJ: Inferior joint space arthrography of normal temporomandibular joints: Reassessment of diagnostic criteria. Radiology 1986;*159*:585–589.
36. Westesson P-L, Bronstein SL: Temporomandibular joint: Correlation of single- and double-contrast arthrography. Radiology 1987;*164*:65–70.
37. Westesson P-L, Katzberg RW, Tallents RH, Sanchez-Woodworth RE, Svensson SA, Espeland MA: Temporomandibular joint: Comparison of MR images with cryosectional anatomy. Radiology 1987;*164*:59–64.
38. Westesson P-L, Katzberg RW, Tallents RH, Sanchez-Woodworth RE, Svensson SA: CT and MR of the temporomandibular joint: Comparison with autopsy specimens. AJR 1987;*148*:1165–1171.
39. Schellhas KP, Wilkes CH: Temporomandibular joint inflammation: Comparison of MR fast scanning with T1- and T2-weighted imaging techniques. AJNR 1989;*10*:589–594.
40. Schellhas KP, Wilkes CH, Fritts HM, Omlie MR, Lagrotteria LB: MR of osteochondritis dissecans and avascular necrosis of the mandibular condyle. AJR 1989;*152*:521–560.

CHAPTER NINE

Trauma

GENERAL CONSIDERATIONS

Traumatic injuries to the temporomandibular joint (TMJ) region are suspected to be a major cause of internal derangement related to disk dysfunction. Trauma can also cause direct damage to both soft and hard tissues, resulting in fibrous or bony ankylosis, or both. The relationship among condylar fractures, dentofacial deformity, and associated clinical dysfunction has been systematically evaluated by Lindahl.[1] This chapter provides an overview of the characteristics of condylar fractures, their relationship to signs and symptoms of internal derangement, their sequelae, and their management. Condylar fractures were classified by Lindahl as condylar head, condylar neck, and subcondylar, as shown in Figure 9–1.[2]

Clinical Aspects

The most common cause of condylar fracture in childhood is bicycle accident. With increasing age, this changes to injuries in connection with sports and, later, assault and motor vehicle accidents.[2] Injury from a fall results in an axial force against the chin that proceeds along the mandibular body to the condylar process and the TMJ. In a blow to the face, the force is horizontally directed and more or less perpendicular to the mandibular body. This can result in a fracture at the site of impact and possibly a fracture of the condylar neck on the opposite side. When injuries to teeth occur in connection with a blow, an individual is probably subjected to more complex traumatic insults, such as might occur in an automobile accident or from repeated blows in an assault.[2]

Table 9–1 summarizes some of the associated characteristics of condylar fractures.[1] The majority are unilateral and occur at the condylar neck, subcondylar region, or superior part of the ramus. Injuries to the teeth occur in 30 per cent of cases. Bilateral condylar fractures and subcondylar fractures have a high association with other concomitant mandibular fractures. Since the skeleton in growing individuals is much more elastic than in adults, fracture without override ("greenstick") is typical in children, whereas complete fracture with lateral override is typical in adults.[2, 3]

Restitutional remodeling leads to a normal relationship between the condylar head and fossa, whereas functional (or adaptive) remodeling leads to an adaptation to a new anatomic position and function.[4] The remodeling process in children is generally of the restitutional type and in adults of the functional

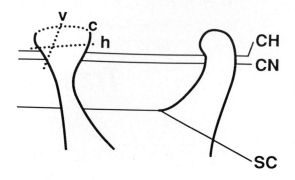

Figure 9–1
As described by Lindahl,[1] the fracture levels can be classified as (1) condylar head (CH), (2) condylar neck (CN), and (3) subcondylar (SC). Fractures within the condylar head can be subclassified as horizontal (h), vertical (v), or compression (c).

type, in which the condylar head frequently remains in the anteromedial position relative to the glenoid fossa. Teenagers occupy an intermediate position; they respond more like children in their early teens and more like adults in their late teens.[5]

Immediately after fracture, a deviation of the chin toward the fracture site is common in children, especially in cases of condylar head dislocation.[6] However, deviation toward the nonfractured side, indicating overgrowth of the fracture, is a frequent sequela after healing occurs.[6, 7]

During clinical follow-up, it has been noted that children are not usually aware of any disturbance of their masticatory system, as is also the case with a great majority of teenagers and adults.[1] However, this low frequency of awareness of dysfunction does not correspond to the findings afforded in the clinical evaluations. This is especially true in adults, in whom a high frequency of clinical signs of dysfunction of the TMJ has been noted.[4, 8] In adults, the palpable translation of the condyle generally did not return after fracture when associated condylar head dislocation had been documented. Clinical signs of persistent dysfunction of joints and muscles have been noted to be very frequent in adults.[8] The main signs reported were tenderness in the muscles of mastication and TMJ clicking detected by palpation.

Skeletal asymmetry caused by condylar fracture is quite frequent but is usually too small to be observed by casual inspection. In adults, deviation of the chin toward the fractured side is frequent as a sequela.[6]

CLASSIFICATION OF CONDYLAR FRACTURES

Fracture levels can be classified as (1) condylar head; (2) condylar neck; and (3) subcondylar (Fig. 9–1).[1, 2] Fractures within the condylar head can be subclassified as horizontal, vertical, or compression[1, 2] (Fig. 9–1). A horizontal fracture through the head of the condyle is noted in the CT scan in Figure 9–2. The plain film tomograph did not demonstrate the subacute fracture margins,

Table 9–1
CHARACTERISTICS OF CONDYLAR FRACTURES

Majority (90%) are unilateral.
Majority (90%) occur at the condylar neck, subcondylar region, or superior part of the ramus.
The condylar fragment is typically displaced anteromedially.
Injuries to the teeth occur in 30% of cases.
Uni- and bilateral condylar fractures have a high association with other mandibular fractures.
Fracture without override ("greenstick") is typical in children.
Fracture with lateral override is typical in adults.

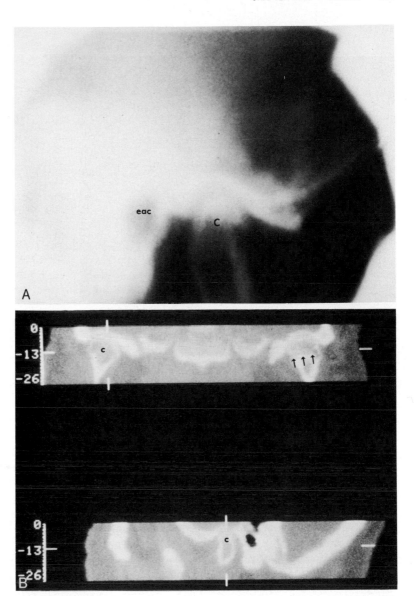

Figure 9–2
A, *Multidirectional tomogram of a patient who sustained a blow to the chin and was evaluated 6 weeks after the injury. C, Condyle; eac, external auditory canal. B, Axial CT of the same patient with reformatting in the coronal (top) and sagittal (bottom) planes. The multidirectional tomogram did not demonstrate the horizontal fracture through the head of the condyle, whereas the coronal CT demonstrated the healing fracture (arrows).*

whereas the reconstructed coronal image through the condyle clearly demonstrated the healing fracture line. A compression fracture of the condylar head demonstrated by magnetic resonance (MR) (Fig. 9–3) is shown in an 8-year-old boy who sustained a blow to the chin following a bicycle accident. The plain film radiographs were negative, but the MR scan clearly depicts the compression injury, with associated blood or edema, or both, in the upper joint space. Note that the TMJ disk is not displaced. A condylar neck fracture is shown by plain film radiography in Figure 9–4, and bilateral subcondylar fractures are shown by coronal computed tomography (CT), transcranial radiography, and panoramic radiograph in Figure 9–5.

The fracture relationships can be defined as lateral override, medial condylar displacement without override (greenstick type in children), medial override, and linear or "hairline" (Fig. 9–6).[1] The typical medial condylar fracture without override is shown in Figure 9–5. The linear type of fracture without displacement is shown in Figure 9–2. Medial angulation of the condylar

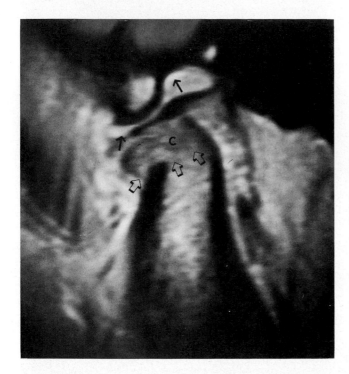

Figure 9–3
MR sagittal image of the TMJ in an 8-year-old child, demonstrating a compression fracture (open arrows) of the condyle (C). The plain film radiographs were negative, but the MR scan clearly depicts the compression injury to the condyle (open arrows), with associated blood and/or edema in the upper joint space (black arrows). The TMJ disk is not displaced.

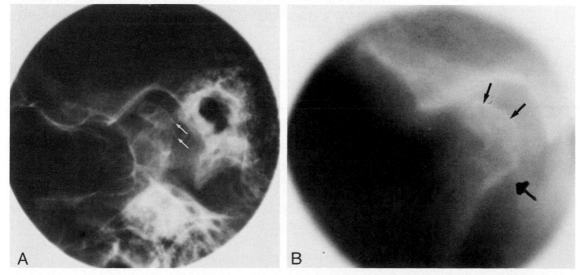

Figure 9–4
A, Transcranial radiograph showing a condylar neck fracture (arrows) with anterior displacement of the condylar fragment. B, Tomogram of the same patient showing displacement of the condylar head (arrows) anteriorly. The region of the fracture is indicated by a hand-drawn arrow. (Courtesy of Dr. Bo Rosenquist, Department of Oral and Maxillofacial Surgery, University of Lund, Lund, Sweden.)

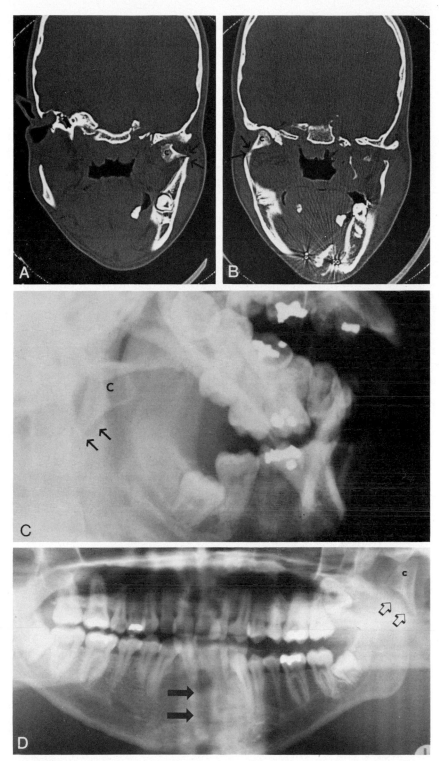

Figure 9–5

Bilateral subcondylar fractures associated with a fracture of the mandibular symphysis resulting from an automobile accident. The findings are demonstrated by coronal CT (A and B), an oblique mandible view of the left side (C), and a panoramic radiograph (D). The coronal CT demonstrates the left and right bilateral subcondylar fractures (arrows). There is a 90° angulation (medial tilt) of the condyle and condylar neck on the left side with condylar dislocation. The condyle on the right side is angulated (also medial tilt) but not dislocated. The left transcranial radiograph (C) also demonstrates the subcondylar fracture (arrows) and dislocation. The panoramic radiograph (D) depicts the left subcondylar fracture/dislocation (open arrows) and the mandibular symphyseal fracture (arrows). The right condylar fracture is not well depicted on this image.

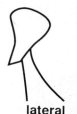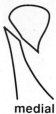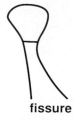

lateral   **no override**   **medial**   **fissure**

Figure 9–6
As described by Lindahl,[1] the fracture relationships can be defined as lateral override, medial condylar displacement without override ("greenstick type"), medial override, and simple linear (fissure, or "hairline"). A simple linear fracture without displacement is shown in Figure 9–2. Bilateral fractures with no override are shown in Figure 9–5.

fragment, with or without lateral override at the fracture site, is the typical fracture in adults (Figs. 9–5 and 9–7), and angulation without override is the characteristic fracture in children (Fig. 9–8). Medial override occurs both in children and adults and appears to be related to a more severe injury to the chin than noted with the other classifications of fracture.

The condylar head relationships to the glenoid fossa can be classified as no displacement, slight displacement, moderate displacement, and frank dislocation (Fig. 9–9).[1] The condylar head usually also displaces in a medial direction, probably secondary to the anteromedial vector of the inferior belly of the lateral pterygoid muscle. Figure 9–10 is an MR scan in a patient with a prior subcondylar fracture and demonstrates the medial and rotational displacement of the condylar head.

Immediately after a fracture, deviation of the chin toward the fractured side is frequent in children; this abnormality is depicted in the diagram in Figure 9–11.[6] A reference line defined by the anterior nasal spine and the base of the crista galli is constructed and extended over the mandible.[6, 9] This line is used as a reference point when studying the horizontal deviation of the mandibular symphysis from the estimated normal position for each individual. This measurement can be used as a baseline at the time of presentation and for comparison following healing. The healing process is often less effective in adults in re-establishing normal anatomic relationships of the mandible to the rest of the face, as depicted in the patient with a healed left condylar fracture (Fig. 9–12A and B).

SEQUELAE OF CONDYLAR FRACTURES

The major sequelae of condylar fractures are (1) mandibular asymmetry, (2) unilateral or bilateral internal derangement due to disk displacement, (3) fibrous or bony joint ankylosis, (4) muscle atrophy, and (5) the occlusal

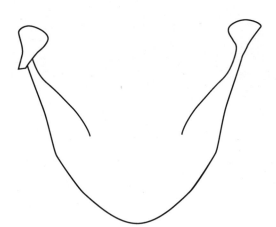

Figure 9–7
Medial tilt or angulation of the condylar fragment with lateral override at the fracture site is a typical fracture encountered in adults.[1]

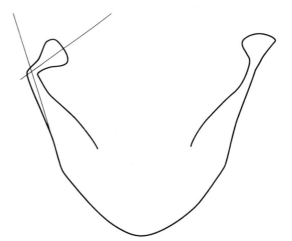

Figure 9–8
A typical fracture noted in children is the medial tilt of the condylar fragment without override, as depicted in this diagram. Medial override occurs both in children and in adults and appears to be related to a more severe injury to the chin than noted with the other types of fractures.[1]

 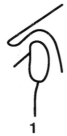 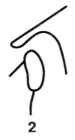 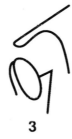

0   **1**   **2**   **3**

Figure 9–9
Condylar head relationships to the articular fossa, which can be classified as no displacement (0), slight displacement (1), moderate displacement (2), and frank dislocation (3). The condylar head usually also displaces in a medial direction, probably secondary to the anteromedial vector of the inferior belly of the lateral pterygoid muscle.[1]

Figure 9–10
Sagittal MR scan in a patient with a prior subcondylar fracture, demonstrating both a medial and rotational displacement of the condylar (C) head. This image is acquired deep within the medial structures of the TMJ, indicating that the condylar head is displaced medially. In addition, the posterior aspect of the condylar head is visualized en face, even though this is a true sagittal image. The lateral pole of the condyle is facing anteriorly (large arrows), and the medial pole of the condyle is facing posteriorly (single arrow).

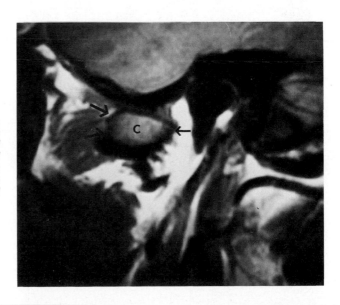

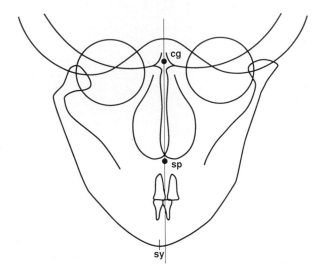

Figure 9–11

As described by Lindahl,[1] mandibular asymmetry is frequent following condylar fractures. This figure depicts a deviation of the chin from the midline (sy, mandibular symphysis) toward the fractured side. A reference line defined by the anterior nasal spine and the base of the crista galli is constructed and extended over the mandible. This line is used as a reference point when studying the horizontal deviation of the mandibular symphysis from the estimated normal position for each individual. This measurement is convenient to use as a baseline at the time of presentation and for comparison following healing. sp, Nasal spine; cg, crista galli.

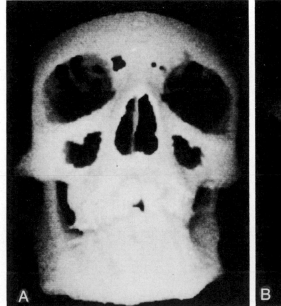
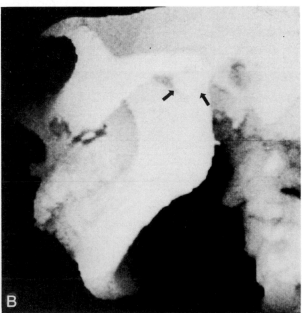

Figure 9–12

A three-dimensional CT scan of an adult patient who sustained a complex left condylar fracture that is now healed. In A, the frontal view, the mandible is deformed and the mandibular midline is shifted to the left, toward the side of the previous fracture. In B, a lateral view of the left side, note the deformed, healed condylar head and neck (arrows), which have resulted in shortening of the left side, accounting for the chin deviation to this side. There was also a fibrous ankylosis of the TMJ, with loss of the normal translatory motion of the condyle and disk. This patient has limited mandibular range of motion and even greater deviation of the mandibular midline to the left with attempted maximal jaw opening.

abnormalities of open bite and retrognathia.[1, 2, 5-13] Recent studies indicate that disorders seem to be frequent, especially in adults.[8, 14-17]

In children, the remodeling processes result in straightening of the condylar fragment, in restitution of the shape and distance of angulation of the condylar head to the reference line defined by the bones of the middle ear, and in restoration of the normal joint space[4, 5] (Fig. 9–13A and B). In adults, these extensive remodeling processes have not been observed (Fig. 9–13C). These changes in adults have been regarded as an adjustment to the position achieved at the time of trauma. After condylar head dislocations in the adult, this adjustment seems to result in the long axis of the condylar head becoming parallel to the frontal plane.

Figure 9–14A through E shows the multidirectional tomograms, the MR scan, and the three-dimensional CT reconstructions in an adult who sustained bilateral condylar fractures 2 years previously. The sagittal MR scan shows the adjustment of the position of the condyle anterior to the glenoid fossa and with a normally positioned disk. The extensive abnormalities of the condylar head following severe, bilateral injuries are nicely depicted by the three-dimensional CT scan. This patient complained of marked limitation of jaw opening—only to 2 cm—with chronic muscle aching. Imaging was performed to determine whether the patient's signs and symptoms were related to disk displacement, which they were not, as clearly demonstrated by these images. Figure 9–15 shows a patient who sustained mandibular symphysis fractures and a right-sided condylar fracture with displacement of the condylar fragment anteriorly and medially. Tomography clearly demonstrates the bony relationships. Arthrography of the lower joint space was performed and showed the disk to remain in a normal superior position (Fig. 9–16).

In a study by Christiansen and coworkers, CT scans of 43 patients who had suffered craniofacial trauma and who had complaints of TMJ pain and dysfunction were assessed.[16] Of the 43 patients, 15 (34 per cent) had sustained fractures, 16 (37 per cent) had documented articular disk derangements without associated fractures, and 32 (74 per cent) had degenerative joint changes. The types of injuries sustained resulted from motor vehicle accidents (42 per cent), falls (19 per cent), assault (14 per cent), industrial accidents (4 per cent), and a miscellaneous group that included gunshot wounds and attempted suicide. Osseous degenerative joint changes were the most frequent findings in this study. The osseous changes in such a high percentage of nonfracture patients were attributed to undetected and untreated soft tissue trauma that resulted in internal derangement. The investigators concluded that TMJ injuries, including subtle fractures and traumatically induced disk derangements, can accelerate osseous changes and should mandate early detection and early treatment.

The clinical and radiologic findings of 30 patients who sustained injuries to the TMJ were retrospectively analyzed by Schellhas.[17] Imaging consisted of conventional radiography, arthrography, CT, and MRI performed 2 days to 24 months after injury. Findings included internal derangement of the TMJ disk, swelling of the retrodiskal tissues, joint effusion, mandibular condyle and condylar neck fractures, degenerative joint disease, and atrophy of muscle. Magnetic resonance was useful in depicting joint effusion and edema in the retrodiskal soft tissues during the acute phase of clinical presentation.

TREATMENT

The general approach to mandibular fractures is as follows: (1) closed reduction primarily utilizing arch bars in patients with adequate dentition, and

Text continued on page 340

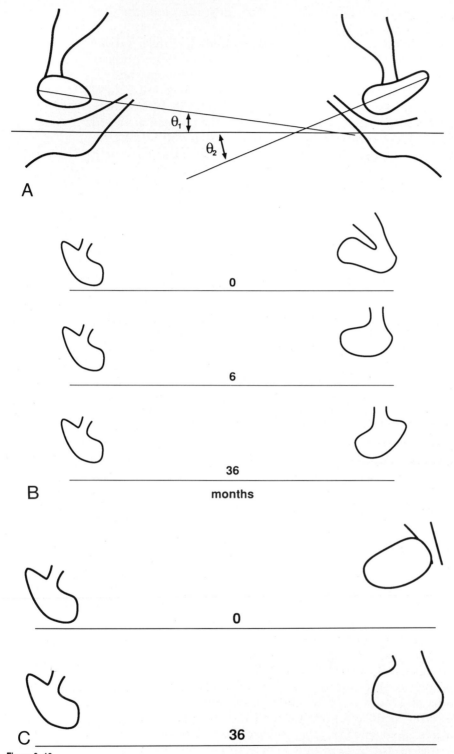

Figure 9–13

Relationships between condylar head angulation and a reference baseline defined by the anatomy of the middle ear structures, as described by Lindahl.[1] In A, the baseline (horizontal line) is constructed and the relationships of the long axes of both condyles are determined by their intersection at angles θ_1 and θ_2. The normal angulation of the condyles relative to the baseline is approximately 15 to 20°. B depicts a left condylar fracture in a child and the healing process over a period of 36 months. This relationship is compared with the horizontal baseline. Typically in children, the healing process is successful in re-establishing normal anatomic relationships. In adults, on the other hand, as depicted in C, the healing process has not resulted in the re-establishment of normal osseous anatomy: the long axis of the left, fractured condyle does not re-establish the normal acute angle with the baseline

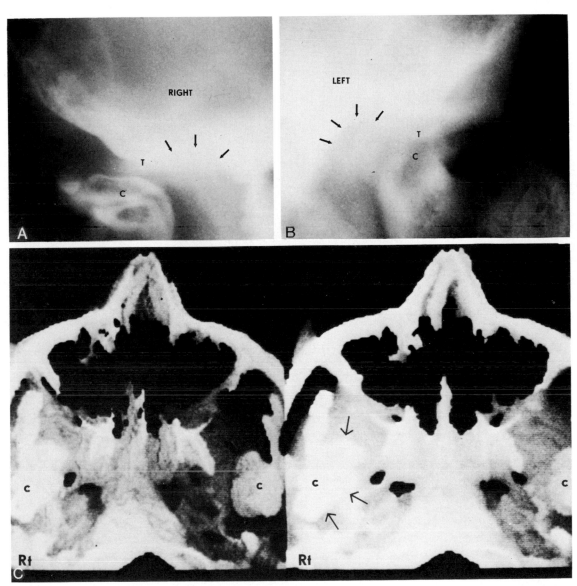

Figure 9–14

Findings in a 28-year-old man who sustained bilateral condylar fractures from a motor vehicle accident 2 years previously. He complained of marked limitation of jaw opening and had an interincisal opening of 2 cm associated with chronic jaw aching. The examination was performed to assess whether a displaced disk was the cause of symptoms. In A and B, multidirectional tomographs of the right and left TMJs with the jaw in the closed position, marked deformity of both condylar heads and fixation of the deformed condylar heads anteriorly away from the glenoid fossa (arrows) are seen. C, A three-dimensional CT scan through the base of the skull that demonstrates the marked deformities of the condyles (arrows).

Illustration continued on following page

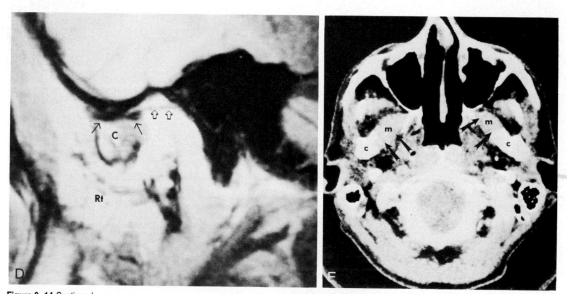

Figure 9–14 Continued

D, *A representative sagittal MR scan of the right TMJ of the patient, acquired in the closed-jaw position, demonstrating that the disk (black arrows) is in a normal relationship to the condyle. Note the linear band of tissue (open arrows) extending posteriorly and possibly representing fibrosis of the elastic tissue of the posterior disk attachment. E, An axial image through the base of the skull of this patient, showing marked shortening and atrophy (arrows) of both lateral pterygoid muscles. C, Condyle; m, muscle; T, tubercle.*

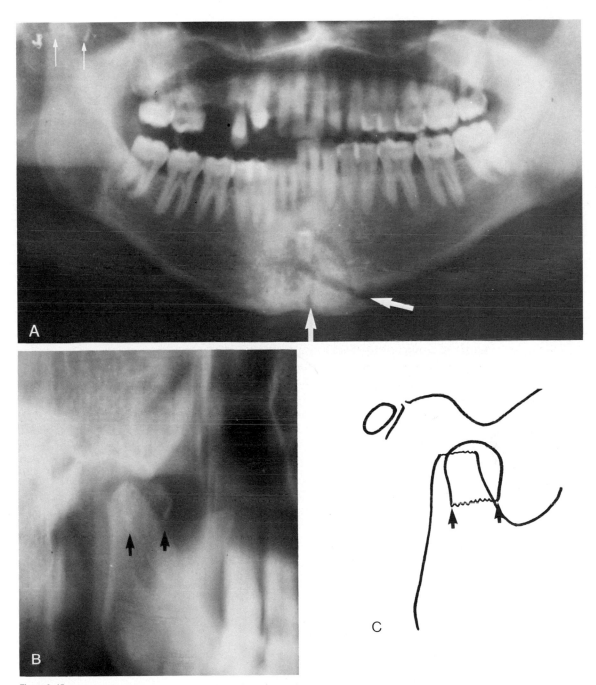

Figure 9–15
Condylar neck fracture with medial displacement of a condylar fragment. A, The patient has a comminuted mandibular symphysis fracture (large arrows) and right condylar fracture (small arrows). B and C, Lateral tomogram shows the condylar fragment (arrows) to be displaced inferiorly.

Illustration continued on following page

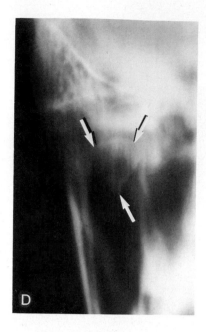

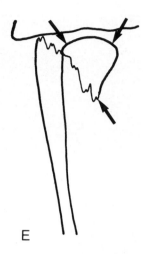

Figure 9–15 Continued
D and E, Frontal tomogram shows the condylar fragment (arrows) medial to the ramus. Arthrograms showed the disk to remain in its normal position over the condyle although the entire condylar fragment has been displaced medially. (Courtesy of Dr. Peter Evans, Johannesburg, South Africa.)

splints or prosthetic devices in other patients; (2) open reduction utilizing stainless steel bars and, less often, bone plates to achieve reapproximation of bone segments; and (3) in selected cases, skeletal pins.[1, 11, 18, 19] Debate continues regarding indications for open reduction of fractures of the mandibular condyles. Most workers agree that when bilaterally displaced condylar fractures are associated with maxillary fractures it is ideal to perform an open reduction of at least one of the condylar fractures in order to establish facial height.[11, 18] Complications with severe bone resorption of the condylar fragment and osteoarthrosis after miniplate fixation of high condylar fractures have been described.[20] According to these workers, the changes were more severe than with transosseous wiring and intramaxillary fixation. The indications for rigid fixation of condyle fracture have to be individually determined until more extensive studies are available.

The principal disadvantages of closed reduction are early dysfunction and malocclusion, along with late arthritic changes secondary to lack of anatomic reduction of the TMJ. Kent and colleagues advocate open reduction of fractured mandibular condyles.[19] Their philosophy is that the absolute indication for open reduction is condyle displacement or dislocation out of the glenoid fossa. These indications are not accepted in the treatment of fractures in children, but their consideration for fractures in adults is currently under evaluation and debate.

IMAGING APPROACH

Transcranial radiographs appear to be the least effective way to visualize the traumatized TMJ.[20] Panoramic radiography, a valuable screening radiograph, is often more sensitive than plain radiographs alone for demonstrating condylar neck fractures but is limited in the evaluation of the TMJ. Linear and multidirectional tomography[21] may show joint fractures, particularly if performed in two imaging planes, but the soft tissues are not depicted, and the

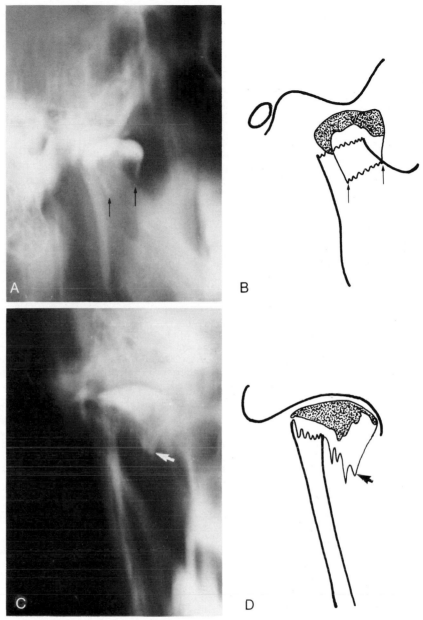

Figure 9–16
Arthrogram of the joint shown in Figure 9–15. A and B, Lateral arthrotomogram showing the condylar fragment (arrows) to be displaced inferiorly. Contrast medium was injected into the lower joint space and shows the disk in normal relationship to the condyle. C and D, Frontal tomogram shows the condylar fragment (arrow) medial to the ramus. There is no evidence of displacement of the disk relative to the condylar fragment. (Courtesy of Dr. Peter Evans, Johannesburg, South Africa.)

Table 9–2
IMAGING APPROACH TO PATIENTS WITH CONDYLAR FRACTURES

Panoramic Radiography	Screening for mandibular fractures
Multidirectional Tomography	Acceptable technique for intra-articular fractures if tomography is performed in two planes
Computed Tomography	Optimal technique for delineation of fractures
Three-Dimensional Computed Tomography	For assessment of spatial relationship between fracture fragments and for planning of reconstructive surgery
Magnetic Resonance Imaging	Optimal for assessment of soft tissue injury to the TMJ

radiation dose is relatively high when compared with plain films.[22] CT is the best method for evaluating the osseous structures of the mandible and face but is not optimal for soft tissue analysis.[16, 20] The advantages of three-dimensional CT for bone have not been fully explored, but this modality does appear very promising. Magnetic resonance imaging is probably the overall best imaging approach to the assessment of the combination of bone and soft tissue damage.[22] Though magnetic resonance is not quite as good as CT for bone, it is adequate. On the other hand, magnetic resonance is unrivaled in its capability for evaluating the soft tissue components of injury. The disk and its attachments are optimally visualized and the multiplanar capabilities of MR allow a depiction of the complex anatomic deformities that are frequently encountered. In addition, the ability of magnetic resonance to depict blood and edema are outstanding. Characteristic features of different imaging modalities are outlined in Table 9–2.

References

1. Lindahl L: Condylar fractures of the mandible; A longitudinal study. Thesis, Göteborg, Sweden, 1977.
2. Lindahl L: Condylar fractures of the mandible. I. Classification and relation to age, occlusion, and concomitant injuries of the teeth and teeth-supporting structures, and fractures of the mandibular body. Int J Oral Surg 1977;6:12–21.
3. Rowe NL: Jaw fractures in children. J Oral Surg 1969;27:467–507.
4. Lundberg M, Ridell A, Öberg T: Mandibular neck fractures. Svensk Tandläkar Tidning 1972;65:363–372.
5. Lindahl L, Hollender L: Condylar fracture of the mandible. II. A radiographic study of remodeling process in the temporomandibular joint. Int J Oral Surg 1977;6:153–165.
6. Lindahl L: Condylar fractures of the mandible. III. Positional changes of the chin. Int J Oral Surg 1977;6:166–172.
7. Jacobsen PU, Lund K: Unilateral overgrowth and remodeling processes after fracture of the mandibular condyle. Scand J Dent Res 1972;80:68–74.
8. Oikarinen KS, Raustia AM, Lahti J: Signs and symptoms of TMJ dysfunction in patients with mandibular condyle fractures. J Craniomandib Pract 1991;9:58–62.
9. Lund K: Mandibular growth and remodeling processes after condylar fracture. Acta Odontol Scand 1974;32:(Suppl 64): 56–70.
10. Lindahl L: Condylar fractures of the mandible. IV. Function of the masticatory system. Int J Oral Surg 1977;6:195–203.
11. Stephens WL: Trauma. *In* Keith DA, ed: Surgery of the Temporomandibular Joint. Boston, Blackwell Scientific Publications, 1988, pp 116–133.
12. Katzberg RW, Tallents RH, Hayakawa K, et al: Internal derangements of the temporomandibular joint: Findings in the pediatric age group. Radiology 1985;154:125–127.
13. Bessette RW, Katzberg RW, Natiella JR, Rose MJ: Diagnosis and reconstruction of the human temporomandibular joint after trauma or internal derangement. Plast Reconstr Surg 1985;75:192–203.
14. Aggarwal S, Mukhopadhyay S, Berry M, Bhargava S: Bony ankylosis of the temporomandibular joint: A computed tomography study. Oral Surg Oral Med Oral Pathol 1990;69:128–132.
15. Harms SE, Wilk RM, Chiles DG, Milam SB: The temporomandibular joint: Magnetic resonance using surface coils. Radiology 1985;157:133–136.
16. Christiansen EL, Thompson JR, Hasso AN: CT evaluation of trauma to the temporomandibular joint. J Oral Maxillofac Surg 1987;45:920–923.
17. Schellhas KP: Temporomandibular joint injuries. Radiology 1989;173:211–216.
18. Zide MF, Kent JN: Indications for open reduction of mandibular condyle fractures. J Oral Maxillofac Surg 1983;41:89.
19. Kent JN, Neary JP, Silvia C, Zide MF: Open reduction of fractured mandibular condyles. Oral Maxillofac Surg Clin North Am 1990;2:69–102.
20. Manzione JV Jr, Katzberg RW: Diagnostic imaging of the temporomandibular joint. *In* Keith DA, ed: Surgery of the Temporomandibular Joint. Boston, Blackwell Scientific Publications, 1988; pp 7–46.
21. Littleton JT: Tomography: Physical Principles and Clinical Application. Baltimore, Williams and Wilkins, 1976.
22. Katzberg RW: State of the art: Temporomandibular joint imaging. Radiology 1989;170:297–307.

CHAPTER TEN

Miscellaneous Conditions

This chapter presents case material of a miscellaneous group of conditions that are uncommonly encountered when imaging the temporomandibular joint (TMJ) of patients presenting with signs and symptoms of temporomandibular internal derangement. The entities described are unrelated and include loose joint bodies of different etiologies, chondrocalcinosis, the asymmetric jaw with etiologies other than trauma, metastatic diseases to the TMJ region, fibrous ankylosis, infection, dislocation of the jaw, and penetrating trauma.

LOOSE BODIES

Loose bodies within the TMJ are very uncommon. The medical literature consists mainly of single case reports.[1–12] Radiographic manifestations include the occurrence of single or multiple calcified or noncalcified densities within the TMJ (Figs. 10–1 and 10–2). Loose bodies may or may not be associated with degenerative arthritis. The range of diseases producing loose bodies in joints includes synovial chondromatosis, osteoarthritis, intracapsular fractures, and osteochondrosis dissecans.

Clinical Presentation

The clinical presentation of loose bodies of any etiology may be that of crepitus within the joint, clicking, or locking of the jaw. Frequently these mechanical symptoms are associated with pain aggravated with function. The mechanical dysfunction of locking may occur during jaw opening or jaw closing. It may also vary within the same patient at different phases of jaw movement. This is probably because the loose body may be moving around within the joint space at different phases of jaw opening. Frequently this leads to confusion in the clinical presentation with mechanical symptoms that are not solely typical of disk displacement. However, in general it is not possible to suspect the presence of loose joint bodies based on the clinical presentation alone since this is not significantly different from that of patients with internal derangement or degenerative joint disease. Indeed, these conditions may coexist at the same time and even be interrelated.

Synovial Chondromatosis

In our experience, synovial chondromatosis and osteochondritis dissecans have been the most common etiologies for loose joint bodies in the TMJ.

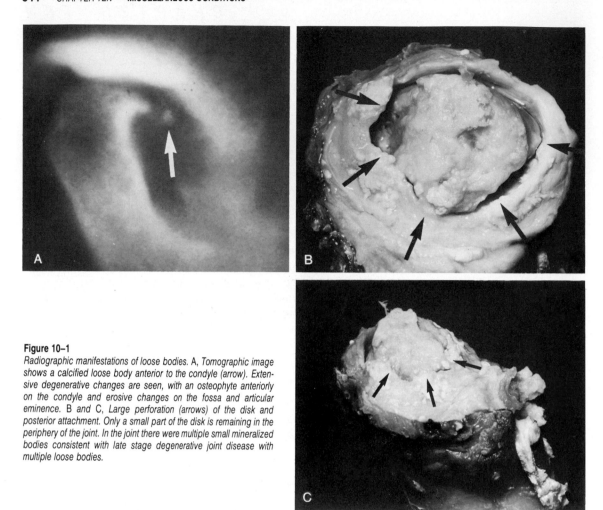

Figure 10–1
Radiographic manifestations of loose bodies. A, Tomographic image shows a calcified loose body anterior to the condyle (arrow). Extensive degenerative changes are seen, with an osteophyte anteriorly on the condyle and erosive changes on the fossa and articular eminence. B and C, Large perforation (arrows) of the disk and posterior attachment. Only a small part of the disk is remaining in the periphery of the joint. In the joint there were multiple small mineralized bodies consistent with late stage degenerative joint disease with multiple loose bodies.

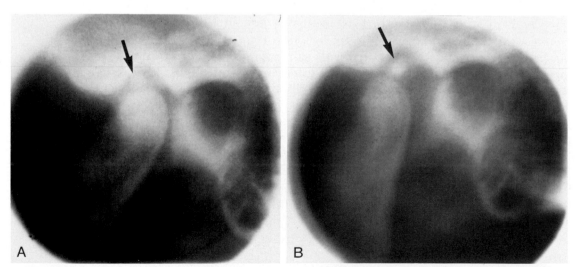

Figure 10–2
Single loose body of the TMJ. Closed (A) and open (B) jaw positions showing a single calcified loose body (arrow) in the joint space. The patient is a young woman with minimal TMJ symptoms. She was found on tomography to have a calcified loose body between the condyle and the glenoid fossa. Upon mouth opening (B), the body is moving, suggesting that it is located within the posterior disk attachment. (No surgical proof.) (Courtesy of Dr. Cecare Fava, Torino, Italy.)

Synovial chondromatosis has been the most commonly reported anomaly associated with loose joint bodies in the literature.[8–10] However, one group of investigators describes a high prevalence of osteochondrosis dissecans in their clinical material without noting synovial chondromatosis.[13]

Synovial chondromatosis represents a cartilaginous metaplasia and is associated with an abnormal synovium.[8–10] One might anticipate that the arthrographic manifestations would include abnormalities in the synovial outline. Synovial chondromatosis is a chronic monoarticular condition that is characterized by metaplastic formation of multiple foci of highly cellular cartilage within the subintimal connective tissue of the synovial membrane.[5–19] The condition is rare and of unknown etiology. It is even uncertain as to whether the process is neoplastic or hyperplastic in nature. The most commonly accepted theory about the origin of synovial chondromatosis is cartilaginous metaplasia of embryonal mesenchymal tissue remnants in the subintimal layer of the synovial membrane. Embryonal synovial mesenchyme gives rise to the synovial tissues and to all intracapsular structures, including ligaments, tendons, and fibrillar cartilage. Some of these metaplastic foci form a spheroid body that has a villous process of the synovium as a pedicle and is thus nourished by the blood supply of the synovial tissue as well as by nutrients in the synovial fluid. The foci form a perichondrium that allows the chondrocytes to grow by proliferation. Calcification of the cartilaginous foci occurs in advanced stages of the disorder, and, as growth continues, the foci detach from the synovial wall and become free-floating bodies within the joint space. Examples of synovial chondromatosis are shown in Figures 10–3 to 10–5.

Imaging and Treatment

The imaging assessment should include a plain radiographic evaluation followed by computed tomography (CT) or magnetic resonance (MR) imaging (Figs. 10–3 to 10–5). The radiographic findings are of calcifications in and around the TMJ, demonstrated best by CT (Fig. 10–4); expansion of the joint space and capsule with multiple low density areas, as manifested by MR (Figs. 10–4 and 10–5); and a slightly increased signal on T2-weighted images within the synovium itself (Fig. 10–4).

There is general agreement that treatment should consist of removal of the affected synovial tissue and of any free particles. Joint lavage is also recommended.[3] Arthroscopy of the TMJ in synovial chondromatosis also shows promise.[19]

Osteochondrosis Dissecans

Osteochondrosis dissecans connotes the development of an osteochondral fragment of articular cartilage from the underlying bone at the superficial surface of a diathrodial joint. The osteochondral fragment may be in situ, incompletely or completely detached from the joint surface. The joints most frequently affected are the knee, ankle, elbow, and hip. It is our feeling that the one to several loose bodies within the TMJ that are not associated with synovial chondromatosis are appropriately classified as osteochondrosis dissecans, as with other joints. This condition has not been widely recognized in the literature until recently.[13] An example of a cadaver joint with morphology

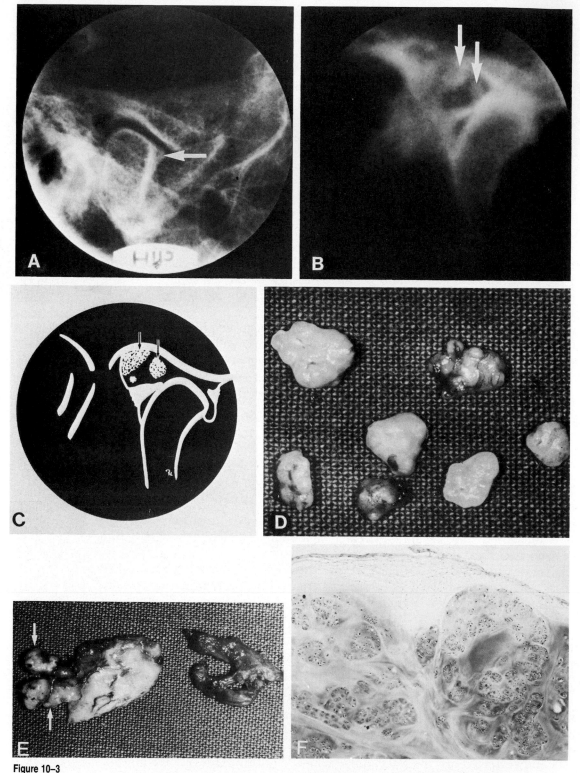

Figure 10–3

Synovial chondromatosis. A, Transcranial projection of the right TMJ, showing flattening of the tubercle and condyle and an osteophyte anteriorly on the condyle (arrow). The condyle is located slightly anteriorly in the fossa. B and C, Double-contrast arthrotomogram and schematic drawing of the joint. Remnants of the disk (in white) are seen anteriorly and posteriorly. Radiopaque structures are seen in the posterior part of the joint (arrows), representing loose bodies. D and E, Seven loose bodies (D) were removed from the joint. The specimen seen in the left in E was removed from the posterior part of the joint and shows two attached bodies (arrows). The disk specimen at right in E was located superior to the condyle and demonstrated a large perforation. F, Confluent nodules of hyaline cartilage in a detached fragment of synovial tissue. (Hematoxylin and eosin, × 27.) (Surgery by Lars Eriksson, DDS, PhD, University Hospital, Lund, Sweden.)

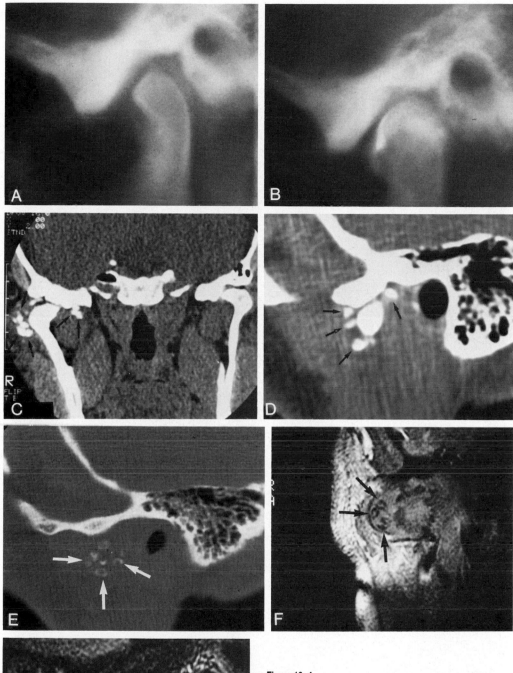

Figure 10–4

Synovial chondromatosis. A and B, Plain tomogram and lower joint space arthrogram were normal in a patient presenting with pain, locking, and swelling of the right TMJ. C, Coronal, and D and E, sagittal CT scans of the right TMJ, with soft tissue and bone settings showing multiple calcific densities (arrows) contained within the right TMJ. F, MR in the coronal, and G, sagittal planes, demonstrating multiple low signal intensity loose bodies (arrows) within the capsule of the right TMJ. The coronal image is a T1-weighted sequence; the sagittal is a T2-weighted sequence.

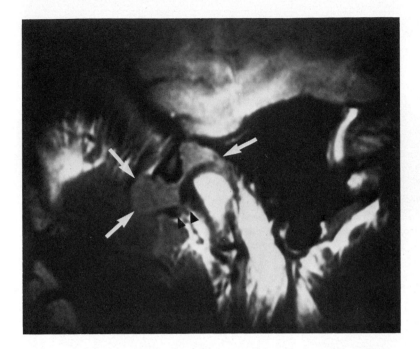

Figure 10–5
Synovial chondromatosis of the temporomandibular joint. Sagittal T1-weighted MR shows a large soft tissue mass in the upper joint compartment (arrows) of the TMJ with downward displacement of the disk (arrowheads). This tissue represented synovial chondromatosis of the upper joint space in a 33-year-old patient with clicking, pain, and swelling of the joint.

consistent with osteochondrosis dissecans is shown in Figure 10–6. The MR image of the TMJ of a 49-year-old patient with significant TMJ pain and dysfunction is shown in Figure 10–7. This image is consistent with the condition of osteochondrosis dissecans. A small piece of the top of the condyle appears to be displaced from the condyle and is located in the joint space.

In osteochondrosis dissecans with or without osteoarthritis, the centers of the loose bodies are composed of dead cancellous bone that represents a detached osteophyte or fibrillated cartilage.[9] The general concept is that osteochondrosis dissecans is a sequela of microtrauma or aseptic necrosis.[13, 15] A fragment of cartilage becomes loose in the joint space and continues to enlarge because of proliferation of cartilage nourished by joint fluid. The fragment of cartilage may also become implanted in the synovium and continue to grow in this manner. In osteochondrosis dissecans, the disk may or may not be abnormal. It is also possible that the fragments of cartilage may actually arise from disk tissue itself.

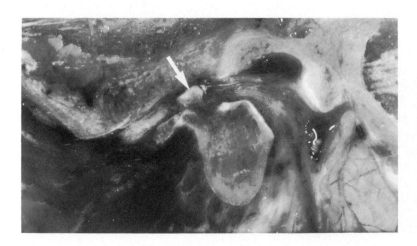

Figure 10–6
Osteochondrosis dissecans. Sagittal cryosection of a joint with morphology consistent with osteochondrosis dissecans. A small piece of the condyle (arrow) has been displaced from the articular surface and is located in the joint space and partly in the posterior disk attachment. The joint shows advanced degenerative joint disease, with an osteophyte on the condyle and extensive flattening and erosive changes of the articular eminence. The disk is anteriorly displaced and severely deformed.

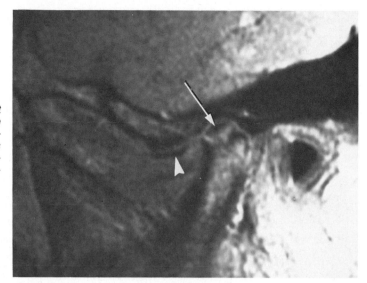

Figure 10–7
Osteochondrosis dissecans. Sagittal MR scan of a patient with significant TMJ pain. A fragment (arrow) from the condyle is dislocated into the joint space, with a corresponding defect in the condylar head. This observation is consistent with osteochondrosis dissecans. The disk (arrowhead) is anteriorly displaced and deformed. (No surgical proof.)

Imaging and Treatment

The first step in the imaging evaluation of a patient with the clinical suspicion of a loose body due to osteochondrosis dissecans includes transcranial radiographs or multidirectional tomograms of the TMJ. Further evaluation might include CT, MR imaging, and/or arthrography to prove that the calcified or noncalcified body or bodies are located within the upper or lower joint space.

The treatment of intra-articular loose bodies resulting from osteochondrosis dissecans is symptomatic and includes surgical exploration and removal of the body.[14] It is believed that the presence of the loose body will lead to progressive symptomatology and to breakdown of the joint surfaces because of the ensuing mechanical dysfunction. In the TMJ we suggest that abnormalities of disk function should be evaluated preoperatively and, if detected, corrected along with extirpation of the cartilaginous fragment.[14]

CHONDROCALCINOSIS

Crystalline arthropathies such as chondrocalcinosis (pseudogout) and gout rarely involve the TMJ and are usually not considered in the differential diagnosis.[20]

Chondrocalcinosis, or calcium pyrophosphate dihydrate deposition disease,[21] occurs when calcium phosphate salt crystals are deposited within fibrocartilaginous tissue. The radiographic pattern of chondrocalcinosis of joints other than the TMJ was first described in 1958 by Zitnan and Sitaj after they observed a linear punctate calcification in the fibrocartilaginous meniscus of the knee.[22, 23] The incidence of chondrocalcinosis increases with age; most cases are observed in the fifth decade of life. Related predisposing factors include systemic conditions such as hyperparathyroidism, hyperphosphatemia, hypomagnesemia, iron storage disorders, gout, hypothyroidism, and chronic arthritic conditions, including rheumatoid arthritis and juvenile rheumatoid arthritis.[20,]

[21, 24–28] The pathogenesis of crystal formation in chondrocalcinosis is not known. The most common location of chondrocalcinosis is in the meniscus of the knee, where 50 per cent of reported cases are seen.[29]

Chondrocalcinosis of the TMJ is rare—only about ten cases have been reported in the medical literature.[20, 30–36] The first case was described by Pritzker and colleagues in 1976 and presented as a pseudotumor of the TMJ.[35] Chondrocalcinosis frequently has been associated with erosion of the cartilage.

We encountered a 45-year-old patient with a several-year history of left TMJ pain. An arthrogram showed normal superior disk position and normal function and the patient was not treated further. Two years later further evaluation was done with a fine section CT scan which revealed minute calcification in the joint space (Fig. 10–8A). The diagnosis was made by a CT-guided fine needle aspiration biopsy that showed multiple pyrophosphate crystals, suggesting the diagnosis of chondrocalcinosis. On retrospect, the arthrogram showed filling defects in the anterior recess of the upper joint space (Fig. 10–8B).

Imaging and Treatment

Definitive treatment for chondrocalcinosis is not known because its cause remains obscure. The cases reported in the medical literature have been treated with surgical therapy and irrigation of the joint.

VILLONODULAR SYNOVITIS

Pigmented villonodular synovitis is a relatively rare, monoarticular, benign tumor-like condition of the synovium of diarthrodial joints.[37] The etiology is

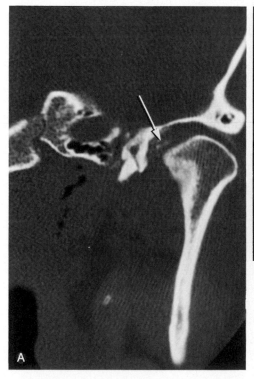
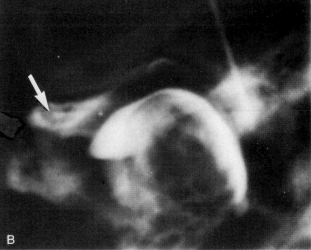

Figure 10–8
Chondrocalcinosis. A, Coronal CT scan shows minute calcifications (arrow) in the joint space. Aspiration showed calcium pyrophosphate crystals consistent with chondrocalcinosis. B, Dual space transcranial arthrogram showing the disk in a normal position. There is a filling defect (arrow) in the anterior recess of the upper joint space.

unknown. It usually affects young adults, with no sex predilection.[38–40] The knee and hip are the most common sites for the tumor.[37, 41–43]

Low-grade pain of long duration is the usual complaint. Pathologically, the thickening of the synovia is characteristic and may sometimes be detected with arthrography. Calcification is not a feature of this entity. Pigmented villonodular synovitis can be seen rarely in the TMJ.[44–51]

ASYMMETRY OF THE MANDIBLE AND FACIAL SKELETON RELATED TO ABNORMALITIES OF THE TEMPOROMANDIBULAR JOINT

Trauma with fracture of the condyle or condylar neck is probably the most common cause of mandibular asymmetry. Other causes of mandibular asymmetry have been relatively poorly understood until recently.[52–54] Mandibular and facial asymmetry is most often of concern in the physical appearance of young women. The most prominent facial features include a shift of the chin to the short side or away from the long side and prominence of the mandibular (gonion) angle on the long side.[55] Dental features may include an open bite on the long side, shift of the mandibular midline away from the long side, crossbite on the short side, and a tilt of the frontal occlusal plane.[55–58]

Previous studies have suggested that the long side has an enlarged condylar head and elongated condylar neck.[53, 56] In some circumstances, histologic examination has been obtained, and this shows abnormal cellular activity of the elongated side.[58–60] Typically, the patients have enlargement of the condyle and elongation of the condylar neck on the long side of the face, i.e., condylar hyperplasia.

Causes of Mandibular Asymmetry

Recent studies with MRI of the TMJ in patients with asymmetry of the mandible have indicated that there are two distinct groups of mandibular asymmetry with different etiologies. One group includes enlargement of the condyle and elongation of the condylar neck on the long side of the face (condylar hyperplasia) (Figs. 10–9 and 10–10). This group has been further subdivided into hemimandibular hyperplasia and hemimandibular elongation.[60] These patients show no evidence of internal derangement or degenerative joint disease. The other group includes patients with uni- or bilateral internal derangement, sometimes associated with degenerative joint disease on the short side but a normal condition on the long side (Fig. 10–11). A patient with a normal facial appearance and a normal TMJ is shown in Figure 10–12 for comparison. The asymmetry related to internal derangement and degenerative joint disease was first reported in children in 1985.[61] Decreased condylar growth or degenerative joint disease, secondary to disk displacement, was documented in a series of pediatric patients to result in facial asymmetry.[61] The association between internal derangement and mandibular and facial asymmetry has been further documented in a recent clinical study.[62] Thus, the etiology of mandibular asymmetry is multifactorial, and modern imaging techniques are invaluable to assess the cause and lead to the appropriate treatment plan.

The condition usually presents as a developing mandibular asymmetry manifested either during the pubertal growth spurt as a result of an abnormal

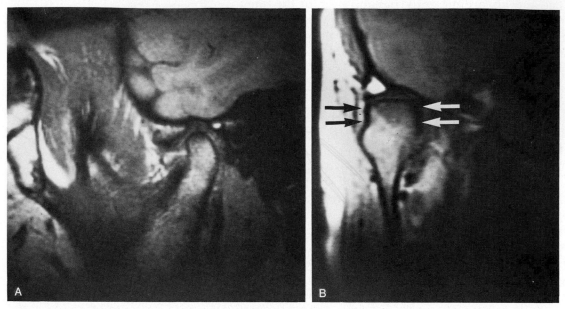

Figure 10–9
Condylar hyperplasia. A, MR image of the hyperplastic condyle in the sagittal plane, using a T1-weighted image. B, The coronal plane of imaging, using a similar pulse sequence. Note the "squaring-off" of the condylar head, both in the sagittal and in the coronal planes of imaging (arrows).

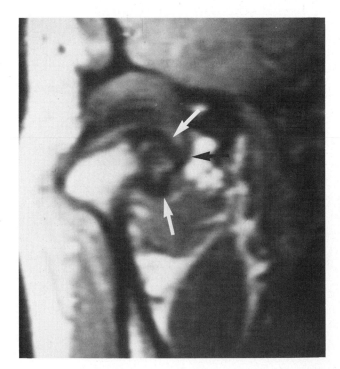

Figure 10–10
Focal condylar hyperplasia. Coronal T1-weighted MR of the right TMJ shows a protuberance (arrows) projecting from the medial aspect of the condyle. This patient presented with a soreness of the TMJ and with a mild mandibular asymmetry. Surgical proof was obtained.

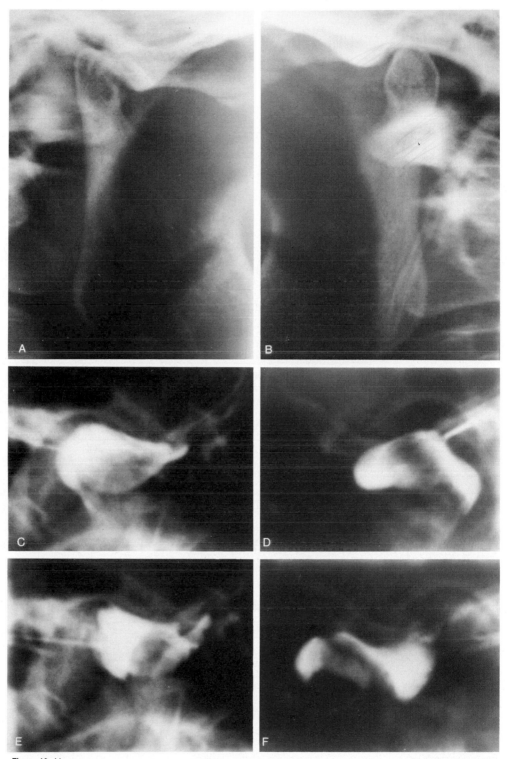

Figure 10–11
Patient with asymmetry secondary to degenerative joint disease in the right TMJ. A and B, Tomograms of left and right TMJ's and mandibular ramus showing evidence of degenerative joint disease and shortening of the ramus height on the right. The left side is normal. C and D, Closed-mouth arthrogram showing perforation irregularities of the outline of the joint space. The left joint (D) is normal. E and F, In the right joint (E), the disk is anteriorly displaced and there is a perforation between the two joint spaces. The outline of the joint compartments is irregular. In the left joint (F), the disk is normal and functions normally on opening.

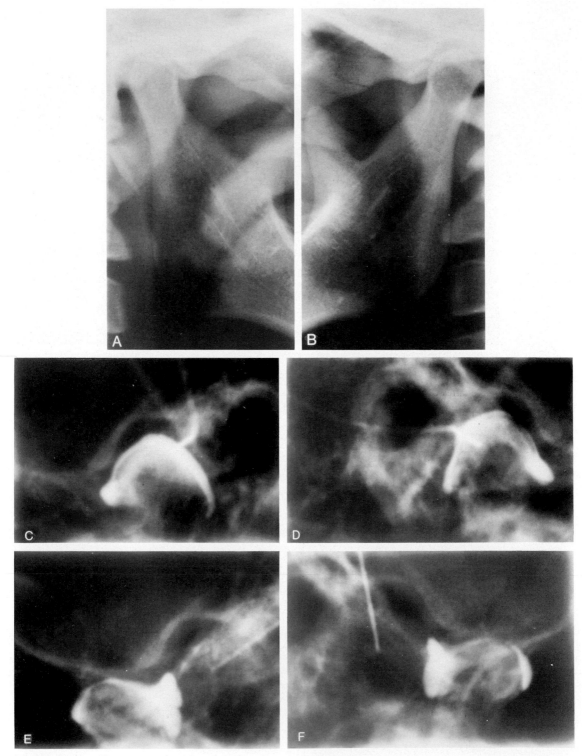

Figure 10–12
Normal patient without asymmetry. A and B, Tomograms of the TMJ and ramus showing joints without evidence of degenerative joint disease and with symmetric ramus heights. C and D, Closed-mouth arthrogram showing normal superior disk position in the left and right joints. E and F, Open-mouth arthrogram showing normal range of motion and normal function of the disk.

hypermetabolic growth center in the affected condyle or at the end of puberty when growth in one condyle persists into adulthood.[63]

The histologic features of condylar hyperplasia are generally accepted as being the presence into adulthood of a continuous germ layer of undifferentiated mesenchymal cells, a hypertrophic cartilage layer, and the presence of cartilage remnants, or "islands," in the bony trabeculae.

The prevalence of mandibular asymmetry is unknown. In a study by Westesson and associates, 11 patients showing clinically obvious mandibular asymmetry were detected over a 2-year period within a TMJ clinic that saw about 300 patients over this time interval.[64]

Diagnostic Imaging

The recommended work-up for patients presenting with mandibular asymmetry (Table 10–1) is a bilateral plain film evaluation of both TMJ in order to assess condylar hyperplasia versus condylar hypoplasia and/or degenerative joint disease, and bilateral sagittal and coronal MRI scans for internal derangement. Arthrography is an alternative imaging method that might be used if MRI is not available. We believe that the status of the soft tissue structures of the TMJ represents a significant component of the asymmetric mandible and that an assessment of this possibility is critical for an understanding of the etiology of the disease and, therefore, for effective treatment planning. Nuclear scanning can be done to assess any asymmetric activity in the joint. This modality is highly sensitive but not specific. Internal derangement or condylar hyperplasia can cause increased skeletal activity, and the nuclear study has to be compared with morphologic studies of the joint.

Condylar hyperplasia must be differentiated from osteochondroma of the mandibular condyle (see Figure 10–13). Osteochondroma has the morphology of a discrete osteocartilaginous exostosis with no cartilage islands seen in the underlying trabeculae. This, however, is a consistent finding in condylar hyperplasia.

Treatment

Some treatment modalities that have been suggested for mandibular asymmetry include resection of the hyperplastic condyle, radiation therapy, sagittal osteotomy, functional orthodontic appliances, or simple observation. Until recently,[11, 62, 64] there has been no consideration in the treatment planning that mandibular asymmetry can be due to degeneration of the short side and that this degeneration or growth deficit in the growing child or adolescent could be related to an internal derangement secondary to long-standing disk displacement.[61, 62, 64–66] If an internal derangement is the cause of a short condyle

Table 10–1
IMAGING STRATEGY FOR PATIENTS WITH MANDIBULAR ASYMMETRY

1. Lateral and anterior posterior cephalograms
2. Lateral tomograms of TMJs, including entire mandibular ramus
3. MRI or arthrography of both left and right TMJs
4. Serial nuclear bone scan to evaluate changes in osseous activity over time

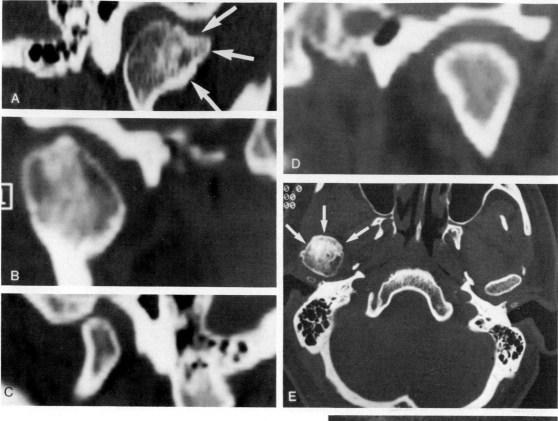

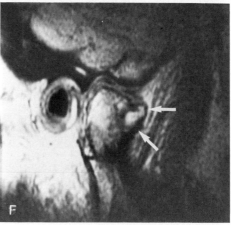

Figure 10–13
Osteochondroma. CT in the sagittal and coronal planes of imaging of the abnormal (A and B) and normal (C and D) TMJ's showed marked irregularity and distortion of the head of the condyle (arrows) in A, indicating osteochondroma. The condyle on the opposite side (B) is normal. E, The axial CT scan showing both the abnormal (arrows) and normal condyles, demonstrating distortion of the condyle in association with a chondroma. F, The sagittal MR scan showed the marked deformity and distortion of the condylar head (arrows) with variable signal intensity from the marrow space on this T1-weighted pulsed sequence.

due to decreased growth during childhood or puberty, this condition must be specifically addressed.

OSTEOCHONDROMA OF THE TEMPOROMANDIBULAR JOINT

An example of osteochondroma of the condyle of the TMJ is shown in Figure 10–13; the patient presented with signs and symptoms suggestive of internal derangement of the TMJ. The patient also had mandibular asymmetry, and clinical examination revealed crepitation in the right joint. A bulbous or cauliflower-like configuration of the right condyle is noted and is typical for this condition.

Loftus and colleagues reported three cases of osteochondroma and reviewed the relevant literature.[67] They indicated that the clinical and histologic presentation was distinctly different from that of condylar hyperplasia. Osteochondroma has the form of a discrete osteocartilaginous exostosis, with no cartilage islands seen in the underlying trabeculae. This, however, is a characteristic finding in condylar hyperplasia. The treatment of osteochondroma is surgical therapy. There is no general consensus of how extensive operation should be. Some surgeons have elected to remove only the excess of the condylar head and then to follow the patient with sequential imaging.

METASTATIC DISEASE TO THE TEMPOROMANDIBULAR JOINT REGION

Figures 10–14 and 10–15 represent metastatic bladder carcinoma and lymphoma, respectively. Fewer than 1 per cent of all tumors metastasize to the maxillofacial area.[68–70] Adenocarcinoma is the most common of all metastatic tumors in the jaws, accounting for 70 per cent of cases. Batsakis and McBurney reviewed 115 cases of mandibular metastases and found the following primary sites: breast, 30.4 per cent; kidney, 15.6 per cent; lung, 14.8 per cent; colon and rectum, 7.8 per cent; prostate, 7 per cent; thyroid, 6.1 per cent; stomach, 5.2 per cent; skin, 4.4 per cent; testis, 2.6 per cent; other sites, less than 1 per cent each.[71] Most metastases to the mandible are found in the molar and premolar regions; only 14 cases of metastases to the mandibular condyle have been reported in the medical literature.

Neoplastic lesions occurring in the condyle are most often either benign tumors or local primary malignancies. Osseous and cartilaginous tumors are the most common benign neoplasms arising in the condylar area. Malignant tumors involving the TMJ are usually a result of direct extension from neoplasms of the skin, parotid, ear, or nasopharynx.[72] The rarity of condylar metastases may be the result of the isolated nature of the condyle's blood supply. Another theory relates to the paucity of red marrow in the jaw bones. Most of the red marrow is found in the mandibular third molar region, and this is the region most often involved in metastatic disease.

In approximately 50 per cent of the reported cases of metastasis involving the condyle, the presenting symptom was TMJ-related. The cases presented here also had symptomatology related to the possibility of TMJ internal derangement, including pain, limited mandibular opening, or mandibular deviation and trismus.

The patient shown in Figure 10–15 demonstrates the unique capability of bone regeneration. This has been described previously.[73]

The radiographic findings of a lytic lesion in or around the bony structures of the TMJ should raise the suspicion of metastasis. Thus, a search for a primary site of tumor, if not already known, should be initiated.

Surgical therapy is rarely possible in the treatment of metastatic tumors of the TMJ; usually, symptomatic or palliative treatments, such as radiotherapy or chemotherapy or both, are used.

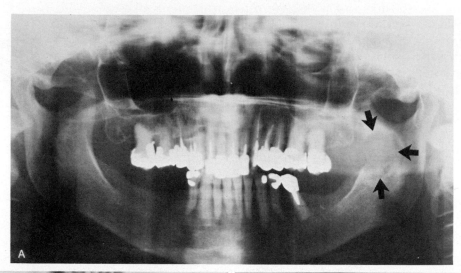

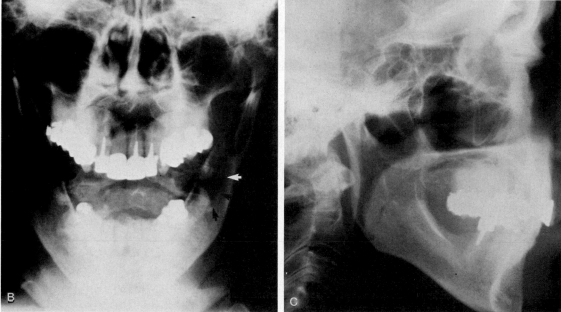

Figure 10–14

Metastatic bladder carcinoma in a 71-year-old woman with bladder carcinoma, now presenting with pain on the right side of the face and TMJ region. A, Panoramic radiograph shows destruction measuring 3 × 2.5 cm (arrows) of the anterior aspect of the ramus, which could explain her pain. Based on assessment of the osseous components, the TMJ is normal. B, AP radiograph shows that the destruction (arrows) also involves the medial compacted bone of the ramus of the mandible. C, The lateral view is presented for comparison. (Courtesy of Arne Petersson, DDS, PhD, University of Lund, Lund, Sweden.)

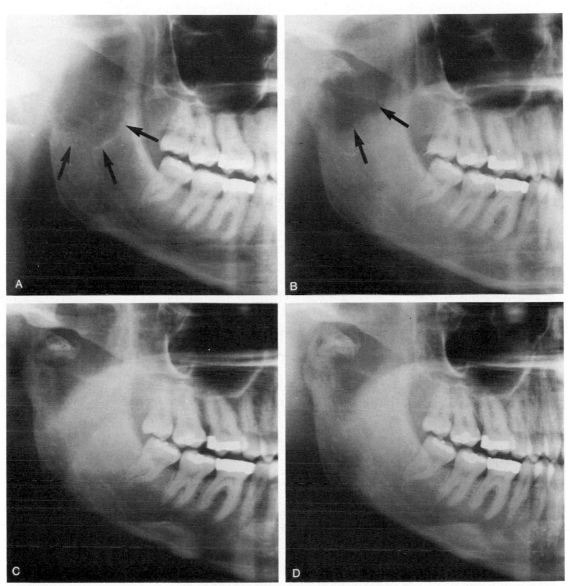

Figure 10–15
Metastatic lymphoma in a 29-year-old patient with pain from the right TMJ region. A, Panoramic radiograph demonstrates extensive destruction of the posterior part of the ramus (arrows). Histology demonstrated a malignant lymphoma of histologic type 4. B, The patient was treated with chemotherapy, and on this radiograph obtained 3 months after the radiograph in A, the bone destruction (arrows) is smaller than seen on the previous radiograph, indicating mandibular regeneration. C, Chemotherapy continued. The radiograph in this figure was obtained 2 months after the radiograph in B and demonstrates further regeneration of the mandible. D, A radiograph of the mandible obtained 2 months after the radiograph in C demonstrates further regeneration of the osseous components. Further examination of the histologic material showed malignant histiocytosis. During the following months additional metastases were noted to the head, hip, ribs, and left hand, indicating generalized disease. The patient died 1 year later. (Courtesy of Lars-Göran Hansson, DDS, Department of Radiology, University Hospital of Sweden, Stockholm, Sweden.)

FIBROUS ANKYLOSIS

The main causes of fibrous ankylosis of the TMJ are prior operation, trauma, and extensive childhood miliary infection with spread to the TMJ. Fibrous ankylosis from trauma and prior operation is probably related to intra-articular hemarthrosis and healing to fibrosis. Figure 10–16 is an MR scan of a patient with a fibrous ankylosis of the TMJ. It shows complete obliteration of the joint space, with low-signal intensity tissue on these T1-weighted images. This low-signal intensity tissue represents dense fibrous tissue. With attempted maximal opening of the jaw, there was only a hinge articulation of the joint. More severe changes from fibrous ankylosis to bony ankylosis can occur, as discussed in Chapter 7.

DISLOCATION OF JAW

Patients with dislocation of the jaw are usually seen clinically in the emergency department. Dislocation can create moderate to severe pain and distress to the patient. These patients are not commonly seen for imaging. Imaging may be obtained later to determine the status of the joint.

Reduction of jaw dislocation manually involves forceful downward and then retrusive manipulation of the mandible to overcome the hindrance created by the forward and upward locked position of the condyle. Muscle relaxants or local anesthesia or both are sometimes necessary to reduce the open locked mandible. Recurrent dislocations of the jaws may require surgical intervention. A multitude of surgical procedures have been described, but no standard technique has been established. Techniques include plication of the joint capsule, reducing the height of the articular eminence, augmentation of the articular eminence with bone grafting, detachment of the external pterygoid muscle, ligating the condyle to the zygomatic arch, diskectomy, fracture of the zygomatic arch, and condylectomy.[74–76] Some clinicians recommend less invasive procedures, including muscle exercises, injection of sclerosing solutions into

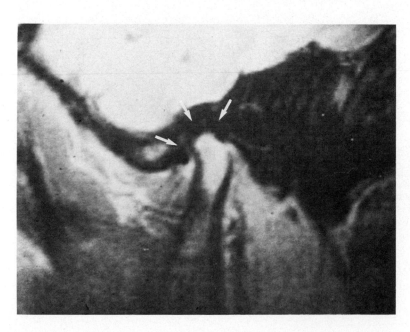

Figure 10–16
A 31-year-old female with post-traumatic fibrous ankylosis of the TMJ. This MR scan was obtained with a T1-weighted sequence and showed complete obliteration (arrows) of the joint spaces due to a fibrous ankylosis.

the inferior joint compartment, and jaw immobilization. These techniques have met with variable degrees of success.

Postulated causes of jaw dislocations include the TMJ pain dysfunction syndrome, trauma, psychologic factors (mental retardation), overclosure of the mandible (especially in edentulous patients), familial etiology, and idiopathic etiologies.[76] It appears that once displacement of the condyle occurs in front of the articular eminence, the dysfunction is accentuated by spasm of the muscles of mastication and that faulty muscular coordination is the mechanism of dislocation.

In a description of the plain film and arthrographic findings in six patients, the findings ranged from a concave depression (Fig. 10–17) on the posterior surface of the condyle to severe degenerative arthritis.[77] The arthrotomographic findings varied from disk displacement with reduction to virtually complete destruction of the disk itself and its attachments. These findings suggest that the mechanism of jaw dislocation is related to entrapment of the condyle when it translates beyond the articular eminence, rather than to condyle-disk incoordination (Fig. 10–17).

The plain tomographic findings following dislocation of the jaws may be nonspecific and might include degenerative changes resulting from severe damage to the disk and its attachments. A diagnosis of acute dislocation of the condyle can be accurately made if it is known that the patient has attempted to close the jaw and the mandibular condyle is noted to be forward of the articular eminence. The grooved defect on the posterior condylar surface (Fig. 10–17) appears analogous to the Hill-Sachs deformity that has been described in patients with recurrent dislocations of the humeral head of the shoulder.[78]

Acute dislocation of the jaw is usually not related to disk-condyle incoordination but to the physical dysfunction between the bony eminence and the bony condyle (Fig. 10–17). However, we have also seen a few cases where the condyle gets locked in front of the anterior band of the disk. In these cases the condyle is inferior to the articular eminence or is still within the glenoid fossa, and the patient is unable to close. The plain film or tomographic

Figure 10–17
Dislocation of the jaw with a defect in the posterior aspect of the condyle. The concave depression (arrows) on the condyle is analogous to the Hill-Sachs deformity, noted for recurrent dislocations of the shoulder joint in this patient with over 30 episodes of complete dislocation of the jaw. (a, Anterior band of the disk.)

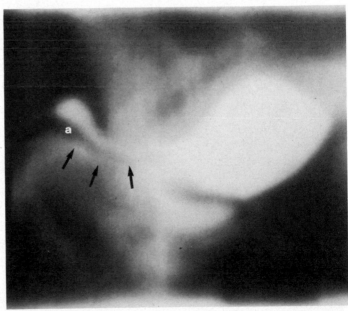

assessment may be enough to differentiate between locking due to dislocation anterior to the articular eminence or due to dislocation anterior to the anterior band of the disk. An example of a condyle dislocated anterior to the articular eminence and also dislocated anterior to the anterior band of the disk is seen in Figure 10–18. Thus there are two etiologies of the open lock situation. One is the condition in which the disk is displaced posterior to the condyle and prevents the condyle from moving into the glenoid fossa (Fig. 10–18). The other is when the complex of condyle and disk gets locked in front of the articular eminence (Fig. 10–19). The clinical presentations of these two conditions are similar, and imaging with soft tissue depiction is the only way to differentiate the cause of the open lock situation. Figure 10–19 shows an example of an open lock situation where the condyle is articulating against the anterior aspect of the articular eminence but the disk is in normal superior position.

INFECTION OF THE TEMPOROMANDIBULAR JOINT

Acute and chronic infections of the TMJ are exceedingly rarely encountered.[79–82] The most common causes of infection in the TMJ are external and middle ear infections and postsurgical complications. Two cases of gonococcal arthritis of the TMJ have been reported.[81, 82]

Figure 10–20 is of a 23-year-old man with severe pain and swelling over the left TMJ and inability to close the mouth on the left side. The plain tomographic radiograph with the jaw in the closed position shows downward

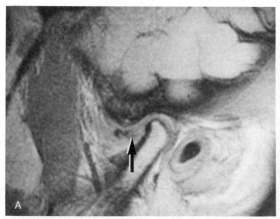
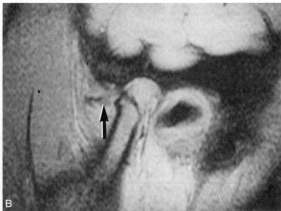
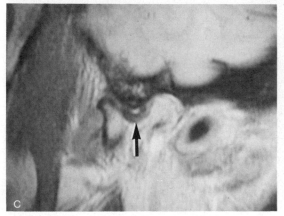

Figure 10–18
Dislocation of jaw with disk displacement. A, MRI scan with mouth closed shows the disk (arrow) anterior to the condyle. B, MRI scan with open mouth. The disk (arrow) is located anterior to the condyle. C, MRI scan at maximal mouth opening in the locked position. The disk (arrow) is now posterior to the condyle. The disk and articular eminence are blocking posterior translation of the condyle.

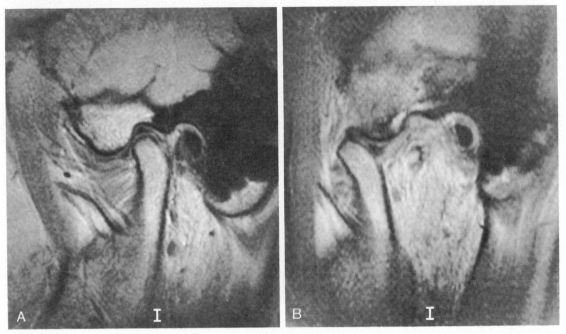

Figure 10–19
Dislocation of jaw without disk displacement (A), MR scan at closed-mouth position shows normal osseous condition and normal position of disk. B, MR scan at maximal mouth opening in open lock position shows condyle and disk complex articulating against the anterior slope of the articular eminence. There is normal relationship between disk and condyle. The condyle–disk complex is locked in front of the articular eminence.

Figure 10–20
Infection of the TMJ. This plain radiograph shows anterior and downward displacement of the condyle in a patient with an infection involving the posterior attachment of the disk but without direct bony involvement. The findings are nonspecific.

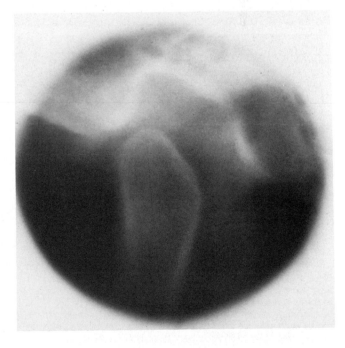

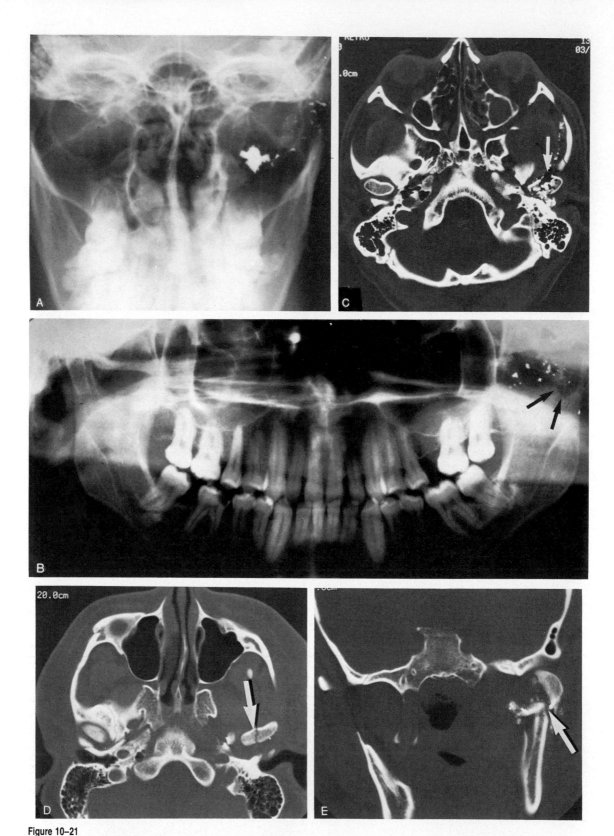

Figure 10–21

Bullet wound to the TMJ. A, Towne's projection of the mandible and face shows metallic fragments from a left-sided bullet wound to the face. B, Panorex examination shows the metallic bullet fragments and a fracture through the base of the condyle and coronoid process (arrows). C, Axial CT scan demonstrates a fracture through the long axis of the condyle (arrow) associated with the bullet wound to the face. Multiple metallic bullet fragments and gas are noted within the soft tissues. D, Axial CT of another patient showing a sagittal fracture (arrow) of the condyle following a gunshot wound to the face. E, Coronal CT scan shows the comminuted fracture and a metallic fragment (arrow) in the area of the fracture.

and forward displacement of the condyle from acute swelling of the posterior disk attachment. Arthrography (not shown) was performed but no pus could be aspirated, and the patient was treated successfully with antibiotics. No changes occurred in the appearance of the osseous structures.

PENETRATING TRAUMA

Penetrating trauma to the TMJ region is occasionally encountered and can lead to severe bone and soft tissue injury. Figure 10–21A to C demonstrates the radiographic findings of a patient suffering from a gunshot wound to the left TMJ, causing condylar fracture. Figure 10–21A and B shows the plain film and Panorex images of this patient, demonstrating the metallic missile fragments and a fracture of the condylar neck. The axial CT scan demonstrates a comminuted fracture of the left condyle, vertically directed along its long axis and the bullet path. Air is noted in the soft tissues and bony structures. Debridement of the foreign material is often necessary, and infection can be a complication.

References

1. Trevor D: A case of synovial chondromatosis of the temporomandibular joint. Postgrad Med J 1952;28:408.
2. Feist JH, Gibbons TG: Osteochondromatosis of the temporomandibular joint. Radiology 1960;74:291.
3. Kusen GJ: Chondromatosis: Report of a case. J Oral Surg 1969;27:735.
4. Schulte WC, Rhyne RR: Synovial chondromatosis of the temporomandibular joint. Oral Surg 1969;28:906.
5. Ballard R, Weiland LH: Synovial chondromatosis of the temporomandibular joint. Cancer 1972;30:791.
6. Alling CC, Rawson DW, Staats OJ, Middleton RA: Synovial chondromatosis of the temporomandibular joint. J Oral Surg 1973;31:604.
7. Tasanen A, Lamberg MA, Kotilainen R: Osteochondromatosis of the temporomandibular joint: Report of a case. Oral Surg 1974;38:845.
8. Rosen PS, Pritzker KPH, Greenbaum J, et al: Synovial chondromatosis affecting the temporomandibular joint. Case report and literature review. Arthritis Rheum 1977;20:736.
9. Blenkinsopp PT: Loose bodies of the temporomandibular joint; Synovial chondromatosis or osteoarthritis. Br J Oral Surg 1978,16.21.
10. Olley SF, Leopard PJ: Osteochondritis dissccans affecting the temporomandibular joint. Br J Oral Surg 1978;16:12.
11. Fee WE Jr, Windhorst P, Wiggins R: Synovial chondromatosis of the temporomandibular joint. Otolaryngol Head Neck Surg 1979;87:741.
12. Stoneman DW, Speck JE, Weinberg S, Mock D: Chondrometaplasia involving the temporomandibular joint. Oral Surg 1980;49:556.
13. Schellhas KP, Wilkes CH, Fritts HM, et al: MR of osteochondritis dissecans and avascular necrosis of the mandibular condyle. AJR 1989;152:551–560.
14. Anderson QN, Katzberg RW: Loose bodies of the temporomandibular joint: Arthrographic diagnosis. Skeletal Radiol 1984;11:42–46.
15. Pappas AM: Osteochondrosis dissecans. Clin Orthop 1981;158:59.
16. Blankenstijn J, Panders AK, Vermey A, Scherpbier AJ: Synovial chondromatosis of the temporomandibular joint. Report of 3 cases and a review of the literature. Cancer 1985;55:479–485.
17. DeBont LGM, Blankenstijn J, Panders AK, Vermey A: Unilateral condylar hyperplasia combined with synovial chondromatosis of the temporomandibular joint. J Oral Maxillofac Surg 1985;17:32–36.
18. Eriksson L, Westesson P-L, Henrikson H: A 66-year-old man with limited jaw opening and temporomandibular joint pain, clicking, and crepitation. J Craniomandib Pract 1985;3:184–188.
19. McCain JP, de la Rua H: Arthroscopic observation and treatment of synovial chondromatosis of the temporomandibular joint. Report of a case and review of the literature. Int J Oral Maxillofac Surg 1989;18:233–236.

20. Magno WB, Lee SH, Schmidt J: Chondrocalcinosis of the temporomandibular joint: An external ear canal pseudotumor. Oral Surg Oral Med Oral Pathol 1992;*73:*262–265.
21. Ryan M, McCarthy D: Calcium pyrophosphate dihydrate crystal deposition disease: Pseudogout and articular chondrocalcinosis. *In* McCarthy DJ, ed: Arthritis and Allied Conditions. 10th ed. Philadelphia, Lea & Febiger, 1985, pp 1515–1546.
22. Zitnan D, Sitaj S: Mnohopocetna familiarlia kalcifkacie artikularnych chrupiek. Bratisl Lek Listy 1958;*28:*217–224.
23. Zitnan D, Sitaj S: Chondrocalcinosis articularis: Clinical and radiological study. Ann Rheum Dis 1963;*22:*142–152.
24. Brasseur J, Huaux J, Devogelaer J, et al: Articular chondrocalcinosis in seropositive rheumatoid arthritis. J Rheumatol 1987;*26:*51–52.
25. Doherty M, Dieppe PA: Pyrophosphate arthropathy as a late complication of juvenile chronic arthritis. J Rheumatol 1984;*11:*219–221.
26. Huaux J, Geubel A, Koch M, et al: The arthritis of hemochromatosis. Clin Rheumatol 1986;*5:*317–324.
27. McGill P, Grange A, Royston C: Chondrocalcinosis in primary hyperparathyroidism. Scand J Rheumatol 1984;*13:*56–58.
28. Resnick D, Rausch J: Hypomagnesemia with chondrocalcinosis. J Can Assoc Radiol 1984;*35:*214–216.
29. McCarty DJ, Hogan JM, Gatter RA, et al: Studies on pathological calcifications in human cartilage. J Bone Joint Surg [Am] 1966;*48:*309–325.
30. De Vos RAI, Brants J, Kusen GJ, et al: Calcium pyrophosphate dihydrate arthropathy of the temporomandibular joint. Oral Surg Oral Med Oral Pathol 1981;*51:*497–502.
31. Good AE, Upton LG: Acute temporomandibular arthritis in a patient with bruxism and calcium pyrophosphate deposition disease. Arthritis Rheum 1982;*25:*353–355.
32. Gross B, Williams R, DiCosimo C, Williams S: Gout and pseudogout of the temporomandibular joint. Oral Surg Oral Med Oral Pathol 1987;*63:*551–554.
33. Hutton C, Doherty M, Dieppe P: Acute pseudogout of the temporomandibular joint: A report of three cases and review of the literature. Br J Rheumatol 1987;*14:*40–41.
34. Mogi G, Kuga M, Kawauchi H: Chondrocalcinosis of the temporomandibular joint: Calcium pyrophosphate dihydrate disease. Arch Otolaryngol Head Neck Surg 1987;*113:*1117–1119.
35. Pritzker K, Phillips H, Luk SC, et al: Pseudotumor of the temporomandibular joint: Destructive calcium pyrophosphate arthropathy. J Rheumatol 1976;*3:*770–781.
36. Zemplenyi J, Calcaterra T: Chondrocalcinosis of the temporomandibular joint: A parotid pseudotumor. Arch Otolaryngol 1985;*111:*403–405.
37. Jaffe HL, Lichenstein L, Sutro CJ: Pigmented villonodular synovitis, bursitis and tendosynovitis: A discussion of the synovial and bursal equivalents of tendosynovial lesion commonly denoted as xanthoma, xanthogranuloma, giant cell tumor or myeloplaxoma of tendon sheath, with some consideration of this tendon sheath lesion itself. Arch Pathol 1941;*31:*731–765.
38. Greenfield MM, Wallace KM: Pigmented villonodular synovitis. Radiology 1950;*54:*350–356.
39. Larmon WA: Pigmented villonodular synovitis. Med Clin North Am 1965;*49:*141–150.
40. Nilsonne U, Moberger G: Pigmented villonodular synovitis of joints. Histological and clinical problems in diagnosis. Acta Orthop Scand 1969;*40:*448–460.
41. Breimer CW, Freiberger RH: Bone lesions associated with villonodular synovitis. AJR 1958;*79:*618–629.
42. Scott PM: Bone lesions in pigmented villonodular synovitis. J Bone Joint Surg [Br] 1968;*50:*306–311.
43. Smith JH, Pugh DG: Roentgenographic aspects of articular pigmented villonodular synovitis. AJR 1962;*87:*1146–1156.
44. Geiger S, Pesch HJ: Synovitis pigmentosa villonodularis, eine seltene Kiefergelenkerkrankung. Fortschr Kiefer Gesichtschir 1980;*25:*129–132.
45. Takagi M, Ishikawa G: Simultaneous villonodular synovitis and synovial chondromatosis of the temporomandibular joint. Report of a case. J Oral Surg 1981;*39:*699–701.
46. Rickert RR, Shapiro MJ: Pigmented villonodular synovitis of the temporomandibular joint. Otolaryngol Head Neck Surg 1982;*90:*668–670.
47. Lapayowker MS, Miller WT, Levy WM, Harwick RD: Pigmented villonodular synovitis of the temporomandibular joint. Radiology 1973;*108:*313–316.
48. Barnard JDW: Pigmented villonodular synovitis in the temporomandibular joint: A case report. Br J Oral Surg 1975;*13:*182–187.
49. Miyamoto Y, Tasaburo T, Hamaya K: Pigmented villonodular synovitis of the temporomandibular joint. Plast Reconstr Surg 1977;*59:*283–286.
50. Raibley SO: Villonodular synovitis with synovial chondromatosis. Oral Surg Oral Med Oral Pathol 1977;*44:*279–284.
51. Dawiskiba S, Eriksson L, Elner Å, et al: Diffuse pigmented villonodular synovitis of the temporomandibular joint diagnosed by fine-needle aspiration cytology. Diagn Cytopathol 1989;*5:*301–304.
52. Jonck LM: Facial asymmetry and condylar hyperplasia. Oral Surg Oral Med Oral Pathol 1975;*40:*567–573.

53. Markey RJ, Potter BE, Moffett BC: Condylar trauma and facial asymmetry. An experimental study. J Oral Maxillofac Surg 1980;*8*:38–51.
54. Wang-Norderud R, Ragab RR: Unilateral condylar hyperplasia and the associated deformity of facial asymmetry. Scand J Plast Reconstr Surg 1977;*11*:91–96.
55. Lineaweaver W, Vargervik K, Tower BS, Ousterhout DK: Post traumatic condylar hyperplasia. Ann Plast Surg 1989;*22*:163–171.
56. Kessel LJ: Condylar hyperplasia—case report. Br J Oral Surg 1970;*7*:124–128.
57. Matteson SR, Proffit WR, et al: Bone scanning with [99m]technetium phosphate to assess condylar hyperplasia. Oral Surg Oral Med Oral Pathol 1985;*60*:356–367.
58. Norman JED, Painter DM: Hyperplasia of the mandibular condyle: A historical review of important early cases with a presentation and analysis of twelve patients. J Oral Maxillofac Surg 1980;*8*:161–175.
59. Egyedi P: Aetiology of condylar hyperplasia. Aust Dent J 1969;*14*:12–17.
60. Obwegeser HL, Mahek MS: Hemimandibular hyperplasia—hemimandibular elongation. J Oral Maxillofac Surg 1986;*14*:183–208.
61. Katzberg RW, Tallents RH, Hayakawa K, et al: Internal derangements of the temporomandibular joint: Findings in the pediatric age group. Radiology 1985;*154*:125–127.
62. Schellhas KP, Piper MA, Omlie MR: Facial skeleton remodeling due to temporomandibular joint degeneration: An imaging study of 100 patients. AJNR 1990;*11*:541–551.
63. Gray RJM, Sloan P, Quayle AA, Carter DH: Histopathological and scintigraphic features of condylar hyperplasia. Int J Oral Maxillofac Surg 1990;*19*:65–71.
64. Westesson P-L, Tallents RH, Katzberg RW, Guay JA: Radiographic assessment of asymmetry of the mandible. AJNR, in press.
65. Nickerson JW Jr, Boering G: Natural course of osteoarthrosis as it relates to internal derangement of the temporomandibular joint. Oral Maxillofac Surg Clin North Am 1989;*1*:27–45.
66. Boering G: Arthrosis Deformans van het Kaakegewricht. Thesis, Rijksuniversiteit te Groningen, 1966.
67. Loftus MJ, Bennett JA, Fantasia JE: Osteochondroma of the mandibular condyles. Oral Surg Oral Med Oral Pathol 1986;*61*:221–226.
68. Bhasker SN: Synopsis of Oral Pathology. St. Louis, CV Mosby, 1973, p 304.
69. Ruben MM, Jui B, Cozzi GM: Metastatic carcinoma of the mandibular condyle presenting as temporomandibular joint syndrome. J Oral Maxillofac Surg 1989;*47*:511–513.
70. Zachariades N: Neoplasms metastatic to the mouth, jaws and surrounding tissues. J Craniomaxillofac Surg 1989;*17*:283–291.
71. Batsakis JG, McBurney TA: Metastatic neoplasms to the head and neck. Surg Gynecol Obstet 1971;*133*:675.
72. Own DG, Stelling CB: Condylar metastasis with initial presentation as temporomandibular joint syndrome. J Oral Med 1985;*40*:198.
73. Ruggiero SL, Donoff RB: Bone regeneration after mandibular resection: Report of two cases. J Oral Maxillofac Surg 1991;*49*:647–651.
74. Cherry CQ, Frew AL: Bilateral reductions of articular eminence for chronic dislocation: A review of eight cases. J Oral Surg 1977;*35*:598.
75. Irby WB, ed: Current Advances in Oral Surgery. St. Louis, CV Mosby, 1974, p 189.
76. Lawlor MG: Recurrent dislocation of the mandible: Treatment of ten cases by the Dautrey procedure. Br J Oral Surg 1982;*20*:14.
77. Katzberg RW, Anderson QN, Manzione JV, et al: Dislocation of jaws. Skeletal Radiol 1984;*11*:38–41.
78. Hill DA, Sachs MD: The grooved defect of the humeral head. A frequently unrecognized complication of dislocations of the shoulder joint. Radiology 1940;*35*:690.
79. Thomson HG: Septic arthritis of the temporomandibular joint complicating otitis externa. J Otolaryngol Otol 1989;*103*:319–321.
80. Hilbert L, Peters WJ, Tepperman PS: Temporomandibular joint destruction after a burn. Burns 1984;*10*:214–216.
81. Alexander WN, Nagy WW: Gonococcal arthritis of the temporomandibular joint. Report of a case. Oral Surg Oral Med Oral Pathol 1973;*36*:809–813.
82. Chue PW: Gonococcal arthritis of the temporomandibular joint. Oral Surg Oral Med Oral Pathol 1975;*39*:572–577.

PART FOUR

Arthroscopy

CHAPTER ELEVEN

Ralph G. Merrill

Arthroscopy of the Temporomandibular Joint

Arthroscopy has long been accepted as an important method to treat disorders of the knee. The introduction of the small-diameter needlescope by Watanabe[1] in 1970 paved the way for arthroscopy of smaller joints. Ohnishi in 1975 described its use in arthroscopy of the temporomandibular joint (TMJ).[2] Since then, international TMJ arthroscopists have rapidly developed applications and expanded knowledge of diagnosis and treatment. The ability to visualize the internal structures of the joint under magnification has added to the understanding of the pathologic and physiologic processes taking place in this unique articulation.

Arthroscopy is a conservative and safe tool needing minimal access to visualize the internal structure of a joint for diagnosis and treatment of arthropathy. The temporomandibular superior joint compartment is about the size of a 50-cent piece, and the inferior space is approximately the size of a 25-cent piece. The viewing field is about one fourth the size of a postage stamp (0.75 cm²). Orderly movements of the arthroscope and magnified viewing in living color throughout the joint facilitate diagnoses.

The diagnostic information arthroscopy can provide is unique. It is an excellent complement to clinical and radiologic diagnostic methods. One can visualize the surface structures within the joint and evaluate either normality or pathology, but radiology is needed to evaluate subarticular bone and extracapsular structures. Pertinent information can be obtained by direct and magnified arthroscopic visualization of the synovium, the capsule, and the fibrocartilage of the disk, eminence, and condyle. The abnormalities of the articular structures can be appreciated in a manner not possible by other methods. Early articular and lining surface changes are seen that are not appreciated by radiologic and clinical examination. The location of soft tissue lesions, synovial hyperplasia, inflammation, diskal lesions, tears, and perforations can be readily identified and localized by arthroscopy. Magnetic resonance (MR) imaging is not accurate in identifying diskal and retrodiskal perforations and tears (Fig. 11–1A and B). False-negatives are not uncommon. Arthrography is accurate in the identification of a perforation but not in its location, size, and character. Not only is arthroscopy unsurpassed for evaluating intra-articular lesions, but fluid from the joint is readily obtained for analysis. Biopsy of lesions of synovium and fibrocartilage can easily be performed for histopathologic diagnosis.

The information obtained from viewing the internal joint structures is impressive. The 25° and 30° arthroscopes with a wide angle lens and magnifi-

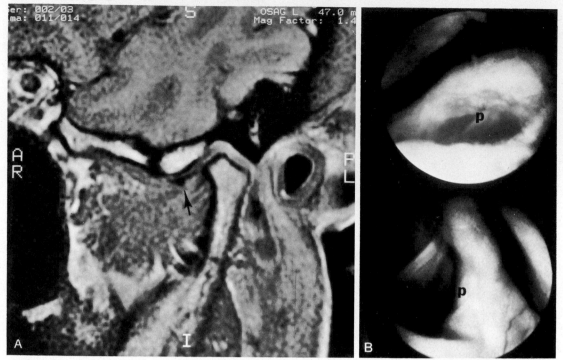

Figure 11-1
A, *This MRI scan did not reveal a perforation that was found at arthroscopy. A medial perforation surrounded by fibrillations was present at the junction of the posterior discal band and the oblique protuberance. B, Examples of perforations found at arthroscopy. (Courtesy of Dr. Nobuo Inoue, Associate Professor, Department of Oral Surgery II, School of Dentistry, Hokkaido University, Sapporo, Japan.)*

cation up to 30 times provide the ability to study intra-articular pathology in great detail. The experienced arthroscopist can determine disk position[3] and the presence of synovitis,[4, 5] grade chondromalacia,[6] evaluate adhesions,[7] identify loose bodies, and localize perforations with a high degree of accuracy. A recent study comparing arthroscopy, arthrography, and MR imaging demonstrated that arthroscopy was superior to arthrography and MR imaging in detecting and localizing perforations, adhesions, and articular degenerative changes.[8]

The arthroscopist strives to perform established arthrotomy procedures in a conservative manner using arthroscopic techniques and to develop procedures unique to arthroscopy. Therapeutic procedures by arthroscopic access are often those that traditionally have been performed by open dissection. It is apparent, however, that relatively conservative arthroscopic surgery is usually sufficiently effective to eliminate the need for complex arthroscopic and arthrotomy procedures. Arthrocentesis and arthrolysis have been effective for relief of symptoms and improving joint function in patients with internal derangements.[9-19] Arthroscopy-assisted manipulation has improved overall results by improving disk mobility and eliminating lateral capsular impingements.[20] Sclerotherapy of retrodiskal and collateral ligament tissues using chemicals, cautery, or laser has improved outcomes in selected cases of hypermobile and dislocating joints.[21-23] Disk suturing is used by some arthroscopists.[24-26] Abrasion arthroplasty[27] for chondromalacia and shaving of fibrillations and surface irregularities are advocated by others. The relatively new holmium:YAG laser is excellent for vaporization of adhesions and for performing other procedures by arthroscopy. The small size of TMJ compartments, especially the inferior

Table 11–1
INDICATIONS FOR TMJ ARTHROSCOPY

Internal derangement	Vacuum phenomenon
Osteoarthritis	Hemarthrosis
Hypermobility syndrome	Inflammatory arthritides
Recurrent mandibular dislocation	Avascular necrosis
Articular fibrosis	Articular trauma

space, is a limiting factor with arthroscopy, which tends to favor conservative procedures. Further refinement and development of the needlescope and arthroscopic equipment will undoubtedly broaden the spectrum of diagnoses and surgical therapy for both compartments of the articulation. Kondoh and Westesson described a 0.7-mm needlescope that is small enough to fit inside an 18-gauge spinal needle.[28]

It has become apparent in recent outcome studies that the repositioning and suturing procedures for disk dislocation by open and arthroscopic techniques do not necessarily secure the disk in a normal anatomic position for the long term.[11, 18, 29, 30] The arthrolysis and lavage procedure does not by definition reposition and maintain normal disk position for dislocated and deformed disks. Inherent and acquired articular laxity and disk deformity further complicate the ability to maintain an anatomic disk position. Acute dislocated disks that have not deformed can be reduced by arthroscopic manipulation, but it is not yet established that a normal disk position can be maintained. A dilemma exists in that disk position and morphology are not normal in most patients who have had arthroscopic and arthrotomy procedures, yet most individuals have successful relief of pain and improved function. The assumption that an anatomic disk position is highly desirable for the long-term health and stability of the articulation, facial skeleton, and dental occlusion is now in question. Wilkes' recent long-term study compared outcomes of patients with internal derangement not having surgical treatment with those having either reconstructive arthroplasty or disk removal.[30] His study indicated that in those who had disk preservation surgery, disk position was maintained and there was less progression to arthrosis. This study gives support to the notion that disk position improved by operation is more desirable than treatment that accepts an abnormal position of the disk.

INDICATIONS FOR ARTHROSCOPIC SURGICAL TREATMENT

Surgical treatment is reserved for patients with arthropathy who are for the most part resistant to nonsurgical treatment. Indications for arthroscopy are much the same as for arthrotomy procedures. Many of the arthropathies, including rheumatoid arthritis, may have an indication for arthroscopic treatment. Traumatic arthritis, neoplastic disease, and pyogenic arthritis are some of the conditions. Most TMJ surgical treatment, however, is performed for internal derangement and its sequelae. Sequelae may include osteoarthrosis, ankylosis, and avascular necrosis. Internal derangement with or without osteoarthritis is by far the predominant disorder for which diagnostic and surgical techniques have been developed (Table 11–1). An accurate diagnosis of joint pathology must be made. The arthropathy must be the basis for the signs, symptoms, and dysfunction interfering with the person's quality of life in order to require surgical treatment. Some individuals adapt to their internal derangement without experiencing disability and symptoms significant enough to interfere with quality of life. This should be considered when recommending treatment of any kind. Certain individuals may adapt and learn to tolerate their joint disease without invasive and other methods of nonreversible therapy.

Internal derangement of this articulation is thought to be a progressive disease;[31] signs and symptoms tend to be episodic. Staging of progression provides valuable information for decision making not only for surgical treatment and its category but also in diagnosis, other treatment, and prognosis. A convenient staging was developed by Wilkes from clinical, radiologic, surgical anatomic, and pathologic observations.[32] He noted three broad categories with early, intermediate, and late characteristics but found it useful to separate the derangements into five stages: I, early; II, early intermediate; III, intermediate; IV, late intermediate, and V, late. This staging can be adapted and enhanced by arthroscopic observations. Bronstein and Merrill modified Wilkes' staging from arthroscopic observations[55] (Table 11–2).

Skeletal deformity can occur from loss of condylar substance in the adult or by interference in development from disk dislocation in the child.[56, 57] Mandibular asymmetry from a unilateral shortened ramus from late stage internal derangement, articular degeneration, disk deformity, and perforation is sometimes a finding in a patient without knowledge of the disorder. Some internal derangements progress without signs and symptoms. An asymptomatic internal derangement seldom needs treatment. The threshold of adaptation in any stage of internal derangement may be exceeded to produce signs and symptoms due to a variety of factors, including external trauma and increased joint loading. Mediators of pain and inflammation from the degradation products of chondromalacia and synovitis appear to play a role in symptomatology. The appreciation of this is due in part to observations and to analysis of synovial fluid obtained at arthroscopy.[36, 40]

Patients with painful mandibular hypermobility, mandibular subluxation, and recurrent dislocation, control of which cannot be achieved by nonsurgical means, can be successfully treated by arthroscopic surgery. Hypermobility of the mandible associated with an internal derangement is common; however, the incidence of recurrent mandibular dislocation is only 3 per cent of all temporomandibular disorders. Condylar subluxation is an incomplete dislocation in which articular surfaces maintain partial contact and the patient is able to return the condyle to the glenoid fossa by shifting the mandible or self-manipulation. A transient subluxation can occur when the condyle becomes temporarily blocked in its path of closure, either in front of the disk or by a deformation of the disk along with altered coordination in the timing of muscular contraction and relaxation. Degenerative disease with rough articular surfaces also can contribute to condylar subluxation and luxation. Joints may be predisposed to subluxations and dislocations and to internal derangements by virtue of their hypermobility. Hypermobility without symptoms can be considered normal for a large segment of the population. This is characterized by a strong forward movement of the condyle at full capacity of mouth opening without symptoms or strain in either opening or closing movements. Such an individual does not have a disk derangement. The condyle is situated anterior to the articular eminence when imaged with the mouth wide open. The mouth can be closed without locking, clicking, or other signs and symptoms. Hypermobility becomes clinically important when signs and symptoms and disk

Table 11-2
ARTHROSCOPIC STAGING OF TMJ INTERNAL DERANGEMENT

Staging Classification of Bronstein and Merrill[55]

I. Early Stage

Roofing, 80 (closed position) to 100 per cent (open or protrusive positions); incipient bilaminar zone elongation; normal disk flexure at junction of diskal eminence and superior lamina; normal synovium; incipient loss of articular surface smoothness; normal superior compartment recesses and vascularity

II. Early/Intermediate

Roofing, 50 (closed) to 100 per cent (open or protrusive); bilaminar elongation with decreased flexure; early adhesive synovitis with beginning adhesion formation; slight lateroanterior capsular prolapse

III. Intermediate

Advanced bilaminar elongation wtih accordion-shaped redundancy and loss of flexure; prominent synovitis; diminished lateral recess; advanced adhesion formations; anterior pseudowall formation in substage B

Substage A: Roofing, 5 (closed) to <15 per cent (open or protrusive); chondromalacia grades I–II (softening, blistering, or furrowing)

Substage B: No roofing, more severe anterior recess changes; chondromalacia grades II–III (blistering, furrowing, ulceration, fraying, fibrillation, surface rupture)

IV. Intermediate/Late

Increase over intermediate stage disease; hyalinization of posterior attachment; chondromalacia grades III–IV (ulceration, fraying, furrowing, fibrillation, surface rupture, cratering, bone exposure)

V. Late Stage

Prominent fibrillations on articular surfaces, perforation, retrodiskal hyalinization, false-capsule formation anteriorly, generalized adhesions, advanced synovitis; chondromalacia grade IV (cratering, bone exposure)

Staging Classification of Wilkes

I. Early Stage

    A. Clinical: No significant mechanical symptoms other than opening reciprocal clicking: no pain or limitation of motion
    B. Radiologic: Slight forward displacement, good anatomic contour of the disk, negative tomograms
    C. Anatomic/pathologic: Excellent anatomic form, slight anterior displacement, passive incoordination demonstrable

II. Early/Intermediate Stage

    A. Clinical: One or more episodes of pain; beginning major mechanical problems consisting of mid to late opening loud clicking, transient catching, and locking
    B. Radiologic: Slight forward displacement, beginning disk deformity of slight thickening of posterior edge, negative tomograms
    C. Anatomic/pathologic: Anterior disk displacement, early anatomic disk deformity, good central articulating area

III. Intermediate Stage

    A. Clinical: Multiple episodes of pain; major mechanical symptoms consisting of locking (intermittent or fully closed), restriction of motion, and difficulty with function
    B. Radiologic: Anterior disk displacement with significant deformity/prolapse of disk (increased thickening of posterior edge), negative tomograms
    C. Anatomic/pathologic: Marked anatomic disk deformity with anterior displacement, no hard tissue changes

IV. Intermediate/Late Stage

    A. Clinical: Slight increase in severity over intermediate stage
    B. Radiologic: Increase in severity over intermediate stage, positive tomograms showing early to moderate degenerative changes: flattening of eminence, deformed condylar head, sclerosis
    C. Anatomic/pathologic: Increase in severity over intermediate stage, hard tissue degenerative remodeling of both bearing surfaces (osteophytosis), multiple adhesions in anterior and posterior recesses, no perforation of disk or attachments

V. Late Stage

    A. Clinical: Characterized by crepitus, variable and episodic pain, chronic restriction of motion and functional difficulty
    B. Radiolgic: Disk or attachment perforation, filling defects, gross anatomic deformity of disk and hard tissues, positive tomograms with essentially degenerative arthritic changes
    C. Anatomic/pathologic: Gross degenerative changes of disk and hard tissues, perforation of posterior attachment, multiple adhesions, osteophytosis, flattening of condyle and eminence, subcortical cystic formation

pathology are present. It is rare to see patients with either painful hypermobility or recurrent dislocation who do not have an associated internal derangement.

The intra-articular injection of sclerosing agents was commonly advocated in the 1940s and 1950s for painful TMJ hypermobility. The new technology of arthroscopy allows accurate injection of the sclerosant under direct vision into retrodiskal tissues and not into the joint space. The sclerosed tissue is confined to the subsynovial tissue in the posterior disk attachment. Sclerosis is also accomplished arthroscopically by cautery and laser. Ohnishi and coworkers reported an arthroscopic technique, using either electrocautery or laser (ND:YAG), for scarification of the posterior attachment of the disk, for 120 joints in 75 patients with hypermobility or recurrent mandibular dislocation.[22, 23] The arthroscopic procedure produces posterior scarring with a subsequent decrease in forward motion of the condyle.

Conditions other than internal derangement with or without hypermobility and osteoarthritis with surgical indications are treatable by arthroscopic techniques. Adhesiveness and arthrofibrosis from prior articular surgical treatment and trauma can be lysed. Persistent hypomobility after orthognathic surgery can be improved by arthrolysis and lavage.[10] Septic arthritis can be drained and lavaged aided by arthroscopy. Arthroscopy as an adjunct to the diagnosis and treatment of articular fractures can improve condylar and disk relationship and position.[33, 34] Articular injuries can be identified, hemarthrosis evacuated, and intra-articular manipulations carried out without resorting to an arthrotomy procedure.

Arthroscopic procedures are usually not indicated when articular disease is so extreme that access is limited for placement of instruments, as in extensive fibrous and bony ankylosis. Many joints with arthrofibrosis can be successfully treated by arthroscopic debridement aided by power shavers and by laser techniques. The holmium:YAG laser has expanded the capability in treating joints limited by fibrosis. It is effective in vaporizing pathologic tissue without damage to adjacent normal tissue. A debridement arthroplasty by arthrotomy is usually needed for ankyloses and for destructive implant arthropathy cases, especially when interpositional grafts are needed for reconstruction.[46] Pseudotumors such as osteochondromatosis may be treated by arthroscopic debridement, laser evaporation, and lavage. True neoplasms require arthrotomy for adequate excision. Adjacent infections of the ear, parotid gland, and preauricular skin are contraindications for arthroscopy.

ARTHROSCOPIC FINDINGS

Information obtained from arthroscopic observations has definitely improved our knowledge of TMJ articulation. The adaptive and pathologic changes that occur are similar to those in other synovial joints. Accuracy was high for findings of synovitis and osteoarthritis in a study by Holmlund and Hellsing.[5] Comparisons between arthroscopic observation and histologic findings in a study by Merrill, Yih, and Langan disclosed that the arthroscopic diagnoses of intra-articular tissue abnormalities were 89.6 per cent accurate.[4] It is reasonable that internal derangements can be more clearly identified and understood by directly observing the changes in synovium and articular surfaces by arthroscopy. The early stages of chondromalacia can be observed by arthroscopy but not by radiology.

Chondromalacia

Quinn has noted progressive stages of articular cartilage degeneration on articular surfaces at arthroscopy.[6] The same stages, graded I through IV, are seen when observing chondromalacia of the patella. There is softening of the cartilage in Grade I, which can be felt and observed by arthroscopic probing. Grade II chondromalacia is characterized by furrowing, the result of disruption of the deep zone collagen fibrils at the calcified and noncalcified cartilage attachment. There is hydrated swelling of proteoglycan-depleted areas among the collagen fibrils, resulting in so-called blistering. Grade III is characterized by fibrillation and ulceration. This condition is due to rupture of deeper collagen fibrils from their cartilage attachments and disruption of the parallel articular surface fibrils. Fibrillar strands hanging from articular surfaces are seen on arthroscopic examination. Grade IV is characterized by crater formation and subchondral bone exposure. Progressive breakdown of superficial and intermediate cartilage fibrils exposes the subchondral bone. Chondromalacia may produce arthralgia by friction, by compression and impingement of degenerating articular cartilage, and through the production of chemical mediators of pain and inflammation, resulting in synovitis. Stegenga, DeBont, and Boering described a relationship between internal derangement and osteoarthrosis and noted that chondromalacia often precedes osteoarthrosis.[35] Israel and associates studied TMJ synovial fluid and found a significant increase in keratin sulfate in patients with early osteoarthritis.[36] The osteoarthritis was not appreciated from preoperative clinical and radiologic examinations.

Vacuum Phenomenon

Nitzen and coworkers have proposed the existence of an adhesive phenomenon in the superior joint compartment when there is painful, stubborn, limited mandibular opening of 25 mm or less.[11, 37] This phenomenon may be due to articular adhesiveness as a consequence of a vacuum effect and increased synovial fluid viscosity.[38] The flexible, concave temporal surface of the disk under increased joint loading may be pressed against the eminence to displace synovial fluid. The pull of the disk from the eminence upon release of pressure may create a vacuum, thus preventing the gliding motion that normally takes place in the superior joint compartment. A flexible biconcave disk without deformity is most conducive to producing this vacuum effect. This adherence may be released by arthroscopic insufflation and arthrocentesis.[39] An increase in joint loading by clenching and bruxism or by other mechanisms probably plays a role in producing this phenomenon. Nitzen and associates used superior joint compartment hydraulic pumping and arthrocentesis in 17 patients for the treatment of sudden, severe, and persistent limited mouth opening.[37] This simple treatment was found to be effective in re-establishing normal opening and relieving pain for a follow-up period of 14 months.

Synovitis

The diagnosis of synovitis (Fig. 11–2) has been shown to be accurate by arthroscopic observations. [4, 5] Early signs of synovitis are detected by observing

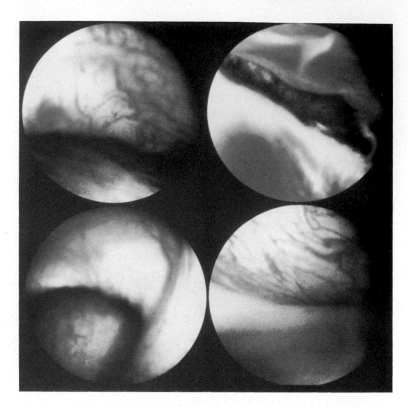

Figure 11–2
Moderate to severe examples of synovitis observed during arthroscopy. (Courtesy of Dr. Nobuo Inoue, Associate Professor, Department of Oral Surgery II, School of Dentistry, Hokkaido University, Sapporo, Japan.)

surface vascularity of the synovium. Variations in degree and location of hypervascularity are found. Sensory nerves and blood vessels are present in the subintimal layer of the synovial membrane. Trauma to this tissue produces pain as well as an inflammatory tissue exudate with debris that cannot be adequately ingested and removed by the phagocytic action of the synovial membrane. Trauma elicits mediators of inflammation and pain to produce synovitis. Some pain mediators in the mandibular joint have been identified by Quinn and Bazan: prostaglandin E_2, leukotriene B_4, and platelet-activating factor.[40] Arthroscopic debridement with washing out of the inflammatory components has effectively decreased pain.

A pathway in the pathogenesis of adhesions is related to the progression of synovitis, cellular injury, and necrosis, and a disruption of synovial tissue. The normal synovial coating of hyaluronic acid is replaced by a layer of inflammatory fibrinous exudate. Synovitis in this way may contribute early to disk hypomobility. The deposition of a layer of fibrin with a decrease in lubrication of the articulating surfaces can enhance an adhesive response. As the surfaces heal, fibrous tissue may mature into adhesions.

Adhesions

Variations in fibrous adhesions are observed at arthroscopy. It is questionable whether adhesions can be accurately identified by imaging techniques. Adhesions contribute to pain by mechanical limitation of the disk at the diskotemporal interface. Kamanishi and Davis have described several types of adhesions identified at arthroscopy.[7] Variations of fibrosis were categorized as

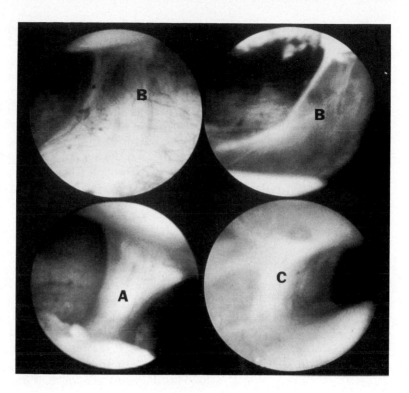

Figure 11–3
Arthroscopic views of superior space adhesions. A, Fibrosynovial band. B, Fibrous C, Pseudowall. (Courtesy of Dr. Nobuo Inoue, Associate Professor, Department of Oral Surgery II, School of Dentistry, Hokkaido University, Sapporo, Japan.)

fibrous bands, fibrosynovial bands, intracapsular fibrosis, capsular fibrosis, diskal osseous bands, and pseudowalls (Fig. 11–3). A number of conditions appear to contribute to the formation of intracapsular fibrosis. Synovitis with cellular injury may create surface fibrin rather than hyaluronic acid for lubrication. An increase in loading with synovitis present contributes to pain and probably the "suction cup" effect of the disk to the eminence, as described by Murakami and associates,[43] and the "vacuum phenomenon" described by Nitzen and associates.[37] Persistent adhesiveness may lead to fibrosis and chronic immobility. Traumatic intracapsular hemorrhage with hematoma can also contribute to adhesion formation. It is evident from arthroscopic observation that intracapsular adhesions play a role in pain, hypomobility, and progression of disk pathology. The success of superior joint compartment arthrolysis with lavage is evidence that superior space adhesions are important in limiting translational motion. The release of adhesions in the anterior superior synovial pouch is often dramatic in immediate mobilization of the joint. This is an important component of arthroscopic surgery. It is accomplished by one or a combination of hand instruments, motorized shavers, cautery, or laser.

Lateral Impingement Phenomenon

Moses described a condition of lateral impingement of the TMJ from observations made from arthroscopic endaural views and coronal magnetic resonance imaging.[20] Pain and decreased mobility of the acromioclavicular joint show striking similarities to lateral impingement seen in the TMJ. It has been noted in intermediate to late stage internal derangement that significant pathology exists in the lateral one third of the joint. Anteromedial disk displacement, disk deformity, and adhesions in the anterosuperior synovial pouch are often components of this pathology. Early changes of lateral synovitis and decreased lubrication with weakening of the lateral diskal attachment may lead to lateral negative remodeling of bone, then anteromedial rotation of the disk. This process probably precedes the anterior and medial pathologic changes. Lateral capsular prolapse, fibrosis, and proliferative synovitis are likely components of this process. The lateral release and capsular stretch procedure described by Moses significantly improves disk and joint mobility.[20] It is an important concept of internal derangement that was not adequately appreciated prior to arthroscopy and coronal MRI views of this articulation.

Perforations

Perforations are readily identified and observed at arthroscopy (Fig. 11–1B). They are pathognomonic of late stage internal derangement. Large perforations allow easy access and visualization of the posterior synovial pouch and collateral recesses of the inferior joint space. The perforations are most commonly located posterior and lateral but not in the disk itself. Perforations occur after chronic prolapse of the disk with condylar loading on anteriorly stretched bilaminar retrodiskal tissues. At arthroscopic examination, it is common to find fibrillations, sometimes described as crabmeat, surrounding the perforation. Once fibrillations are observed in the retrodiskal tissue, it is probable that a perforation is present. Chondromalacia is present on the opposing articular surfaces. An effort is made to study and characterize the perforation. Late intermediate internal derangement has changes in articular bone that are identifiable on imaging. The derangement becomes late stage when perforation occurs. Small perforations with surrounding fibrillations have been found in joints that do not have articular bony changes on imaging; therefore, exceptions are possible. However, late stage chronic internal derangements often have perforations with smooth and rounded edges. The irregular articular surface of the condyle adjacent to the chronic perforation is often covered by fibrous tissue and not exposed bone. This is probably due to remodeling of articular surfaces that were previously involved in an active osteoarthritic process. The discovery of a perforation, multiple adhesions, and a deformed, prolapsed disk does not mean that arthrotomy and disk removal are automatically indicated. Most patients with late stage internal derangement do well with arthroscopic arthrolysis and debridement. Debridement and contouring of the periphery of the perforation can be done with a laser or shaver. Debridement using the holmium laser will undoubtedly improve outcomes. A positive outcome in late stage internal derangement is probably attributed not only to arthrolysis, lavage, disk manipulation, lateral release, and capsular stretch but also to decreasing functional load and increasing capacity for articular remodeling. Postarthroscopic surgical and physical therapy, diet restriction, and occlusal therapy are all important in this respect.

ARTHROSCOPIC TECHNIQUE AND DIAGNOSTIC EXAMINATION

General anesthesia in the hospital operating room has been the preference for arthroscopy procedures, to ensure an aseptic technique and to gain adequate

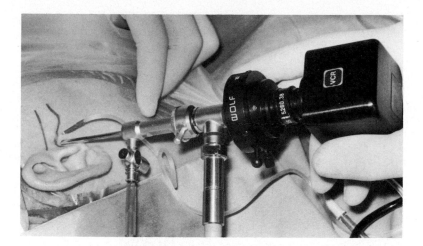

Figure 11–4
Arthroscopic 2.7-mm cannula and 25° scope in place from an inferolateral approach to the superior compartment in the mid-preauricular pouch. A puncture site for the anterior working cannula is placed several millimeters anterior to the outflow 19-gauge needle.

muscle relaxation for the necessary arthroscopic maneuvers and mandibular manipulation. The patients are admitted and discharged on the same day of the procedure. Outpatient diagnostic and surgical arthroscopy can be done with the patient under local anesthesia or local anesthesia with sedation. However, the use of general anesthesia facilitates surgical treatment and is well accepted by the patients. Adequate mandibular traction is difficult to attain under local anesthesia. Prior to the operative procedure an examination is carried out with the patient relaxed and under anesthesia. Range of mandibular motion is evaluated and measured. Joint laxity, noise, and articular mechanical disturbances are evaluated as well. It is advantageous at this time to perform an oropharyngeal examination to rule out lesions or abnormalities that may contribute to pain and dysfunction.

The draping is done with transparent plastic drapes in such a way to enable the assistant to manipulate the mandible intraorally through the sterile drapes. The mandible can be manipulated to evaluate abnormalities and to facilitate placement of the arthroscope and operating instruments. An alternative method for manipulation is an extraoral technique using a large, towel-like clamp at the angle of the mandible.

The midfossa puncture site is used most commonly for the arthroscope. The anterior puncture site is used for the working cannula in triangulation techniques. Switching the working cannula to the fossa puncture site and the scope anteriorly can be done with compatible cannulas and scopes to facilitate operative procedures. The inferolateral approach into the mid preauricular pouch is most commonly used for diagnosis and surgical procedures (Fig. 11–4). A triple technique has been described by Moses and Poker[41] and by Ohnishi.[23] A third site is endaural and is used for improved viewing of the lateral structures of the superior joint compartment. The appreciation of lateral impingement, prolapse, and fibrosis was due to observations by Moses using the endaural approach.[41]

A meticulous puncture technique and an appreciation of the unique periarticular anatomy are very important to perform arthroscopy properly and to avoid injury to significant neurovascular and otologic structures. Important extracapsular structures completely surround the joint. The temporal and zygomatic branches of the facial nerve, the parotid gland, auriculotemporal branches of the trigeminal nerve, and the superficial temporal vessels are important lateral structures. The ear and its contents are only a few millimeters

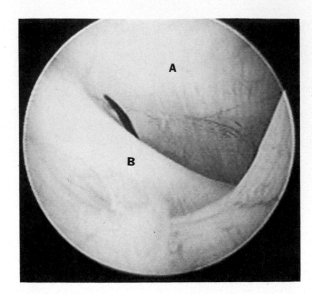

Figure 11–5
View of the posterior synovial pouch of the superior compartment. A, Medial wall. B, Oblique protuberance of retrodiscal attachment.

away posteriorly. The very thin bony partition between the glenoid fossa and the middle cranial fossa is only a few millimeters. Anteriorly, an abundance of vessels is found. A venous plexus surrounds the articulation. Few other articulations are in such hostile territory.

Prior to placement of the arthroscope, the superior compartment is insufflated with a compatible solution. Viewing and working cannulas are placed with the aid of trocars. Inflow and outflow of normal saline or Ringer's lactate allow for joint expansion, clear viewing, and lavage.

The arthroscope with camera and light source is inserted, and the joint space is examined. The examination of the superior joint compartment is made in a systematic way. The assistant distracts the mandible in a forward position. It has been convenient to start the examination and video recording at the posterosuperior attachment of the superior lamina of the retrodiskal tissue (Fig. 11–5). The entire posterosuperior synovial pouch is then inspected. Observation of the posterior slope of the eminence and the posterior diskal band in open and closed positions allows for the assessment of disk position and function (Fig. 11–6). Catching, interferences, and the degree of roofing of the disk over the condyle are observed. The medial capsule, followed by the lateral capsule, lateral articular eminence, disk, and paradiskal groove, is then examined. The scope is advanced to the anterolateral pouch for examination. Capsular fibrosis and adhesions may limit examination of this area and the entire anterior synovial pouch. Adhesiveness and fine adhesions are usually lysed by the insufflation and during the arthroscopic examination by passing the instruments through the recesses and articular parts of the joint.

Arthroscopic Procedures

Arthroscopic surgeons utilize one or a combination of procedures for disorders of the TMJ: biopsy, arthrolysis, lavage, and debridement; disk manipulation; capsular release, anterior release; posterior disk pexis by chemical, cautery, or laser sclerotherapy; abrasion arthroplasty; synovectomy by shaving, cautery, or laser; and partial or complete meniscectomy using a

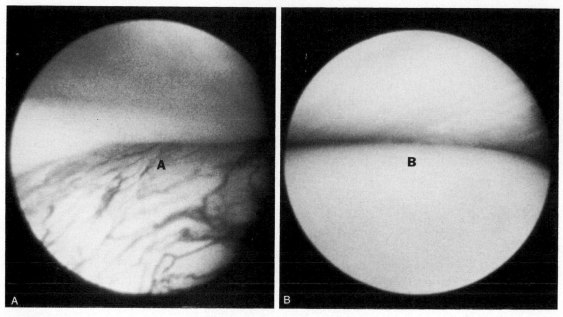

Figure 11–6
Arthroscopic views of the interface between the posterior slope of the eminence and retrodiscal tissue, with the condyle in forward translation. A, Posterior discal band not "roofing" the condyle, with only inflamed retrodiscal tissue showing at the interface. B, Complete roofing of the posterior band. Fibrocartilage of the disk and the eminence are normal in appearance.

motorized shaver or laser. Arthrolysis and lavage was the first surgical procedure used in temporomandibular arthroscopy. This is a conservative procedure that restores joint mobility and reduces pain. The addition of intracapsular disk manipulation and lateral capsular stretch improves disk position and joint mobility. Lavage with Ringer's solution removes debris responsible for pain and inflammation. Areas of moderate to severe synovitis are often injected under direct vision with betamethasone.

Intra-Articular Steroids

Intra-articular injections of glucocorticosteroids are used to control inflammation and pain independent of surgical treatment and presently as an adjunct in arthroscopic surgery. The injection of intra-articular steroids has been questioned owing to the concern of contributing to degenerative changes in cartilage, bone, and other articular structures. Wenneberg, Kopp, and Grondahl followed 16 patients for 8 years after intra-articular injections of glucocorticosteroids.[42] The subjective symptoms as well as the clinical signs were significantly reduced. The patients each had three intra-articular injections of 0.5 ml of betamethasone with an equal volume of lidocaine into the TMJ at 1-week intervals. Erosions of articular bony margins observed before treatment were found to be remineralized with improved remodeling. The long-term results were encouraging, and articular degeneration was not found upon radiologic evaluation.

Betamethasone is injected into the superior compartment or into the subsynovial tissue as the last step in the arthroscopic procedure when inflammation is present. There is no clinical or radiographic evidence of a negative

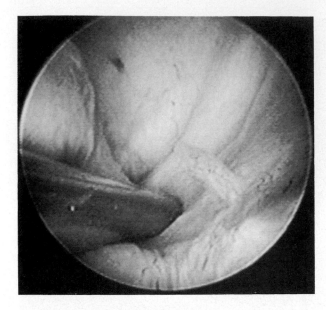

Figure 11–7
An 18-gauge spinal needle directed into subsynovial tissue of retrodiscal tissue for injection of sclerosant.

effect using steroids in this manner in over 1000 of our procedures. Observation at arthroscopy has revealed that synovitis can be present at any stage of internal derangement. Pain, particularly with chewing or function, correlates with the clinical and arthroscopic finding of synovitis.[43] It is probable that the steroid is a safe and helpful adjunct to arthroscopic surgical treatment when used judiciously.

Chemical Sclerotherapy for Hypermobility and Recurrent Dislocation

Arthroscopic examination, arthrolysis, lavage, manipulation, and lateral stretch are completed prior to the injection of a sclerosant for painful hypermobility and recurrent dislocation. Subsynovial injection of the sclerosant into the posterior attachment area is accomplished under direct vision (Fig. 11–7*A* and *B*). The conservative amount of sodium tetradecyl sulfate injected is up to 1 ml of a 1 per cent solution in painful hypermobility and 1 ml of a 3 per cent solution for patients with recurrent mandibular dislocation.

POSTARTHROSCOPIC SURGICAL CARE

Excessive joint loading and mouth opening are thought to be deleterious to healing after any arthroscopic procedure. The patient is instructed to avoid daytime clenching and bruxism. Some joint protection is accomplished with an occlusal appliance. The patient is instructed to use the appliance in the early postoperative period, removing it only for cleaning. Thereafter, using it only during sleep may be continued up to 3 months. Reduction of joint loading is further accomplished by avoidance of heavy chewing and 3 or more months of a soft diet. Activities that stress the articulation or put it at risk for injury are avoided during the 3 months following the arthroscopic procedure. Wide opening as in yawning is to be avoided.

Physical therapy to relax masticatory muscles and to promote healing of joint tissues is indicated. One needs to be specific when prescribing care by a physical therapist. A biconcave disk that has been successfully freed, manipulated into position, and stabilized by posterior pexis can be dislocated by overzealous manipulation and stretching. Ultrasound to the joint and to the associated muscles and other modalities to relax musculature are beneficial. Range of motion exercise after muscle relaxation will promote healing and minimize restricted motion. The arthrolysis, lavage, and manipulation procedure is successful in relieving symptoms for joints in which the disk is deformed and cannot be reduced. Release of superior compartment adhesiveness increases translation and joint mobility. This improvement can be maintained by exercise and physical therapy. More vigorous stretching procedures for advanced internal derangements are recommended except when associated hypermobility has been treated by sclerotherapy. All patients should continue to use physical therapy techniques directed by the surgeon and therapist. Heat or cold packs or both to masticatory muscles prior to range of motion exercises are recommended four to six times a day for 2 weeks or longer after surgery. Continuous passive motion (CPM) and other exercise devices are individualized and can be very beneficial for healing and improving range of mandibular motion.

Postoperative care for patients with the hypermobility syndrome or recurrent dislocation stresses greater limitation of motion of the mandible. The patients with active recurrent dislocation are placed in maxillomandibular elastic fixation for 4 weeks. Then a soft, nonchew diet is started and continued for at least 2 months. Progressive range of motion exercise is initiated after release of fixation. The patients with hypermobility are not placed into maxillomandibular fixation but are instructed in restraint of mouth opening no greater than 25 mm. Multiple mouth-opening exercises up to 25 mm four times a day are advised. The extremes of vertical and horizontal mandibular motion are restricted, and prolonged opening needed in dental treatment or with imaging is avoided during the healing period. Medications used are narcotic analgesics for the early postoperative days, a nonsteroidal anti-inflammatory drug for 2 weeks; and a muscle relaxant for those with a significant myofascial component to their disorder. Work and activities that place the joint at risk for injury are avoided. The hypermobility patients are instructed to use a soft diet for 3 months and are not placed in fixation.

COMPLICATIONS OF ARTHROSCOPY

All surgical procedures carry with them the risk of complication. Each procedure has inherent risks and general risks. Complications occur predominantly at the time of surgery. Infections occur mainly in the postoperative period. An improper diagnosis followed by an inappropriate procedure can be considered a preoperative complication. Complications are either temporary or permanent. Morbidity is variable, but permanent complications obviously are of greater concern. Fortunately, permanent complications of temporomandibular arthroscopy are rare, and temporary complications are infrequent. The surgeon and surgical team must be aware of possible complications, their prevention, and treatment. This joint is one of the smallest treated by arthroscopy and some complications are inherent in this. Some of the arthroscopic complications also apply to arthrography and arthrotomy.

Sprague categorized complications of general arthroscopy into three categories. That of *general medical* includes sepsis, aseptic synovitis, thromboembolism, and anesthetic and reflex sympathetic dystrophy. The second category is *general technique–related* injuries to ligament, bone, nerve, vessel, and soft tissue. A third category is *specific procedure–related* complications.[44] Carter and Schwaber categorized complications of temporomandibular arthroscopy differently, into anesthetic, infectious, neurologic, vascular, instrument failure, otologic, and inflammatory.[45]

Local and general anesthetic techniques are appropriate for arthroscopic surgery. Patient acceptance of general anesthesia is high, and it is not surprising that it is the most commonly used technique. A national survey in 1983 and 1984 on the incidence of complications of arthroscopy, not including the TMJ, reported an anesthetic complication incidence of 0.038 per cent in 118,590 procedures.[44] An incidence of 0.12 per cent was found in a temporomandibular arthroscopy survey (see Table 11–5). Cardiac asystole, bradycardia, and other dysrhythmias can occur with head and neck surgery. Gomez and Van Gelder reported a case of profound bradycardia reversed by atropine occurring during arthroscopy of the TMJ in a 31-year-old woman under general anesthesia.[47] The cause was an increase in intra-articular pressure during insufflation of the joint. Arthroscopy has the unique possibility of airway obstruction from extravasated fluids into the fascial planes medial to the joint.[45] Irrigating fluids most likely gain access through defects in the thin anteromedial wall of the joint capsule by penetration of instruments. A large volume of irrigant may enlarge the lateral pharyngeal space and tonsillar fossa, with edema of the soft palate and uvula. Early extubation can lead to airway compromise.

Vascular injury can occur with injections of local anesthetics and insufflation fluids. Trocars may tear a vessel. Penetration or cutting with instruments beyond the capsule anteriorly and medially may initiate hemorrhage. A 1992 survey revealed few vascular complications, but in one instance open ligation of the masseteric artery was necessary.[59] Tamponade or suturing at the portal site usually controls bleeding, which usually originates from the superficial temporal vessels, without resorting to an open ligation. Moses and Toper reported an unusual postoperative complication of an arteriovenous fistula between the superficial temporal vein and artery in the path of the preauricular puncture site, which eventually required resection.[49]

Neurologic injury of the trigeminal and facial cranial nerves is the most common category of morbidity from arthroscopy.[50] Traction from instruments, fluid extravasation, and punctures with trocars and needles are mechanisms of neurologic injury. Fluid extravasation results in transient neuropraxia. Nerve injury from instruments and needles is neuropraxia, axonotmesis, or neurotmesis. The most devastating injury is seventh cranial nerve neurotmesis (see Table 11–5). Auriculotemporal neuropraxia is the predominant injury and is rarely more than transient.

Otologic complications as a result of TMJ arthroscopy may involve any component of the ear. Otitis, tympanic membrane perforation, and damage to the ossicular chain and other middle ear structures can occur. Van Sickles, Nishioka, and Hegewald reported an arthroscopic case with tympanic membrane perforation and partial dislocation of the malleus.[51] There was conductive hearing loss and tinnitus in the affected ear. The structures healed, but mild conductive loss was present after 3 months. Applebaum and colleagues reported three cases of otologic injury, and in two of the cases there had been prior arthrotomies.[52] Severe sensorineural hearing loss occurred in two cases and conductive loss occurred in the third case. They speculated that the sensori-

Table 11–3
COMPLICATIONS OF 2225 TMJ ARTHROSCOPY PROCEDURES: CARTER AND TESTA, 1987

	Per Cent
Vascular	1.7
Neurologic	3.8
Infectious	0.4
Mechanical	3.3
Inflammatory	0.3
TOTAL	9.5

Data from Carter JB, Testa L: Complications of TMJ arthroscopy: A review of 2,225 cases. J Oral Maxillofac Surg 1988;46:M14–M15.

neural loss may have resulted from increased irrigation pressure in the middle ear causing damage to the oval or round window. One patient had transient seventh nerve paralysis, attributed to nerve damage within the middle ear. The most probable site of entrance to the ear is at the bony and cartilaginous junction of the external auditory canal. Interruption of the external auditory canal from deflection of an instrument at the postglenoid tubercle takes place only several millimeters from the tympanic membrane and middle ear. Studies by Jones and Horn[53] and by McCain, Goldberg, and de la Rua[54] using pre- and postoperative audiometry tests confirmed that arthroscopy does not cause ear dysfunction.

The incidence of broken instruments during arthroscopy is low. The instruments used are delicate and have the potential to break. The option of leaving a fragment of an instrument in place is not desirable. A lost object may be perceived as dangerous owing to its location, or it may be blamed for a poor result. One option is removal at a second arthroscopy, which certainly is not as desirable as removal at the time of breakage. The advantage of arthroscopic retrieval is the ability to visualize joint recesses under light and magnification. Retrieval is usually accomplished by triangulation and a grasping forcep or by a magnetic retriever. A broken needle tip in the joint from arthrography could best be retrieved by arthroscopy.

Arthroscopic procedures are done under strict aseptic conditions. The likelihood of infection of the joint and adjacent structures as a complication of a procedure is rare. Wound infection and joint sepsis apparently are not a material complication of TMJ arthroscopy, for in three large surveys, a combined incidence for infection was only 0.13 per cent, or 12 infections in 8799 procedures (see Table 11–6).

The first survey on complications in temporomandibular arthroscopy was completed by Carter and Testa in 1987[48] (Table 11–3). This was early in the experience of most surgeons surveyed. The total incidence was 9.5 per cent. Neurologic and instrument failures were more common than vascular, infectious, and inflammatory complications. Greene and Van Sickles surveyed 38 training programs in 1989, finding a 2.5 per cent total incidence of complications in 897 procedures (Table 11–4).[58] Again, neurologic injury was the most common category of morbidity. Ear canal perforation occurred in four patients. A survey of experienced members of the International Study Group on TMJ Arthroscopy was done in 1992 (Table 11–5). The incidence of complications in 5677 procedures was 4 per cent. Neurologic morbidity again was most common, accounting for 2 per cent, or half of all complications. This survey identified temporary and permanent complications. All but four complications were temporary and short-term. The four permanent complications include

Table 11–4
COMPLICATIONS OF 897 TMJ ARTHROSCOPY PROCEDURES: GREENE AND VAN SICKLES, 1989[58]

	Number	Per Cent
Sensory nerve injury	7	0.78
Facial nerve injury	5	0.58
Ear canal perforation	4	0.45
Fluid extravasation	4	0.45
Bleeding requiring ligation	1	0.11
External otitis	1	0.11
TOTAL	22	2.5

two cases of hearing loss, one case of total facial paralysis, and one case of Frey's syndrome. An incidence of long-standing complications of only 0.07 per cent in 5677 procedures speaks well for the safety of temporomandibular arthroscopy.

The complication rate when combining the three surveys but not separating temporary and permanent morbidity was 5.2 per cent of 8799 procedures (Table 11–6). The incidence of 3.93 per cent temporary complications and 0.07 permanent complications in the 1992 survey is probably the most accurate for arthroscopic procedures now being performed by experienced surgeons. The most serious and permanent complications reported in the surveys were two cases of hearing loss and one case of facial nerve paralysis in 8799 procedures. It is the opinion of the arthroscopists surveyed that sensorineural hearing loss with vertigo, total facial paralysis, and conductive hearing loss, in that order, are the most serious long-standing complications of arthroscopy.

OUTCOMES OF ARTHROSCOPIC PROCEDURES

The diagnosis of internal derangement in 1000 joints in 790 patients was confirmed by history, physical diagnosis, arthrotomography, or MR imaging, and by arthroscopic observation.[60] All stages of internal derangement were represented except early stage. All the patients in this series had nonsurgical care that did not adequately correct their condition. Elimination or a marked reduction of symptoms and a significant improvement in mandibular range of motion were accomplished in the majority of the patients treated by arthroscopic lysis, joint lavage, and manipulation of the disk and capsule (LLM).

Table 11–5
COMPLICATIONS OF 5677 TMJ ARTHROSCOPY PROCEDURES: INTERNATIONAL STUDY GROUP SURVEY, MERRILL, 1992[59]

	Temporary	Permanent	Per Cent
Anesthetic	7	0	0.12
Infectious	3	0	0.05
Neurologic	120	2*	2.1
Vascular	47	0	0.83
Instrument	15	0	0.26
Otologic	31	2†	0.58
TOTAL	223 (3.93%)	4 (0.07%)	4

*Total VII, Frey's syndrome.
†Hearing loss.

Table 11–6
COMPLICATION INCIDENCE IN THREE SURVEYS OF 8799 TMJ ARTHROSCOPY PROCEDURES

	Procedures	Complications	Per Cent
Carter and Testa (Table 11–3)	2225	211	9.5
Greene and Van Sickles (Table 11–4)	897	22	2.5
Merrill (ISG) (Table 11–5)	5677	227	3.94
TOTAL	8799	460	5.2

A detailed evaluation of the outcome of LLM was completed in the first 98 patients 1 to 3 years after surgery.[60] There were 157 joints in this group. Eighty-five per cent of the patients were women, with a mean age of 31 years. Thirty-four joints were stage II internal derangement. Seventy-seven joints were stage III. Twenty-six joints were stage IV. Twenty joints were judged to be stage V. The outcome evaluation was done by comparing pre- and postoperative conditions by means of detailed questionnaires that included a pain analog scale, historical information, physical examination, and radiology of soft and hard tissue.

There was minimal morbidity and high positive acceptance of the procedure by the patients. The success rate in this group of 98 patients was adjudged better, the same, or worse 2 to 3 years after the surgery. No patients in this group were worse. Seventy-six were judged to be better and thirty-five were the same or not improved by LLM. This translates to a 78 per cent success and 22 per cent failure rate in this early group of 98 patients (Table 11–7). These results are comparable to the results reported by others.[9–19]

The results of LLM were further broken down related to the staging of internal derangement. Twenty-two joints (65 per cent) were significantly improved and twelve (35 per cent) were not improved in stage II internal derangement. The best results were found in patients' stage III joints, which by definition have deformed, prolapsed disks that were not returned to an anatomically normal state by the procedure. Sixty-five joints (85 per cent) were improved and twelve (15 per cent) were not. Twenty-one (80 per cent) were better, and five (20 per cent) the same in stage IV. Thirteen (67 per cent) were better and seven (33 per cent) were with stage V internal derangement. There were no permanent complications in this group of patients. Six per cent of the patients who were not improved continued to experience debilitating symptoms after limited additional nonsurgical therapy failed. Subsequently, arthrotomy procedures were performed on them. Most of the cases requiring arthrotomy had either early/intermediate stage or late stage internal derangement. Disk repair procedures were done for the joints with early/intermediate stage disease, and diskectomy with or without an interpositional autogenous graft for late/intermediate and late stage cases. A graft was not used if bony surfaces were judged to have sufficient fibrocartilage covering them. The graft

Table 11–7
RESULTS OF LLM IN 98 PATIENTS (157 JOINTS)

	Patients	Per Cent
Better	76	78
Same	22	22
Worse	0	0

Table 11–8
RESULTS OF SCLEROTHERAPY AND LLM IN 53 PATIENTS (95 JOINTS)[60]

	Patients	Per Cent
Better	48	91
Same	5	9
Worse	0	0

most commonly used was auricular cartilage. A planned temporary Silastic sheeting was interposed between the cartilage graft and condyle to reduce adhesion formation and to maximize joint recesses.

Results of arthroscopic LLM with the addition of chemical sclerosis of the posterior attachment were studied in 95 joints in 53 patients an average of 2 years after surgery.[60] There were 9 men and 44 women, with a range in age from 15 to 76 years. The mean age was 36 years. Thirty-seven (70 per cent) had a significant history of macrotrauma. The duration of symptoms ranged from 0.5 year to 22 years, with an average of 5.5 years. There were 42 patients with hypermobility and 11 with recurrent mandibular dislocation. Eight of the patients with painful hypermobility had a history of mandibular dislocation. The patients were judged to have hypermobility by radiographic and clinical evidence of the condyle translating anterior to the articular eminence, clinical evidence or history of a wide range of mandibular motion, and laxity of the disk and capsule observed during the arthroscopic diagnostic examination. All of the patients with hypermobility and recurrent dislocation had internal derangement. There were 24 patients with early/intermediate (II) stage, 57 with intermediate (III) stage, 8 with late/intermediate (IV) stage, and 6 with late (V) stage internal derangement. The intermediate stage patients either were not yet in a chronic fixed disk prolapse or had chronic disk prolapse but the ability to open the mouth wide. Frequently the condyle would translate anterior to the dislocated and deformed disk. Subjective pain and dysfunction were present in all patients.

The general success rate was 48 joints better, 5 joints the same, and none worse for a 91 per cent success rate. The results of LLM with sclerotherapy compared with a similar group of 98 patients who had LLM without sclerotherapy are shown in Tables 11–7 and 11–8. The most impressive improvement in results with the addition of sclerotherapy compared with not using sclerotherapy was seen in early/intermediate and those approaching intermediate stage internal derangement. There was a 91 per cent success rate in the sclerotherapy patients and a 78 per cent success rate in patients who had only LLM. There were no complications in patients who had LLM and chemical sclerotherapy. Range of mandibular motion has not been functionally restricted by the sclerotherapy.

Discussion

Arthroscopic surgery of the TMJ has come a long way since 1985. It is now an accepted method of surgical treatment. Complications are uncommon and usually transient. Health care providers and the public have recognized its value as a conservative and effective method of surgical treatment. Indications and arthroscopic techniques continue to evolve. Arthroscopic surgery is indicated when joint pathology is the source of persistent signs and symptoms that interfere with the person's quality of life. An accurate diagnosis of an arthropathy must be made. Strictly myofascial and referred pain conditions must be recognized so an inappropriate procedure will not be done. The predominant arthropathy is internal derangement. The signs and symptoms of most arthropathies improve with nonsurgical care; however, surgical treatment should not be considered only as a last resort for patients in whom other treatment fails. The diagnostic benefits are important, and arthroscopy should not be considered only as a surgical tool.

Arthroscopic surgery has become an effective method of treatment for specific articular disorders (Table 11–1). The objectives, indications, and techniques are similar to those relating to other synovial joints. The preoperative diagnosis, patient selection, imaging studies, choice of surgical procedure, skill and experience level of the surgeon, postoperative care, and patient compliance all influence surgical outcome. Surgery ordinarily should not be performed without imaging studies, including basic radiographs, and arthrography or magnetic resonance imaging or both that clearly define the joint pathology. Arthroscopic diagnosis enhances the clinical and imaging diagnosis, thereby providing a sound basis for improved treatment and prognosis.

References

1. Watanabe M: Arthroscopy of Small Joints. Tokyo, Igaku-Shoin, 1985, p 3.
2. Ohnishi M: Arthroscopy of the TMJ (Japanese; English abstract). J Stomatol Soc Jpn 1975;42:207–213.
3. McCain JP, de la Rua H, LeBlanc WG: Correlation of clinical, radiographic and arthroscopic findings in internal derangements of the TMJ. J Oral Maxillofac Surg 1989;47:913–921.
4. Merrill RG, Yih WY, Langan MJ: A histologic evaluation of the accuracy of TMJ diagnostic arthroscopy. Oral Surg Oral Med Oral Pathol 1990;70:393–398.
5. Holmlund A, Hellsing G: Arthroscopy of the TMJ. Occurrence and location of osteoarthrosis and synovitis in patient material. Int J Oral Maxillofac Surg 1988;17:36–40.
6. Quinn, JH: Arthroscopic and histologic evidence of chondromalacia in the TMJ. Oral Surg Oral Med Oral Pathol 1990;70(3):387–392.
7. Kaminishi RM, Davis CL: Temporomandibular joint arthroscopic observations of superior space adhesions. Oral Maxillofac Surg Clin North Am 1989;1(1):103–109.
8. Roa VM, Farole A, Karasick D: Temporomandibular joint dysfunction: Correlation of MR imaging, arthrography, and arthroscopy. Radiology 1990;174:663–667.
9. Sanders BS, Buoncristiani R: Diagnostic and surgical arthroscopy of the TMJ: Clinical experience with 137 procedures over a 2-year period. J Craniomandib Disorders Facial Oral Pain 1987;1(3):202–213.
10. Sanders B, Kaminishi R, Buoncristiani R, Davis C: Arthroscopic surgery for treatment of temporomandibular joint hypomobility after mandibular sagittal osteotomy. Oral Surg Oral Med Oral Pathol 1990;69:539–541.
11. Nitzen DW, Dolwick MF, Heft MW: Arthroscopic lavage and lysis of the temporomandibular joint: A change in perspective. J Oral Maxillofac Surg 1990;48:798–801.
12. White RD: Retrospective analysis of 100 consecutive surgical arthroscopies of the temporomandibular joint. J Oral Maxillofac Surg 1989;47:1014–1021
13. Perrott DH, Alborzi A, Kaban LB, Helms CA: A prospective evaluation of the effectiveness of temporomandibular joint arthroscopy. J Oral Maxillofac Surg 1990;48:1029–1032.
14. Indresano AT: Arthroscopic surgery of the temporomandibular joint: Report of 64 patients with long-term follow-up. J Oral Maxillofac Surg 1989;47:439–441.
15. Goss A, Bosanquet A: Temporomandibular joint arthroscopy. J Oral Maxillofac Surg 1986;44:614–617.
16. Montgomery MT, Van Sickle JE, Harms SE, Thrash WJ: Arthroscopic TMJ surgery: Effects on signs, symptoms, and disc position. J Oral Maxillofac Surg 1989;47:1263–1271.
17. Israel H, Roser SM: Patient response to temporomandibular joint arthroscopy: Preliminary findings in 24 patients. J Oral Maxillofac Surg 1989;47:570–573.
18. Moses JJ, Poker I: TMJ arthroscopic surgery. J Oral Maxillofac Surg 1989;47:790–794.
19. Taro AW: Arthroscopic diagnosis and surgery of the temporomandibular joint. J Oral Maxillofac Surg 1988;46:282–289.

20. Moses JJ: Lateral impingement syndrome and endaural surgical technique. Disorders of TMJ I: Diagnosis and arthroscopy. Oral Maxillofac Clin North Am 1989;*1*:165.
21. Merrill RG: Arthroscopic lysis, lavage, manipulation and chemical sclerotherapy of the TMJ for hypermobility and recurrent dislocation. Proceedings, Fourth International Symposium of TMJ Arthroscopy, Hawaii, 1989.
22. Ohnishi M, Nakayama E, Kino K: Arthroscopic surgery for habitual dislocations of temporomandibular joint (Japanese; English abstract). Arthroscopy 1987;*12*:103–105.
23. Ohnishi M: Arthroscopic surgery for hypermobility and recurrent mandibular dislocation. Oral Maxillofac Surg Clin North Am 1989;*1*(1):153–164.
24. Tarro AW: Arthroscopic treatment of anterior disc displacement. J Oral Maxillofac Surg 1989;*47*:353–358.
25. McCain JL: Arthroscopic suturing techniques for TMJ disc displacement. Proceedings, Fourth International Symposium on TMJ Arthroscopy, Hawaii, 1989.
26. Kondoh T, Westesson P-L: Diagnostic accuracy of TMJ lower compartment arthroscopy using an ultra thin arthroscope. J Oral Maxillofac Surg 1991;*49*:619–626.
27. Quinn JH: Arthroscopic TMJ abrasion arthroplasty. Proceedings, Fifth International Symposium on TMJ Arthroscopy, New York, 1990.
28. Kondoh T, Westesson P-L: TMJ lower compartment arthroscopy with an ultrathin scope. Proceedings, Fifth International Symposium on TMJ Arthroscopy, New York, 1990.
29. Moses JJ, Sartoris D, Glass R, et al: The effect of arthroscopic surgical lysis and lavage of the superior joint space on TMJ disc position and mobility. J Oral Maxillofac Surg 1989;*47*:674–678.
30. Wilkes CH: Surgical treatment of internal derangements of the temporomandibular joint: A long-term study. Arch Otolaryngol Head Neck Surg 1991;*117*:64–72.
31. Nickerson JW, Boering G: Natural course of osteoarthrosis as it relates to internal derangement of the temporomandibular joint. Oral Maxillofac Surg Clin North Am 1989;*1*(1):27–45.
32. Wilkes CH: Internal derangements of the temporomandibular joint. Arch Otolaryngol Head Neck Surg 1989;*115*:469–477.
33. Goss AN, Bosanquet AG: The arthroscopic appearance of acute TMJ trauma. J Oral Maxillofac Surg 1990;*48*:780–783.
34. Jones JK, Van Sickles JE: A preliminary report of arthroscopic findings following acute mandibular trauma (abstract). Proceedings, AAOMS Annual Meeting, New Orleans, 1990.
35. Stegenga B, DeBont LGM, Boering G: Osteoarthrosis as the cause of craniomandibular pain and dysfunction. J Oral Maxillofac Surg 1988;*47*:249–256.
36. Israel HA, Ratcliffe A, Fatemeh SN: Synovial fluid keratin sulfate concentration in TMJ with arthroscopically diagnosed osteoarthrosis (abstract). Proceedings, AAOMS Annual Meeting, New Orleans, 1990.
37. Nitzen DW, Dolwick FM, Martinez GA: Temporomandibular joint arthrocentesis: A simplified treatment for severe, limited mouth opening. J Oral Maxillofac Surg 1991;*49*:1163–1167.
38. Levick JR, McDonald JN: Synovial capillary distribution in relation to altered pressure and permeability in knees of anesthetized rabbits. J Physiol (Lond) 1989;*419*:477.
39. Murakami K-I, Matsuki M, Izuka T, Ono T: Diagnostic arthroscopy of the TMJ: Differential diagnosis in patients with limited jaw opening. J Craniomandib Pract 1986;*4*(2):117–126.
40. Quinn JH, Bazan NG: Identification of prostaglandin E$_2$ and leukotriene B$_4$ in the synovial fluid of painful, dysfunctional TMJ. J Oral Maxillofac Surg 1990;*48*:968–971.
41. Moses JJ, Poker ID: TMJ arthroscopy: The endaural approach. Int J Oral Maxillofac Surg 1989;*18*:347–351.
42. Wenneberg B, Kopp S, Grondahl H-G: Long-term effect of intra-articular injections of a glucocorticosteroid into the TMJ: A clinical and radiographic 8 year follow up. J Craniomandib Disorders Facial Oral Pain 1991;*5*:11–18.
43. Murakami K-I, Segami N, Fujimura K, Iizuka T: Correlation between pain and synovitis in patients with internal derangement of the temporomandibular joint. J Oral Maxillofac Surg 1991;*49*:1159–1161.
44. Sprague NF, ed: Complications in Arthroscopy. New York, Raven Press, 1989.
45. Carter JB, Schwaber MK: TMJ arthroscopy complications and management. Oral Maxillofac Surg Clin North Am 1989;*1*(1):185–199.
46. Sanders B, Buoncristiani RD, Johnson L: Silicone rubber fossa implant removal via partial arthrotomy followed by arthroscopic examination of the internal surface of the fibrous capsule. Oral Surg Oral Med Oral Pathol 1990;*70*:369–371.
47. Gomez TM, Van Gelder J: Reflex bradycardia during TMJ arthroscopy. J Oral Maxillofac Surg 1991;*49*:543–544.
48. Carter JB, Testa L: Complications of TMJ arthroscopy: A review of 2,225 cases. J Oral Maxillofac Surg 1988;*46*:M14–M15.
49. Moses JJ, Toper D: Arteriovenous fistula: An unusual complication associated with arthroscopic TMJ surgery. J Oral Maxillofac Surg 1990;*48*:1220–1222.
50. McCain JP: Arthroscopy of the human TMJ. J Oral Maxillofac Surg 1988;*46*:648–655.
51. Van Sickles JE, Nishioka GJ, Hegewald MD: Middle ear injury resulting from TMJ arthroscopy. J Oral Maxillofac Surg 1987;*45*:962–965.
52. Applebaum EL, Berg LF, Kumar H: Otologic complications following TMJ arthroscopy. Ann Otol Rhinol Laryngol 1988;*97*:675–679.

53. Jones JL, Horn KL: The effect of temporomandibular joint arthroscopy on ear function. J Oral Maxillofac Surg 1989;47:1022–1025.
54. McCain JP, Goldberg HM, de la Rua H: Preoperative and postoperative audiologic measurements in patients undergoing arthroscopy of the TMJ. J Oral Maxillofac Surg 1989;47:1026–1027.
55. Bronstein SL, Merrill RG: Clinical staging for TMJ internal derangement: Application to arthroscopy. J Craniomandib Disorders Facial Oral Pain 1992;6(1).
56. Schellhas KP, Piper MA, Omlie MR: Facial skeleton remodeling due to temporomandibular joint degeneration: An imaging study of 100 patients. AJR 1990;155:373–383.
57. Bocring G: Arthrosis deformans van het kaakgewrect. Een klinisch en rontgenologisch onderzoch (dissertation). Groningen, The Netherlands, Ryksuniversiteit te Groningen, 1966.
58. Greene MW, Van Sickles JF: Survey of TMJ arthroscopy in oral and maxillofacial surgery residency programs. J Oral Maxillofac Surg 1989;47:574–576.
59. Merrill RG: Indications and morbidity in TMJ arthroscopy. Proceedings, American Association Oral and Maxillofacial Surgery Clinical Congress, San Antonio, Texas, Feb 1992.
60. Merrill RG: Arthroscopic lysis, lavage, manipulation and chemical sclerotherapy of the TMJ for hypermobility and recurrent dislocation. Advances in Diagnostic and Surgical Arthroscopy of the Temporomandibular Joint. Philadelphia, WB Saunders, 1993, pp 75–84.

PART FIVE

Putting It All Together

CHAPTER TWELVE

Selection of Diagnostic Tests

There are many philosophies regarding the selection of diagnostic modalities for the evaluation of patients with signs and symptoms of temporomandibular joint (TMJ) disorders. Many of these philosophies are based upon the availability of clinical and imaging expertise, imaging systems that are readily available, and economic considerations. The preceding pages have presented a series of different imaging modalities that can be used to study patients presenting with signs and symptoms of TMJ internal derangement and other musculoskeletal disorders affecting the joint. Our goal in this chapter is to provide our recommendation on the appropriate flow chart combining clinical presentation with optimal imaging assessments. We have taken into account our own unique logistical and economic environment. There are many variations from our recommendations that will work well as they are adapted to different clinical settings.

CLINICAL EXAMINATION

The clinical examination is the single most important component in the evaluation of patients presenting with orofacial pain or symptoms of a TMJ disorder. Selection of the optimal diagnostic modality should be based on the findings of the clinical examination and determined by the special clinical need for additional information.[1] The overall objective of the imaging assessment is to detect and define specific anatomic abnormalities that account for the patient's signs and symptoms. Some patients may have asymptomatic internal derangement as incidental findings in the contralateral joints. These patients should be informed of these findings as a potential risk factor, but they may not necessarily require treatment. At the present time, there are no indications that specific treatments can prevent the development of symptoms later or prevent progression of the disease. For this reason, we do not recommend preventive treatment of an asymptomatic internal derangement. A careful clinical and imaging evaluation can help exclude the referred pain from sources other than the TMJ.[2] Therefore, evaluation of symptoms related to the TMJ is mandatory, since numerous other causes of facial pain in and around the TMJ region exist.

Accuracy of Clinical Examination

There is controversy in the literature over the accuracy of clinical diagnosis to determine the status of the TMJ in patients with symptoms and signs of internal derangement and arthrosis. Several studies[3-10] have reported accuracy rates of the clinical examination for different stages of internal derangement at between 43 and 90 per cent; one single study reported a 100 per cent accuracy rate on a selected group of patients.[11] However, our experience is that the clinical examination is not exacting with respect to the status of the joint, and our studies suggest that the accuracy of the clinical examination is between 50 and 60 per cent in a consecutive series of patients with TMJ symptoms.[12] If only those patients with characteristic signs and symptoms are considered, the overall diagnostic accuracy of the clinical examination would be higher, but this is not relevant for the clinical situation, in which patients cannot be preselected.

SCREENING MODALITIES

Plain Film and Tomography

Though plain films of the TMJ evaluate the osseous structures of the joint, they provide no direct information regarding any of the soft tissue anatomy. One must also keep in mind that the radiographic plain film is only a two-dimensional representation of a three-dimensional object (see Chapter 4). The osseous components of the joint are three-dimensional structures, yet the surface seen on the radiographs represents only those portions of the cortical bone under the articular surface that are tangential to the x-ray beam. Therefore, on any given plain film projection, only a small portion of the cortex beneath the joint surface is represented on the radiographic image. The joint surface is never entirely visualized with the plain film technique. With this limitation in mind, one can understand why there are a multitude of plain film projections for assessment of the TMJ.

Despite the relative simplicity of the anatomy obtainable with single projections, plain film radiographs continue to be a useful screening method for detecting gross osseous abnormalities of the TMJ (Fig. 12–1). They are readily performed and inexpensive. Some of the routine techniques include the transcranial radiograph, linear or multidirectional tomography, and the panoramic radiograph. The transcranial radiograph has an overall positive yield for osseous abnormalities of around 5 to 8 per cent of patients presenting with symptoms of internal derangement, and the tomographic radiograph has a yield of approximately 10 to 15 per cent positive findings in patients with clinical symptoms of TMJ disorders.[13] If these simple screening modalities are negative, there is no assurance of whether an internal derangement does or does not exist. Even when positive for degenerative disease, the etiology of this condition is not specific for internal derangement.

Radionuclide Imaging

If the patient has rather diffuse and poorly localized facial pain around the TMJ region, we recommend radionuclide skeletal imaging as a sensitive test for skeletal pathology (see Chapter 7). This imaging modality has a proven high sensitivity for a wide variety of osseous lesions.[14, 15] In many osseous conditions, the bone scintigram will demonstrate an abnormality long before any change can be detected on conventional radiographs. Thus, even early cellular changes in the bony structures may result in a demonstrable lesion with

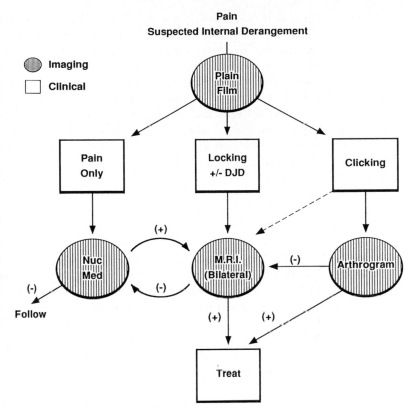

Figure 12–1
Flow chart of a recommended imaging approach for a patient with facial pain and internal derangement in the differential diagnosis. The plain film is a standard screening modality for all patients with suspected internal derangement. If the patient has diffuse pain, without clicking or locking, a screening evaluation using radionuclide skeletal imaging is recommended. In a patient with pain and locking of the TMJ, with or without degenerative joint disease by plain film imaging, a bilateral MR examination with surface coils is the modality of choice. If the patient has pain and clicking of the TMJ, either arthrography or a bilateral MR examination is recommended. The arthrogram is the procedure of choice if protrusive splint therapy is the treatment modality anticipated. A positive radionuclide scan for TMJ pathology or a negative arthrogram should plead further for the diagnostic evaluation with a bilateral MR. A simplified and also very effective imaging protocol is from plain film to MR in all cases.

scintigraphy before such changes become morphologically suspicious by radiography.[16–19]

Determining the origin of facial pain from clinical examination can be difficult at times.[12] Many different diseases may produce pain that can mimic TMJ pain. Among these are Paget's disease of bone, fibrous dysplasia, bone cysts, sinusitis, osteomyelitis, neoplasm, fractures, inflammatory disease, dental and periapical disease, and cervical spine disease. Many of these conditions have a typical appearance on bone scintigraphy, and thus utilization of these techniques can be of value in establishing an early diagnosis. If the radionuclide scintigram is positive in the TMJ region, we recommend that the patient be evaluated by a bilateral magnetic resonance TMJ imaging study (Fig. 12–1). If the nuclear medicine scan is negative, the patient may then be followed clinically in anticipation of a resolution of the problem or for the development of more specific signs or focal symptoms.

Soft Tissue Imaging

In patients with plain film findings for degenerative joint disease or in those experiencing painful locking of the jaw, we recommend magnetic resonance (MR) imaging using bilateral surface coil technology as the first choice for the principal imaging evaluation. MR with surface coils is a proven method for the assessment of internal derangement of the TMJ and has rapidly surpassed arthrography and computed tomography as the imaging modality of choice.[1, 20–23] The major advantages of MR compared with arthrography are

(a) it is noninvasive; (b) it requires no ionizing radiation for image acquisition; (c) it permits a direct visualization of the disk and associated joint structures; (d) the multiplanar imaging is readily obtained and more easily interpretable; (e) it allows visualization of the soft tissue structures around the joint; and (f) a multitude of different pulse sequences can be utilized for tissue characterization. Comparative studies using cryosectional cadaver material in conjunction with multiplanar imaging have demonstrated the high accuracy of MR.[24–26] The disadvantages of MR are the high initial costs of such imaging systems, the necessity for special site planning and shielding, and patient claustrophobia in the magnet.

If the MR examination is negative, the patient can be assessed for other causes of facial pain with radionuclide imaging (Fig. 12–1). If the MR scan is positive, treatment can be effectively implemented. MR is also excellent for the evaluation of the clicking patient and could prove to be the procedure of choice for all patients with suspected internal derangement.

We have significantly decreased the use of TMJ arthrography during the last few years because of the excellent capabilities and ease of performance of MR. However, if the patient presents with pain from clicking of the TMJ and the referring clinician is an advocate of protrusive splint therapy (see Chapter 5), the arthrogram is the most effective modality for this assessment.[27, 28] The video dynamics of the arthrogram can depict the displaced disk clearly and allow for a precise mandible position to be determined for the initiation of protrusive splint therapy.[28] This technique is easy to perform and has been shown to be an efficacious component in the diagnosis and treatment of disk displacement with reduction. If the arthrogram is negative for internal derangement, we recommend an MR scan to assess whether there is a rotational or sideways disk displacement.[26] These are not easily depicted by the two-dimensional nature of the arthrographic anatomic assessment. Arthrography has been invaluable in the general assessment of the TMJ internal derangement and can still be used as a primary imaging modality for all patients suspected of having internal derangement if high quality MR surface coil–assisted imaging is not available.

Postoperative MR Imaging

MR imaging after treatment is indicated in patients who continue to have symptoms or impaired function that might be related to intra-articular changes. Before MR was available, plain films, tomograms, and arthrography were used to evaluate these patients. Plain films and tomograms are relatively nonspecific because only the osseous structures are seen. Arthrography may be difficult to perform in surgically treated patients because of peripheral adhesions; therefore, MR is the method of choice for most postoperative imaging of the TMJ.[29–32] Arthrography is recommended after surgical treatment only when MR and CT are inconclusive. If bony ankylosis is suspected, CT might be complementary to MR.

IMAGING STRATEGIES FOR PATIENTS WITH CHRONIC ARTHRITIC DISEASE AND TEMPOROMANDIBULAR JOINT SYMPTOMS

Initial TMJ imaging in this patient group should be focused on osseous abnormalities. Plain film or panoramic radiographs will show moderate to advanced osseous changes. In patients with severe disease, these methods may be sufficient. For the assessment of minor cortical erosions, tomography or CT might be necessary and should be performed if the initial screening examination is negative or uncertain. If more detailed information is needed for treatment planning, or if osseous ankylosis is suspected, CT is the method of choice.

For assessment of the soft tissue joint anatomy of patients with chronic arthritis, MR is the first choice.[33-35] Disk displacement, joint effusion, and condylar marrow edema can be evaluated, as well as cortical bone abnormalities.[35] Arthrotomography is an alternative method if high quality MR is not available or, in rare circumstances, if MR is not diagnostic.

OTHER DIAGNOSTIC TESTS

Joint sound analysis is considered a screening modality used as a complement to the clinical examination. At its current stage of technology and testing, joint sound analysis is not diagnostic for specific pathologic entities and cannot be considered definitive.[36]

Arthroscopy is discussed in detail in Chapter 11. The primary goal of small joint arthroscopy is therapy of internal derangement. Arthroscopy is also utilized for diagnosis, but it is generally complementary to the imaging modalities depicted in the flow chart (Fig. 12–1).

CONCLUSION

The most important component in the evaluation of patients with TMJ pain and dysfunction is the clinical examination. Findings in the clinical examination and the clinical need for additional information for treatment planning should determine the type of diagnostic modality selected. Screening techniques, such as plain film radiography and radionuclide imaging in patients with diffuse symptoms, could be a routine part of the assessment, but the limitations of these modalities must be kept in mind. The best imaging modality for the most complete assessment of internal derangement of the TMJ is bilateral multiplanar high-resolution surface coil–assisted MR.

References

1. Katzberg RW: Temporomandibular joint imaging. Radiology 1989;*170*:297–307.
2. Dolwick MF: Clinical diagnosis of temporomandibular joint internal derangement and myofascial pain and dysfunction. Oral Maxillofac Surg Clin North Am 1989;*1*:1–6.
3. Roberts CA, Tallents RH, Espeland MA, Handelman SL, Katzberg RW: Mandibular range of motion versus arthrographic diagnosis of the temporomandibular joint. Oral Surg Oral Med Oral Pathol 1985;*60*:244–251.
4. Roberts CA, Tallents RH, Katzberg RW, Sanchez-Woodworth RE, Espeland MA, Handelman SL: Comparison of arthrographic findings of the temporomandibular joint with palpation of the muscles of mastication. Oral Surg Oral Med Oral Pathol 1987;*64*:275–277.
5. Roberts CA, Tallents RH, Katzberg RW, Sanchez-Woodworth RE, Espeland MA, Handelman SL: Comparison of internal derangements of the temporomandibular joint with occlusal findings. Oral Surg Oral Med Oral Pathol 1987;*63*:645–650.
6. Roberts CA, Tallents RH, Katzberg RW, Sanchez-Woodworth RE, Espeland MA, Handelman SL: Clinical and arthrographic evaluation of the location of temporomandibular joint pain. Oral Surg Oral Med Oral Pathol 1987;*64*:6–8.
7. Roberts CA, Katzberg RW, Tallents RH, Espeland MA, Handelman SL: The clinical predict-

ability of internal derangements of the temporomandibular joint. Oral Surg Oral Med Oral Pathol 1991;*71*:412–414.

8. Anderson GC, Schiffman EL, Schellhas KP, Friction JR: Clinical vs. arthrographic diagnosis of temporomandibular joint internal derangements. J Dent Res 1989;*68*:826–829.

9. Kozeniauskas J: Temporomandibular joint: The diagnostic dilemma. Aust Orthod J 1988;*10*:213–216.

10. Kozeniauskas J, Ralph W: Bilateral arthrographic evaluation of unilateral temporomandibular joint pain and dysfunction. J Prosthet Dent 1988;*60*:98–105.

11. Isberg A, Stenström B, Isacsson G: Frequency of bilateral temporomandibular joint disk displacement in patients with unilateral symptoms: A 5-year follow-up of the asymptomatic joint: A clinical and arthrotomographic study. Dentomaxillofac Radiol 1991;*20*:73–76.

12. Paesani D, Westesson P-L, Hatala MP, Tallents RH, Brooks SL: Accuracy of clinical diagnosis for temporomandibular joint internal derangement and arthrosis. Oral Surg Oral Med Oral Pathol, in press.

13. Stanson AW, Baker HL: Routine tomography of the temporomandibular joint. Radiol Clin North Am 1976;*14*:105–127.

14. Lell PJ: Bones and joints. *In* Maisey MM, Button KE, Gilday DL, eds: Clinical Nuclear Medicine. London, Chapman and Hall, 1983, pp 135–165.

15. O'Mara RE: Benign bone disease. *In* Gottschalk A, Hoffer PB, Potchen EJ, eds: Diagnostic Nuclear Medicine. Baltimore, Williams & Wilkins, 1988, pp 1033–1075.

16. Goldstein HA, Bloom CY: Detection of degenerative disease of the temporomandibular joint by bone scintigraphy: Concise communication. J Nucl Med 1987;*21*:928–930.

17. Collier BD, Carrera GF, Messer EJ, et al: Internal derangement of the temporomandibular joint: Detection by single-photon emission computer tomography: Works in progress. Radiology 1983;*149*:557–561.

18. Katzberg RW, O'Mara RE, Tallents RH, Weber DA: Radionuclide skeletal imaging and single-photon emission computed tomography in suspected internal derangements of the temporomandibular joint. J Oral Maxillofac Surg 1984;*42*:782–787.

19. Wilson JA, O'Mara RE: Nuclear medicine imaging. *In* Westesson P-L, Katzberg RW: Imaging of the Temporomandibular Joint. Cranio Clinics International. Baltimore, Williams and Wilkins, 1991, pp 117–126.

20. Harms SE, Wilk RM, Wolford LM, et al: The temporomandibular joint: Magnetic resonance imaging using surface coils. Radiology 1985;*157*:133–136.

21. Katzberg RW, Bessette RW, Tallents RH, et al: Normal and abnormal temporomandibular joint: MR imaging with surface coils. Radiology 1986;*158*:183–189.

22. Helms CA, Jillespy T III, Sims RE, Richardson ML: Magnetic resonance imaging of internal derangement of the temporomandibular joint. Radiol Clin North Am 1986;*24*:189–192.

23. Kaplan PA, Helms CA: Current status of temporomandibular joint imaging for the diagnosis of internal derangement. AJR 1989;*152*:697–705.

24. Westesson P-L, Katzberg RW, Tallents RH, Sanchez-Woodworth RE, Svensson SA, Espeland MA: Temporomandibular joint: Comparison of MR images with cryosectional anatomy. Radiology 1987;*164*:59–64.

25. Westesson P-L, Katzberg RW, Tallents RH, Sanchez-Woodworth RE, Svensson SA, Espeland MA: CT and MRI of the temporomandibular joint: Comparison with autopsy specimens. AJR 1987;*148*:1165–1171.

26. Katzberg RW, Westesson P-L, Tallents RH, Anderson R, Kurita K, Manzione JV, Totterman S: Temporomandibular joint: MR assessment of rotational and sideways disk displacement. Radiology 1988;*169*:741–748.

27. Bell KA, Walters DJ: Video fluoroscopy during arthrography of the temporomandibular joint. Radiology 1983;*147*:879.

28. Manzione JV, Tallents RH, Katzberg RW, Oster C, Miller TL: Arthrographically guided splint therapy for recapturing the temporomandibular joint meniscus. Oral Surg Oral Med Oral Pathol 1984;*57*:235–240.

29. Kaplan PA, Reiskin AB, Tu HK: Temporomandibular joint arthrography following surgical treatment of internal derangement. Radiology 1987;*163*:217–220.

30. Schellhas KP, Wilkes CH, Fritts HM, et al: Temporomandibular joint: MR imaging of internal derangements and postoperative changes. AJNR 1987;*8*:1093–1101.

31. Kneeland JB, Ryan DE, Carrera GF, et al: Failed temporomandibular joint prostheses: MR imaging. Radiology 1987;*165*:179–181.

32. Westesson P-L, Cohen J, Tallents RH: Magnetic resonance imaging of the temporomandibular joint after surgical treatment of internal derangement. Oral Surg Oral Med Oral Pathol 1991;*71*:407–411.

33. Larheim TA: Imaging of the temporomandibular joint in rheumatoid disease. *In* Westesson P-L, Katzberg RW: Imaging of the Temporomandibular Joint. Cranio Clinics International. Baltimore, Williams and Wilkins, 1991, pp 133–154.

34. Larheim TA: Imaging of the temporomandibular joint in juvenile rheumatoid arthritis. *In* Westesson P-L, Katzberg RW. Imaging of the Temporomandibular Joint. Cranio Clinics International. Baltimore, Williams and Wilkins, 1991, pp 155–172.

35. Larheim TA, Smith H-J, Asperand F: Temporomandibular joint abnormalities associated with

rheumatic disease: Comparison between MR imaging and arthrotomography. Radiology 1992;*183*:221–226.

36. Widmalm S-E, Westesson P-L, Brooks SL, Hatala MP, Paesani D: Temporomandibular joint sounds: Correlation to joint structure in fresh autopsy specimens. Am J Orthod Dentofac Orthop 1992;*101*:60–69.

Index

Note: Page numbers in *italics* refer to illustrations; page numbers followed by (t) refer to tables.

Acoustical analysis, of temporomandibular joint, *242*, *242–247*, *244–247*. See also *Temporomandibular joint, sounds made by*.
Adhesions, appearance of, on arthrography, *260*
  on arthroscopy, 378 *379*, *379*
  on arthrotomography, *161*, *272*
  on MRI, *261–263*
  surgical disk repositioning and, 257, *260–263*, 261
Air injection, for double-contrast arthrotomography, 149–150, *150*
Airway obstruction, due to arthroscopy of TMJ, 386
Anesthesia, in arthrography of TMJ, 106, *109*, 146
  in arthroscopy of TMJ, 380–381
  complications of, 386
Ankylosing spondylitis, involving TMJ, 310, *310*, 314
Ankylosis, of temporomandibular joint, 66, *138*, 360, *360*
  postoperative, 261, *263*, *264*, 290–291, *291*
  spondylitis and, 310, *310*
Anterior band of disk, arthrotomographic appearance of, 121, *121*
  displacement of condyle anterior to, 137, *138*, 211, *216*
  magnetic resonance imaging of, *121*
  subluxation and, 211, *216*
Anterior disk displacement, 9, *10*, 26, 27, 29, *31*
  arthrographic findings in, *103*, *114*, 123, *124*, *126*, *127*, *128*, 145
    disk deformation and, *127*, *131*, *132*
  arthrotomographic findings in, *117*, *125*, *145*, *146*, 155, *155*, *156*, 157, 158, *159*
    disk deformation and, *93*, *157*, 158, *158*
    rheumatoid arthritis and, *313*
  disk deformation associated with, *44*, *93*, *127*, *131*, *132*, *157*, 158, *158*
  fibrosis of posterior disk attachment associated with, *48*
  MRI findings in, *189*, 191, *194*, *195*
    splint therapy guided by, 254, *254*
  partial, 28, *32*, *33*
    arthrotomographic findings in, 155, *156*, 157
    MRI findings in, 191, *194*, *195*
    with reduction, 36–37
  perforation accompanying, *50*, *51*
  thickening of posterior disk attachment associated with, *44*
  with incomplete reduction, 37
  with reduction, 34, *35*, 36–37, *37*

Anterior disk displacement *(Continued)*
  arthrotomographic findings in, *125*, 155, *155*
  without internal derangement, 34
  without reduction, 35
    arthrotomographic findings in, 158, *159*
    MRI findings in, *195*
Anterior open bite, rheumatoid arthritis involving TMJ and, *309*
Anteromedial disk displacement, MRI findings in, *212*
Anteroposterior projection, in plain radiography of TMJ, 80, *80–82*, 82–83
Arthritis. See also *Degenerative disease of TMJ*.
  TMJ involvement in, 61, *61*, 303–324. See also *Rheumatoid arthritis, TMJ involvement in*.
    diagnosis of, 142
    imaging in, 323–324, 324(t), 400–401
Arthrocentesis of TMJ, for vacuum phenomenon, 377
Arthrography of TMJ, 101–162, 400
  adhesions on, *260*
  air injection for double-contrast arthrotomography in, 149–150, *150*
  anterior disk displacement on, *103*, *114*, 123, *124*, *126*, *127*, *128*, 145
    disk deformation associated with, *127*, *131*, *132*
  arthrotomographic phase of. See *Arthrotomography of TMJ*.
  cannulation in, 147, *148*
  clicking evaluated by, 123
  complications of, 142, 162
  conditions contraindicating, 104(t), 105
  condylar displacement on, anterior to anterior band of disk, 137, *138*
  contrast aspiration in, 149
  contrast injection in, 111, *112*, 113, *114*, 148–149. See also *Double-contrast* entries.
    addition of epinephrine to agents used in, 111
    adverse reactions to agents used in, 104
      prophylaxis against, 104(t)
    extravasation of agents used in, 111, *112*, 116, *118*
    needle positioning for, 106, 111, *111*, 113, *113*
      errors in, 111, *112*, 116, *118*, 119, *119*
  development of, 101, 143
  disk appearance (normal) on, *354*
  disk deformation on, 126–127, *127*, 131, *131*, *132*
  disk displacement on, 115, 124
    anterior, *103*, *114*, 123, *124*, *126*, *127*, *128*, 145
      disk deformation associated with, *127*, *131*, *132*
    false-negative diagnosis of, 152–154

Arthrography of TMJ *(Continued)*
 medial, *141*
 sideways, 140, *141*, 209, *214*
 with reduction, 123
  vs. displacement on MRI, 191, *192*
 without reduction, *131*, 131–132
  perforation accompanying, 132–133, *132–135*, 135, *207*
 disk recapture on, 124, 127, *128, 253*
 splinting based on, 127, 129, *129*
 double-contrast, 143, 146–151, *147, 148, 150*. See also *Double-contrast arthrotomography of TMJ.*
 edge sign (of sideways disk displacement) on, 140, *141*, 209, *214*
 equipment for, 105, *105*, 106, 146–151, *147, 148, 150*
 errors in, 111, *112*, 116, *118*, 119, *119*
 evaluation of clicking joint by, 123
 history of, 101, 143
 indications for, 102, 102(t), 104
 joint puncture in, 106, *110*, 147
  anesthetic injection for, 106, *109*, 146
  identification and marking of site for, 106, *107, 108*
 joint space injection in, 111, *112*, 113, *114*, 148–149
  extravasation of contrast material following, 111, *112*, 116, *118*
  needle positioning for, 106, 111, *111*, 113, *113*
  errors in, 111, *112*, 116, *118*, 119, *119*
 lower joint space cannulation in, 147, *148*
 lower joint space injection in, 111, *112*, 148
  needle positioning for, *111*
 mandibular positions for double-contrast arthrotomography in, 151
 medial disk displacement on, *141*
 normal findings on, 119, 121, *144, 354*
  vs. normal findings on MR imaging of TMJ, *188*
 objectives of, 102–104, 115
 patient positioning for, 105–106, *106*, 146
  arthrotomography and, 114, *115*
 perforation on, 132–133, *132–135, 207, 353*
  postoperative, *260*
 post-diskectomy, 271
 results of, 119–140, 151–161. See also entries under *Arthrotomography of TMJ.*
 rupture of posterior disk attachment on, 140
 sideways disk displacement on, 140, *141*, 209, *214*
 single-contrast, 105–113, *105–114*
  complications of, 142
  results of, 119–140
  vs. double-contrast arthrotomography of TMJ, *144, 145*, 162
 technique of, 105–113, *105–114*, 146–151, *147, 148, 150*
 tomographic phase of. See *Arthrotomography of TMJ.*
 upper joint space cannulation in, 147, *148*
 upper joint space injection in, 113, *114*, 149
  needle positioning for, 113, *113*
 vagal response during, 105, 142
 vs. magnetic resonance imaging, 178, 186, *188*
  in disk displacement with reduction, 191, *192*
  in TMJ trauma, 138–139
Arthrolysis–joint lavage–disk manipulation, for internal TMJ derangements, 389, 389(t)
 sclerotherapy with, 390, 390(t)
Arthropathy, psoriatic, TMJ involvement in, *306, 308, 314, 315, 322*
Arthroscopy of TMJ, 371–391
 anesthesia in, 380–381

Arthroscopy of TMJ *(Continued)*
 complications of, 386
 approach to and visualization of upper compartment in, 381, *381*, 382, *382, 383*
 cannulation in, 381, *381*, 382
 diagnostic, 371–372, 376–380, 382
  adhesions on, 378–379, *379*
  chondromalacia on, 377
  lateral impingement phenomenon on, 379–380
  perforations on, *372*, 380
  synovitis on, 377–378, *378*
 equipment for, 381, *381*, 382
  breakage of, 387
 staging of internal derangements by, 374, 375(t)
 technique of, 380–382, *381*
 therapeutic, 372–376, 382–391
  care following, 384–385
  complications of, 385–388, 387(t)–389(t)
  indications for, 373(t), 373–374, 376
  lysis-lavage-manipulation (LLM) in, 389, 389(t)
   sclerosant injection with, 390, 390(t)
  results of, 388–390, 389(t), 390(t)
  sclerosant injection in, 376, 384, *384*
   lysis-lavage-manipulation (LLM) with, 390, 390(t)
  steroid injection in, 383–384
Arthrosis of TMJ. See *Degenerative disease of TMJ.*
Arthrotomography of TMJ, 114, 115, 116
 adhesions on, *161, 272*
 ankylosis on, *138*
 anterior band of disk on, 121, *121*
 anterior disk displacement on, *117, 125, 145, 146, 155, 155, 156*, 157, 158, *159*
  disk deformation and, *93, 157*, 158, *158*
  partial, 155, *156*, 157
  rheumatoid arthritis and, *313*
  with reduction, *125*, 155, *155*
  without reduction, 158, *159*
 condylar fracture sequelae on, *341*
 disk deformation on, *93, 157, 157*, 158, *158*
 disk detachment on, 133, *134*
 disk displacement on, anterior, *117, 125, 145, 146, 155, 155, 156*, 157, 158, *159*
  disk deformation and, *93, 157*, 158, *158*
  partial, 155, *156*, 157
  rheumatoid arthritis and, *313*
  with reduction, *125*, 155, *155*
  without reduction, 158, *159*
 false-negative diagnosis of, 152–154
 medial, *140*
 partial, 155, *156*, 157
 sideways, *140*
 with reduction, *125*, 155, *155*
 without reduction, *136*, 158, *159*
 disk recapture on, *125*
 double-contrast. See *Double-contrast arthrotomography of TMJ.*
 loose bodies on, *139, 346*
 medial disk displacement on, *140*
 normal findings on, *89, 92, 95, 120, 144*, 151–152, *152–154*
 partial disk displacement on, 155, *156*, 157
 patient positioning for, 114, *115*
 perforation on, *134*, 158–159, *160, 312*
 post-diskectomy findings on, *266–269*
 psoriatic arthropathy–associated changes on, *315*
 rheumatoid arthritis–associated changes on, 311–312, *312, 313*
  vs. MRI findings in rheumatoid TMJ disease, 314, *315–318*, 316–320, 320(t)

Arthrotomography of TMJ *(Continued)*
  sideways disk displacement on, *140*
  "therapeutic position" on, *252*
    vs. MRI, after surgical disk repositioning, 161
    in rheumatoid arthritis involving TMJ, 314, *315–318*, 316–320, 320(t)
Articular surfaces, of temporomandibular joint, 12
Articular tubercle of temporal bone, 6
  erosion of, after diskectomy with Proplast-Teflon implant, *284, 285, 286*
  incoordination of, with mandibular condyle, 38–39
    and clicking, 135, 137, *137*
  soft tissue cover of, 19
  thickening of, 12
Artifacts, metallic, on postoperative magnetic resonance imaging, 178, *178*, *291*, 291–292
Aseptic necrosis, 62, 64, *64*
  TMJ as possible site of, 62, 64
Aspiration, of contrast medium, in arthrography of TMJ, 149
Asymmetry, craniofacial, 3-D computed tomography of, 233, *234*
  mandibular, 351, *352, 353*, 355(t), 355–356
    condylar fracture and, 332, *334*
Atrophy, of masticatory muscles, 62, *63*
Atropine, for vagal response, during TMJ arthrography, 105, 142
Attenuation coefficients, in computed tomography of TMJ, 231, 231(t)

Betamethasone, intra-articular injection of, as adjunct to arthroscopic TMJ surgery, 383
Bite opening, anterior, rheumatoid arthritis involving TMJ and, *309*
Blood supply, to temporomandibular joint, 18
Bone. See *Osseous* entries.
Bone marrow changes, on MR imaging of TMJ, 199, *201*, 202, *202, 203*
  edematous, *182, 184, 184*, 202, *321, 322*
Bony ankylosis, of temporomandibular joint, 66
  postoperative, 290–291, *291*
  spondylitis and, 310, *310*
Bronstein-Merrill classification, of internal TMJ derangements, 375(t)
Bullet wound, of temporomandibular joint, *364*, 365

Calcification, of disk of TMJ, CT findings in, 226
Calcium pyrophosphate dihydrate deposition disease (chondrocalcinosis), involving TMJ, 61–62, 349–350, *350*
Cancer, metastatic to TMJ, 357, *358, 359*
Cannulation, in arthrography of TMJ, 147, *148*
  in arthroscopy of TMJ, 381, *381, 382*
Capsule of temporomandibular joint, 13
  bulging of, 211, *217*
  edema in, 211, *218*
  enlargement of, after diskectomy with implant, *282, 284, 286–288*
  herniation of, simulating disk, 186, *190*
  magnetic resonance imaging of, 211
    abnormal findings on, 211, *217, 218*
      diskectomy with implant and, *282, 287, 288, 289*
      herniation simulating disk on, 186, *190*
  thickening of, 211, *217*
Capsulitis, on MR imaging of TMJ, 211, *218*

Carcinoma, metastatic to TMJ, 357, *358*
C-arm, in double-contrast arthrography of TMJ, 146, *147*
Cassettes, multifilm, for arthrotomography of TMJ, 151
  for tomography of TMJ, 87, *88*
Catheter placement, in upper and lower compartments of TMJ, 147, *148*
Cephalostat, to orient patient's head, in plain radiography of TMJ, 77, *80, 82*
  in tomography of TMJ, 86, *86, 87*
Children, healing of condylar fractures in, 335, *336*
Chondrocalcinosis (calcium pyrophosphate dihydrate deposition disease), involving TMJ, 61–62, 349–350, *350*
Chondromalacia, involving TMJ, 377
Chondromatosis, synovial, and loose bodies in TMJ, 343, 345, *346–348*
Chronic arthritis, TMJ involvement in, 303–324. See also *Rheumatoid arthritis, TMJ involvement in.*
Circumferential remodeling, 61. See also *Remodeling.*
Clicking, temporomandibular joint. See *Temporomandibular joint, sounds made by.*
"Closed lock," 36, 130, 194
Closing of jaw, muscles acting in, 14–15, 17
Collagen fibers, in disk of TMJ, 19, 21, 43
  in posterior attachment of disk of TMJ, 43
Compartments of temporomandibular joint, 9, 11–12
  arthroscopic approach to, 381, *381*, 382
  arthroscopic visualization of, 382, *382, 383*
  catheter placement in, 147, *148*
  contrast injection into, 111, *112*, 113, *114*, 148–149. See also *Arthrography of TMJ.*
    needle positioning for, 106, 111, *111*, 113, *113*
      errors in, 111, *112*, 116, *118*, 119, *119*
  effusion in, 181, *181, 182*, 204, *204, 205*
    and demonstration of perforation, 205, *207*
    in psoriatic arthropathy, *322*
    in rheumatoid arthritis, *320, 321*
  vacuum phenomenon in, 377
Complete disk displacement, 28. See also *Disk displacement.*
Computed tomography of TMJ, 223–233
  ankylosis on, 310, *310*
    postoperative, 291, *291*
  calcifications on, 226, *350*
  condylar fracture on, *329, 364*
    treatment failure and, *292*
  costochondral graft on, *294, 294*
  disk calcifications on, 226
  disk displacement on, *226*, 231(t)
    false-negative diagnosis of, *230*, 232
    false-positive diagnosis of, *229*, 232
    vs. displacement on MRI, *197, 198, 198*, 228
  elongated coronoid process on, 66, 232, *233*
  loose bodies on, *347*
  normal findings on, *225*, 226, *227*
  osteochondroma on, *356*
  patient positioning for, 224, *224*
  post-diskectomy findings on, Proplast-Teflon implant and, 284, *284–286*, 290
    silicone implant and, 279, *283*
  rheumatoid arthritis–associated changes on, 305, *306*, 307, *307*
  scan parameters for, 225(t)
  significance of attenuation coefficients in, 231, 231(t)
  single-photon emission system in, 238, *239*, 240
  spondylitis-associated changes on, 310, *310*
  subcondylar fracture on, *331*

Computed tomography of TMJ *(Continued)*
technique of, *224,* 224–225, 225(t)
three-dimensional, 232–233, *234–237, 295, 334, 337*
vs. magnetic resonance imaging, 178, 179(t), *227–230,* 231–232, 232(t)
in disk displacement, *197,* 198, *198, 228*
Condylar angle, horizontal, 4–5, *5*
vertical, *5,* 6
Condyle, mandibular. See *Mandibular condyle.*
Congenital anomalies, of temporomandibular joint, 64–65, *65*
Contrast media, addition of epinephrine to, 111
adverse reactions to, 104
prophylaxis against, 104(t)
Contrast studies, of temporomandibular joint, 101–162, 400. See also *Arthrography of TMJ; Arthrotomography of TMJ.*
Coronoid process of mandible, elongation or hyperplasia of, 66, *66,* 232, *233*
interference with zygomatic process by, 66, *66,* 232, *233*
Corticosteroid(s), intra-articular injection of, as adjunct to arthroscopic TMJ surgery, 383–384
pretreatment with, in patient undergoing radiocontrast studies, 104(t)
Costochondral grafts, in temporomandibular joint, 294, *294–296,* 296
CPPD (calcium pyrophosphate dihydrate) deposition disease (chondrocalcinosis), involving TMJ, 61–62, 349–350, *350*
Craniofacial asymmetry, 3-D computed tomography of, 233, *234*
Crepitation, temporomandibular joint, 241, *247*
CT. See *Computed tomography of TMJ.*
Cyst formation, silicone TMJ implant and, 278–279, *280, 283*

Deformation, of disk of TMJ, 40, *42,* 43, *43*
anterior disk displacement and, *44, 93, 127, 131, 132, 157,* 158, *158*
arthrographic findings in, 126–127, *127,* 131, *131, 132*
arthrotomographic findings in, *93,* 157, *157,* 158, *158*
disk displacement and, *197, 200, 201*
anterior, *44, 93, 127, 131, 132, 157,* 158, *158*
medial, 43, *44*
medial disk displacement and, 43, *44*
MRI findings in, *197,* 199, *200, 201*
pathologic changes associated with, 43, 45, *46*
splitting of posterior disk attachment accompanying, *47*
thickening of posterior disk attachment in, 40, *40, 41, 43, 45*
of temporomandibular joint, 65
Degenerative disease of TMJ, 53–54, *54–56,* 56
crepitation accompanying, *247*
definition of, 28(t), 53
disk displacement and, 53, 54, *55,* 56, *59*
experimentally (surgically) created, 54, 56, *58*
fractured silicone implant and, *282*
mandibular asymmetry associated with, *353*
occurrence of, under normally positioned disk, 27, 56, *60*
perforation and, 56, *59*
primary, 54, 56
Proplast-Teflon implant and, *284*

Degenerative disease of TMJ *(Continued)*
secondary, 54, 56
TMJ sounds accompanying, *242, 247*
vs. remodeling, 56, *60,* 61
Dental apparatuses, interference by, in MR imaging of TMJ, 174, 178, *178*
Derangements, internal, of temporomandibular joint. See *Internal TMJ derangements.*
Dermal grafts, in temporomandibular joint, 290
Detachment, of disk of TMJ, arthrotomographic findings in, 133, *134*
Developmental anomalies, of temporomandibular joint, 64–65, *65*
Digastric muscle, 14(t)
Diphenhydramine pretreatment, in patient undergoing radiocontrast studies, 104(t)
Disk, of temporomandibular joint, 7, *7, 8,* 19, *19,* 21
abnormal position of. See *Disk displacement.*
anterior band of, arthrotomographic appearance of, 121, *121*
displacement of condyle anterior to, 137, *138,* 211, *216*
magnetic resonance imaging of, *121*
subluxation and, 211, *216*
anterior displacement of. See *Disk displacement, anterior.*
anteromedial displacement of, MRI findings in, *212*
calcification of, CT findings in, 226
collagen fibers in, 19, 21, 43
complete displacement of, 28. See also *Disk displacement.*
deformation of, 40, *42,* 43, *43*
anterior disk displacement and, *44, 93, 127, 131, 132, 157,* 158, *158*
arthrographic findings in, 126–127, *127,* 131, *131, 132*
arthrotomographic findings in, *93,* 157, *157,* 158, *158*
disk displacement and, *197, 200, 201*
anterior, *44, 93, 127, 131, 132, 157,* 158, *158*
medial, 43, *44*
medial disk displacement and, 43, *44*
MRI findings in, *197,* 199, *200, 201*
pathologic changes associated with, 43, 45, *46*
splitting of posterior disk attachment accompanying, *47*
thickening of posterior disk attachment in, 40, *40, 41,* 43, *45*
detachment of, arthrotomographic findings in, 133, *134*
displacement of. See *Disk displacement.*
function of, in jaw opening, 9, *11, 20,* 21. See also *Jaw opening.*
herniated joint capsule simulating, 186, *190*
ideal position of, 9, *10,* 26, *26*
lateral displacement of, 28, *30, 31*
MRI findings in, *214, 217*
medial displacement of. See *Disk displacement, medial.*
movement of, 7–8
normal position of, 9, 26, *27, 89, 95, 354*
arthrosis under site of, *27,* 56, *60*
variations in, 9, 26, *27*
partial displacement of. See *Disk displacement, partial.*
perforation involving. See *Perforation(s), involving disk or posterior disk attachment.*
position of, 9, *10, 208*

Disk *(Continued)*
 abnormal. See *Disk displacement.*
 ideal, 9, *10,* 26, *26*
 normal, 9, 26, *27, 89, 95, 354*
  arthrosis under site of, *27,* 56, *60*
  variations in, 26, *27*
  rheumatoid arthritis and, 312, 314
 posterior attachment of, 8, 21, 45, 48
  collagen fibers in, 43
  expansion of, on jaw opening, 9, *12,* 21
  fibrosis of, 48, *48*
  magnetic resonance imaging of, *170,* 186, *188,* 204, *206*
   remodeling and, 198–199, *199*
  perforation involving. See *Perforation(s), involving disk or posterior disk attachment.*
  remodeling of, MRI findings in, 198–199, *199*
  rupture of, 140
   arthrographic findings in, 140, *141*
  splitting of, in disk deformation, *47*
  thickening of, in disk deformation, 40, *40, 41,* 43, *45*
   in disk displacement, 43, *44*
  vascularization of, 48, *49*
 posterior displacement of, *31,* 38
  MRI findings in, 211, *216*
 recapture of, 124, *125,* 126, *126, 253*
  arthrographically assisted, 127, *128,* 129, *129*
  MRI in assessment of, 194, *196*
  splinting and. See *Protrusive splint therapy.*
  staging of, 124, 126, *126*
 rotational displacement of, 28, *31,* 209, *209, 211*
 shape of, 8
 sideways displacement of. See *Disk displacement, sideways.*
 surgical removal of, imaging after, 265, *265–275,* 267, *270–272, 274–275,* 276(t)
  implants used after, 275–290. See also *Implant(s), in TMJ.*
 surgical repositioning of, 255, 257
  adhesion (scar tissue) formation after, 257, *260–263,* 261
  fibrous ankylosis as complication of, 261, *263, 264*
  imaging after, 161, 257, *258–264,* 260(t), 261, *264–265*
 thickness of, 8
Disk displacement, 9, 26, 28, 28(t)
 anterior, 9, *10,* 26, *27, 29, 31*
  arthrographic findings in, *103, 114,* 123, *124, 126, 127, 128, 145*
   disk deformation and, *127, 131, 132*
  arthrotomographic findings in, *117, 125, 145, 146,* 155, *155, 156,* 157, 158, *159*
   disk deformation and, *93, 157,* 158, *158*
   rheumatoid arthritis and, *313*
  disk deformation associated with, *44, 93, 127, 131, 132, 157,* 158, *158*
  fibrosis of posterior disk attachment associated with, *48*
  MRI findings in, *189,* 191, *194, 195*
   splint therapy guided by, 254, *254*
  partial, 28, *32, 33*
   arthrotomographic findings in, 155, *156,* 157
   MRI findings in, 191, *194, 195*
   with reduction, 36–37
  perforation accompanying, *50, 51*
  thickening of posterior disk attachment associated with, *44*

Disk displacement *(Continued)*
 with incomplete reduction, 37
 with reduction, *34, 35,* 36–37, *37*
  arthrotomographic findings in, *125,* 155, *155*
 without internal derangement, *34*
 without reduction, *35*
  arthrotomographic findings in, 158, *159*
  MRI findings in, *195*
 anteromedial, MRI findings in, *212*
 arthrographic findings in. See *Arthrography of TMJ, disk displacement on.*
 arthrosis (degenerative joint disease) associated with, 54, *55,* 56, *59*
 arthrotomographic findings in. See *Arthrotomography of TMJ, disk displacement on.*
 complete, 28
 CT findings in, *226,* 231(t)
  false-negative, *230,* 232
  false-positive, *229,* 232
  vs. MRI findings, *197,* 198, *198, 228*
 definition of, 26, 28(t)
 degenerative joint disease (arthrosis) associated with, 54, *55,* 56, *59*
 disk deformation associated with, *44*
  arthrographic findings in, *127, 131, 132*
  arthrotomographic findings in, *93, 157,* 158, *158*
  MRI findings in, *197, 200, 201*
 etiology of, 52, 53
 false-negative diagnosis of, arthrography in, 152–154
  arthrotomography in, 152–154
  computed tomography in, *230,* 232
 false-positive diagnosis of, computed tomography in, *229,* 232
 fibrosis of posterior disk attachment associated with, *48*
 lateral, 28, *30, 31*
  MRI findings in, *214, 217*
 magnetic resonance imaging of. See *Magnetic resonance imaging, disk displacement on.*
 marrow changes associated with, MRI findings in, 199, *201, 202*
 medial, 28, *30*
  arthrographic findings in, *141*
  arthrosis (degenerative joint disease) associated with, *55, 59*
  arthrotomographic findings in, *140*
  clicking due to, *246*
  disk deformation associated with, 43, *44*
 MRI findings in. See *Magnetic resonance imaging, disk displacement on.*
 osseous changes associated with, MRI findings in, 199, *201*
 partial, 28, *32, 33*
  arthrotomographic findings in, 155, *156,* 157
  MRI findings in, 191, *194, 195*
  with reduction, 36–37
 perforation accompanying, 50, *50, 51,* 132–133, *132–135,* 135, *207*
 posterior, *31,* 38
  MRI findings in, 211, *216*
 remodeling associated with, MRI findings in, 198, *199*
 rotational, 28, *31,* 209, *209*
  "empty fossa" sign in, 209
  MRI findings in, 209, *211*
 sideways, 28, 139–140, 209, *209*
  arthrographic findings in, 140, *141,* 209, *214*
  arthrotomographic findings in, *140*
  edge sign in, 140, *141,* 209, *214*

Disk displacement *(Continued)*
   "empty fossa" sign in, 209, *213*
   MRI findings in, 209, *210, 213, 214*
  surgically created, *52,* 52–53, *53*
  terminology applied to, 208(t)
  thickening of posterior disk attachment associated
    with, 43, *44*
  with incomplete reduction, *37,* 37–38
  with jaw dislocation, *362*
  with reduction, *34, 35,* 35–36, *37,* 123
    arthrographic findings in, 123
      vs. MRI findings, 191, *192*
    arthrotomographic findings in, *125,* 155, *155*
    clicking due to, 35, 122, 122(t), 123, *123*
    CT findings in, 231(t)
    definition of, 28(t)
    MRI findings in, 191, *192–194, 212*
    TMJ sounds accompanying, 35, 122, 122(t), 123,
      123, 242, 243, *244*
  without internal derangement, 33, *34*
  without jaw dislocation, *363*
  without reduction, *35,* 36, 129–130, *130*
    arthrographic findings in, *131,* 131–132
    arthrotomographic findings in, *136,* 158, *159*
    clicking due to, 122, 135, *136*
    CT findings in, *226,* 231(t)
    definition of, 28(t)
    MRI findings in, 194, *195, 197,* 198, *198, 199,*
      201, 202, 207
    perforation accompanying, 132–133, *132–135,*
      135, *207*
    TMJ sounds accompanying, 122, 135, *136,* 242,
      243, *244*
Diskectomy, imaging after, 265, *265–275,* 267, 270–
  272, 274–275, 276(t)
  implants used after, 275–290. See also *Implant(s), in*
    TMJ.
Dislocation, of jaw, 39, 360–362, *361–363.* See also
  Displacement, of mandibular condyle, anterior to anterior
  band of disk; Incoordination (interference), between
  condyle and tubercle.
Displacement, of disk of TMJ. See *Disk displacement.*
  of mandibular condyle, anterior to anterior band of
    disk, 137, *138,* 211, *216*
    following fracture. See *Fractures, condylar.*
  of TMJ implant, *282, 285*
Disruption, of temporomandibular joint, 65
Double-contrast arthrography of TMJ, 143, 146–151,
  147, 148, 150. See also *Double-contrast*
  arthrotomography of TMJ.
Double-contrast arthrotomography of TMJ, 149–151
  complications of, 162
  post-diskectomy findings on, *266–269*
  results of, *92, 93, 96, 144–146,* 151–161, *152–161,*
    346
  normal, *89, 95, 144*
  "therapeutic position" on, *252*
  vs. MRI, after surgical disk repositioning, 161
  vs. single-contrast arthrography of TMJ, *144, 145,*
    162
  vs. single-contrast arthrotomography of TMJ, *146*
Dysplasia, of temporomandibular joint, 65

Ear, complications of TMJ arthroscopy involving,
  386–387
Edema, bone marrow, on MR imaging of TMJ, *182,*
  184, *184,* 202, *321, 322*

Edema *(Continued)*
  capsular, on MR imaging of TMJ, 211, *218*
Edge sign, in sideways disk displacement, 140, *141,*
  209, *214*
Effusion, temporomandibular joint, 181, *181, 182,* 204,
  204, 205
  and demonstration of perforation, 205, *207*
  in psoriatic arthropathy, *322*
  in rheumatoid arthritis, *320, 321*
Eminence, articular, of temporal bone. See *Articular*
  tubercle of temporal bone.
"Empty fossa" sign, in sideways or rotational disk
  displacement, 209, *213*
Epinephrine, addition of, to radiocontrast material,
  111
Erosion, condylar, after diskectomy with silicone
    implant, 277, *277, 278*
  in degenerative disease of TMJ, 54, *56, 58, 59*
  in psoriatic arthropathy involving TMJ, *306*
  in rheumatoid arthritis involving TMJ, *305, 307,*
    316, 321, 323
  eminence, after diskectomy with Proplast-Teflon im-
    plant, 284, *285, 286*
  glenoid fossa, after diskectomy with silicone implant,
    279
Extravasation, of contrast material, following joint
  space injection for arthrography, 111, *112,* 116,
  118

Fast scanning, in MR imaging of TMJ, 183(t), 183–184
Fast-setting impression material, in arthrographically
  assisted disk recapture, 127, *129*
Fat suppression, in MR imaging of TMJ, *184,* 184–185
Fibrosis, of posterior disk attachment, 48, *48*
Fibrous ankylosis, of temporomandibular joint, 66,
  360, *360*
  surgical disk repositioning and, 261, *263, 264*
Film cassettes, for arthrotomography of TMJ, 151
  for tomography of TMJ, 87, *88*
Fossa, glenoid (mandibular fossa), 6–7
  condylar position in, 89–91, *90.* See also *Disk, of*
    temporomandibular joint, position of.
    after diskectomy, 267, *268, 269*
    erosion in, after diskectomy with silicone implant,
      279
Fractures, condylar, 327–340, 328(t)
  bullet wound and, *364*
  classification of, 327, 328, *328,* 329, 332, *332, 333*
  clinical aspects of, 327–328
  healing of, in children vs. adults, 335, *336*
    unsuccessful, 292, *292*
  imaging of, *329, 330,* 341(t)
  sequelae of, *330,* 332, *334,* 335, *336–341*
  treatment of, 335, 340
    unsuccessful, 292, *292*
  silicone implant, 278, *281, 282*
  subcondylar, *331*
  sequelae of, *333*
Fragmentation, of Proplast-Teflon TMJ implant, 287,
  288, 289
Frontal tomography of TMJ, 89, *90.* See also
  Tomography of TMJ.

Geniohyoid muscle, 14(t)
Glenoid fossa (mandibular fossa), 6–7

Glenoid fossa (mandibular fossa) *(Continued)*
  condylar position in, 89–91, *90.* See also *Disk, of temporomandibular joint, position of.*
    after diskectomy, 267, *268, 269*
  erosion in, after diskectomy with silicone implant, *279*
Gout, involving temporomandibular joint, 61
Grafts, in temporomandibular joint, 290, 294, *294–296,* 296
Granulation tissue, around TMJ implant, *282,* 284, 287, *287, 288, 289*
Gunshot wound, of temporomandibular joint, *364,* 365

Head orientation, by cephalostat, in plain radiography of TMJ, 77, *80, 82*
  in tomography of TMJ, 86, *86, 87*
Healing, of condylar fractures, in children vs. adults, 335, *336*
  unsuccessful, after treatment, 292, *292*
Hearing loss, due to arthroscopy of TMJ, 386–387
Hemifacial microsomia, graft surgery in treatment of, 295
  3-D computed tomography of, 233, *234*
Herniation, of temporomandibular joint capsule, simulating disk, 186, *190*
Horizontal condylar angle, 4–5, *5*
Hypermobility, temporomandibular, sclerotherapy for, 376, 384, *384*
  lysis-lavage-manipulation (LLM) with, 390, 390(t)
Hyperplasia, condylar, 65–66, *352*
  vs. osteochondroma of mandibular condyle, 355, 357
  coronoid process, 66, *66,* 232, *233*
Hypocyclodial tomography of TMJ. See *Tomography of TMJ.*
Hypoplasia, temporomandibular, congenital, 65, *65*

Imaging, of temporomandibular joint, 6. See also specific modalities, e.g., *Magnetic resonance imaging.*
  diagnostic, 398–401, *399.* See also specific diagnostic aids, e.g., *Arthrography of TMJ.*
  post-treatment, 251–296, 400. See also *Post-treatment imaging.*
Imaging plane, in magnetic resonance imaging, 171(t), 171–172
  oblique vs. straight, *172, 173*
Impingement, of temporomandibular joint, lateral, 379–380
Implant(s), in TMJ, 275–290
  imaging of, 276(t), 279, 290
  Proplast-Teflon, 283–284
    defects in, 283, *284*
    displacement of, *285*
    erosions associated with, 284, *285, 286*
    fragmentation of, 287, *288, 289*
    granulation tissue around, 284, 287, *287, 288, 289*
    imaging of, *219,* 284, *284–289,* 287, 289, 290, *293*
    results of treatment with, 283–284
    wearing of, 283, 284
  silicone, 275, 277
    cyst formation associated with, 278–279, *280, 283*

Implant(s) *(Continued)*
    erosions associated with, 277–278, *277–279*
    fracture of, 278, *281, 282*
    imaging of, 233, *236, 237, 276,* 278, 279, *282*
    results of treatment with, 278, 282(t)
    wearing of, 278, *281*
  total replacement with, 292, *293,* 294
Impression material, fast-setting, in arthrographically assisted disk recapture, 127, *129*
Incomplete reduction. See also *Reduction.*
  disk displacement with, *37, 37–38*
Incoordination (interference), between condyle and tubercle, 38–39
  resulting in clicking, 135, 137, *137*
  between coronoid and zygomatic processes, 66, *66,* 232, *233*
Infection, of temporomandibular joint, 362, *363,* 365
  due to arthroscopy, 387
Inflammatory arthritis, TMJ involvement in, 61, *61,* 142, 303–324. See also *Rheumatoid arthritis, TMJ involvement in.*
Innervation, of temporomandibular joint, 18
Interarticular disk of TMJ. See *Disk, of temporomandibular joint.*
Interference (incoordination), between condyle and tubercle, 38–39
  resulting in clicking, 135, 137, *137*
  between coronoid and zygomatic processes, 66, *66,* 232, *233*
Internal TMJ derangements, 33–38, 374
  clinical staging of, 38, 39(t), 374, 375(t)
  definition of, 28(t), 33
  diagnosis of, 397–401. See also specific diagnostic aids, e.g., *Arthrography of TMJ.*
    clinical examination in, 397–398
    imaging in, 398–401, *399.* See also specific modalities, e.g., *Magnetic resonance imaging.*
  functional classification of, 35–38
  management of. See specific treatments, e.g., *Arthroscopy, therapeutic.*
  objective component of, 102–103
  presenting complaints in, 102, 103(t)
  problems causing or due to. See specific conditions, e.g., *Disk displacement.*
  progression of, 38
  subjective component of, 103
  with reduction. See *Disk displacement, with reduction.*
  without reduction. See *Disk displacement, without reduction.*
Intra-articular steroid injection, as adjunct to arthroscopic TMJ surgery, 383–384

Jaw closing, muscles acting in, 14–15, 17
Jaw dislocation, 39, 360–362, *361–363.* See also *Anterior band of disk, displacement of condyle anterior to; Incoordination (interference), between condyle and tubercle.*
Jaw opening, 9, *11, 20,* 21
  expansion of posterior disk attachment on, 9, *12,* 21
  maximal, and condylar translation, 79, 91, *92*
  on plain radiography of TMJ, *79,* 79–80
  muscles acting in, 15, 17
Joint, temporomandibular. See *Temporomandibular joint.*
Juvenile rheumatoid arthritis, 304. See also *Rheumatoid arthritis.*
  TMJ involvement in, *309, 311, 312, 313, 315, 316, 321*

Lateral disk displacement, 28, *30*, *31*
   MRI findings in, *214*, *217*
Lateral impingement phenomenon, 379–380
Lateral oblique transcranial projection, in plain
   radiography of TMJ, 76, *76–80*, 79
Lateral pterygoid muscle, 14(t), 15–17, *16*, *17*
   magnetic resonance imaging of, 186, *187*
Lateral tomography of TMJ, 88–89. See also
   Tomography of TMJ.
Lead markers, in plain radiography of TMJ, 74, *75*
Lead shield, in plain radiography of TMJ, 75, 76
Lidocaine injection, for joint puncture, in arthrography
   of TMJ, 106, *109*
Ligament(s), sphenomandibular, 13(t)
   stylomandibular, 13(t)
   temporomandibular joint, 13, 13(t)
LLM (lysis-lavage-manipulation), for internal TMJ
   derangements, 389, 389(t)
   sclerotherapy with, 390, 390(t)
Local anesthetic injection, for joint puncture, in
   arthrography of TMJ, 106, *109*, 146
Lock/locking, closed, 36, 130, 194
   loose body in TMJ and, 343
   open, 39, 151, 211, 362
Loose bodies, in temporomandibular joint, 139, *139*,
   343–349, *344*
      osteochondrosis dissecans and, 345, 348–349, *348–*
      349
      synovial chondromatosis and, 343, 345, *346–348*
Lower temporomandibular joint compartment, 11–12
   catheter insertion in, 147, *148*
   contrast injection into, 111, *112*, 148. See also
      Arthrography of TMJ.
   needle positioning for, *111*
Lymphoma, metastatic to TMJ, *359*
Lysis-lavage-manipulation (LLM), for internal TMJ
   derangements, 389, 389(t)
   sclerotherapy with, 390, 390(t)

Magnetic resonance imaging, 167–220
   adhesions (scar tissue) on, postoperative, *261–263*
   ankylosing spondylitis–associated TMJ changes on,
      314
   ankylosis on, *360*
      postoperative, 261, *263*, *264*
   anterior band of disk on, *121*
      condylar displacement anterior to, 211, *216*
   anterior disk displacement on, *189*, 191, *194*, *195*
      partial, 191, *194*, *195*
      splint therapy guided by appearance of, 254, *254*
      without reduction, *195*
   anteromedial disk displacement on, *212*
   comparative quality of 0.3–tesla and 1.5–tesla scans
      in, 169, *170*
   condylar displacement on, anterior to anterior band
      of disk, 211, *216*
   condylar fracture on, *330*
   condylar fracture sequelae on, *338*
   condylar hyperplasia on, *352*
   contraindications to, 174, 177(t), 178
   costochondral graft (at mandibular ramus) on, 294,
      295, 296, *296*
   development of, 167
      recent advances in, 219–220
   disk deformation on, *197*, 199, *200*, *201*
   disk displacement on, 191–199
      anterior, *189*, 191, *194*, *195*

Magnetic resonance imaging *(Continued)*
      partial, 191, *194*, *195*
      splint therapy guided by appearance of, 254,
      254
      without reduction, *195*
      anteromedial, *212*
      disk deformation associated with, *197*, *200*, *201*
      lateral, *214*, *217*
      marrow changes accompanying, 199, *201*, *202*
      osseous changes associated with, 199, *201*
      partial, 191, *194*, *195*
      posterior, 211, *216*
      remodeling associated with, 198, *199*
      rotational, 209, *211*
         "empty fossa" sign in, 209
      sideways, 209, *210*, *213*, *214*
         "empty fossa" sign in, 209, *213*
      vs. CT findings in disk displacement, *197*, 198,
      198, *228*
      with reduction, 191, *192–194*, *212*
      without reduction, 194, *195*, *197*, 198, *198*, *199*,
      201, *202*, *207*
   disk recapture on, 194, *196*
   disk-simulating herniated joint capsule on, 186, *190*
   "empty fossa" sign (of sideways or rotational disk
      displacement) on, 209, *213*
   fibrous ankylosis on, *360*
      postoperative, 261, *263*, *264*
   herniated joint capsule on, simulating disk, 186, *190*
   imaging characteristics in, 171(t), 171–174
   imaging plane in, 171(t), 171–172
      oblique vs. straight, *172*, *173*
   implants (TMJ implants) on, *219*, *276*, 278, 279, *282*,
      284, *285–289*, 287, 289
   jaw dislocation on, *362*, *363*
   joint capsule on, 211
      abnormal, 211, *217*, *218*
      diskectomy with implant and, *282*, *287*, *288*, *289*
      herniated, simulating disk, 186, *190*
   joint effusion on, 181, *181*, *182*, 204, *204*, *205*
      perforation-enhancing effects of, 205, *207*
      psoriatic arthropathy and, *322*
      rheumatoid arthritis and, *320*, *321*
   lateral disk displacement on, *214*, *217*
   lateral pterygoid muscle on, 186, *187*
   limitations of, in demonstrating perforations, 204–
      205, 208
   loose bodies on, *347*
   marrow changes on, 199, *201*, *202*, *202*, *203*
      edematous, *182*, 184, *184*, 202, *321*, *322*
   masticatory muscle atrophy on, 62, *63*
   matrix size in, 171(t), 174
   metallic artifacts on, 178, *178*, *291*, 291–292
   oblique vs. straight planes in, *172*, *173*
   osseous changes on, 199, *201*, 209, *215*
   osteochondrosis dissecans on, *349*
   partial disk displacement on, 191, *194*, *195*
   perforations on, 205, *207*
      limitations of demonstration of, 204–205, 208
   physical principles of, 167–171
   posterior disk attachment on, *170*, 186, *188*, 204,
      206
      remodeled, 198–199, *199*
   posterior disk displacement on, 211, *216*
   postoperative, 400
      graft (at mandibular ramus) on, 294, *295*, 296, *296*
      implants on, *219*, *276*, 278, 279, *282*, 284, *285–*
      289, 287, 289
      metallic artifacts on, 178, *178*, *291*, 291–292

Magnetic resonance imaging *(Continued)*
site of diskectomy on, 272, *272–275*, *274–275*
implants and, *219*, *276*, 278, 279, *282*, 284, *285–289*, 287, 289
surgically repositioned disk on, 161, *258*, *259*, *262*
adhesions (scar tissue) with, *261–263*
fibrous ankylosis with, 261, *263*, *264*
Proplast-Teflon TMJ implant on, *219*, 284, *285–289*, 287, 289
psoriatic arthropathy–associated TMJ changes on, *314*, *322*
pulse sequence in, 171(t), 174, *176*, 177(t), 183
results of splint therapy on, 194, *196*, *256*
rheumatoid arthritis–associated TMJ changes on, *311*, 312, *313*, 314, *317*, *319–321*
vs. other imaging findings in rheumatoid TMJ disease, 314, *315–318*, 316–321, 320(t)
rotational disk displacement on, 209, *211*
"empty fossa" sign in, 209
scanners used in, *168*, *169*
sideways disk displacement on, 209, *210*, 213, *214*
"empty fossa" sign in, 209, *213*
signal averaging and imaging time in, 171(t), 174, *176*
signal intensity determinants in, 168(t)
silicone TMJ implant on, *276*, 278, 279, *282*
site of diskectomy on, 272, *272–275*, *274–275*
implants and, *219*, *276*, 278, 279, *282*, 284, *285–289*, 287, 289
slice thicknesses used in, 171(t), 172, 174, *175*, 220, *220*
splint therapy assisted by, 254, *254*
straight vs. oblique planes in, *172*, *173*
subcondylar fracture sequelae on, *333*
surgically repositioned disk on, 161, *258*, *259*, *262*
adhesions (scar tissue) with, *261–263*
fibrous ankylosis with, 261, *263*, *264*
synovial chondromatosis on, *348*
temporomandibular, 179–220, 399–400
abnormal findings on, 191–211, 314–323. See also such entries as *Magnetic resonance imaging, disk displacement on.*
dental apparatuses interfering with, 174, 178, *178*
fast scanning in, 183(t), 183–184
fat suppression in, *184*, 184–185
future applications of, 219–220
high-resolution thin-section scans in, 220, *220*
implants on, *219*, *276*, 278, 279, *282*, 284, *285–289*, 287, 289
indications for, 186, 191
normal findings on, *95*, *185*, 185–186, *187*, *188*
variations in, *189*
postoperative. See *Magnetic resonance imaging, postoperative.*
pulse sequence in, 177(t), 183
scanning parameters for, 179(t)
technique of, 179, *180*, 181, 183–185
vs. arthrography, 178, 186, *188*
in disk displacement with reduction, 191, *192*
in TMJ trauma, 138–139
vs. arthrotomography, after surgical disk repositioning, 161
in rheumatoid arthritis involving TMJ, 314, *315–318*, 316–320, 320(t)
vs. computed tomography, 178, 179(t), *227–230*, 231–232, 232(t)
in disk displacement, *197*, 198, *198*, *228*
in rheumatoid arthritis involving TMJ, 321

Magnetic resonance imaging *(Continued)*
vs. tomography, in rheumatoid arthritis involving TMJ, 321
Malformations, of temporomandibular joint, 65
Mandible. See also *Mandibular* entries.
coronoid process of, elongation or hyperplasia of, 66, *66*, 232, *233*
interference with zygomatic process by, 66, *66*, 232, *233*
Mandibular asymmetry, 351, *352*, *353*, 355(t), 355–356
condylar fracture and, 332, *334*
Mandibular condyle, 3–6
arthrotic changes in, 54, *54–56*, 59, *60*
experimentally (surgically) created, 54–55, *58*
displacement of, anterior to anterior band of disk, 137, *138*, 211, *216*
following fracture. See *Mandibular condyle, fractures of.*
duplication of, 65
erosion of, after diskectomy with silicone implant, 277, *277*, *278*
in degenerative disease of TMJ, 54, *56*, *58*, *59*
in psoriatic arthropathy involving TMJ, *306*
in rheumatoid arthritis involving TMJ, *305*, *307*, 316, 321, *323*
fractures of, 327–340, 328(t)
bullet wound and, *364*
classification of, 327, 328, *328*, 329, 332, *332*, *333*
clinical aspects of, 327–328
healing of, in children vs. adults, 335, *336*
unsuccessful, 292, *292*
imaging of, *329*, *330*, 341(t)
sequelae of, *330*, 332, *334*, 335, *336–341*
treatment of, 335, 340
unsuccessful, 292, *292*
hyperplasia of, 65–66, *352*
vs. osteochondroma of condyle, 355, *357*
incoordination of, with articular tubercle of temporal bone, 38–39
and clicking, 135, 137, *137*
marrow changes in, on MR imaging of TMJ, 199, *201*, 202, *202*, *203*
edematous, *182*, 184, *184*, 202, *321*, *322*
normal appearance of, in animal model, *57*
osteochondroma of, *356*, 356–357
vs. condylar hyperplasia, 355, *357*
position of, in glenoid fossa, 89–91, *90*. See also *Disk, of temporomandibular joint, position of.*
after diskectomy, 267, *268*, *269*
shape of, 3–4, *5*
size of, 3
spatial orientation of, 4–6
translation of, at maximal mouth opening, 79, 91, *92*
tumors of, 357
Mandibular fossa (glenoid fossa), 6–7
condylar position in, 89–91, *90*. See also *Disk, of temporomandibular joint, position of.*
after diskectomy, 267, *268*, *269*
erosion in, after diskectomy with silicone implant, *279*
Mandibular positions, for double-contrast arthrotomography of TMJ, 151
Mandibular ramus, *354*
costochondral graft at, 294, *294–296*
destruction of, due to metastatic cancer, *358*, *359*
Mandibular trauma, 3-D computed tomography following, 233, *235*
Marrow changes, on MR imaging of TMJ, 199, *201*, 202, *202*, *203*

Marrow changes (*Continued*)
  edematous, *182*, 184, *184*, 202, *321*, *322*
Masseter muscles, 14(t), 15
  atrophy of, *63*
Masticatory muscles, 13–18, 14(t), *14–17*
  atrophic changes in, 62, *63*
  disorders of, 62
Matrix size, in magnetic resonance imaging, 171(t), 174
Maxilla, interference with zygomatic process of, by
    coronoid process of mandible, 66, *66*, 232, *233*
Medial disk displacement, 28, *30*
  arthrographic findings in, *141*
  arthrosis (degenerative joint disease) associated with,
    55, 59
  arthrotomographic findings in, *140*
  clicking due to, *246*
  disk deformation associated with, 43, *44*
Medial pterygoid muscle, 15
Metallic artifacts, on postoperative magnetic resonance
    imaging, 178, *178*, *291*, 291–292
Metastases, to TMJ, 357, *358*, *359*
Microsomia, hemifacial, graft surgery in treatment of,
    295
  3-D computed tomography of, 233, *234*
Mouth opening. See *Opening of jaw.*
MRI. See *Magnetic resonance imaging.*
Multifilm cassettes, for arthrotomography of TMJ, 151
  for tomography of TMJ, 87, *88*
Muscle(s), masticatory, 13–18, 14(t), *14–17*
  atrophic changes in, 62, *63*
  disorders of, 62
Mylohyoid muscle, 14(t)
Myofascial pain-dysfunction syndrome, 62

Necrosis, aseptic, 62, 64, *64*
  TMJ as possible site of, 62, 64
Needle positioning, for joint space injection, in
    arthrography of TMJ, 106, 111, *111*, 113, *113*
  errors in, 111, *112*, 116, *118*, 119, *119*
Nerve injury, due to arthroscopy of TMJ, 386
Nørgaard, Flemming, *102*
  development of TMJ arthrography by, 101

Oblique transcranial projection, lateral, in plain
    radiography of TMJ, 76, *76–80*, 79
Oblique vs. straight planes, in magnetic resonance
    imaging, *172*, *173*
Open bite, anterior, rheumatoid arthritis involving
    TMJ and, *309*
"Open lock," 39, 151, 211, 362
Opening of jaw, 9, *11*, *20*, 21
  expansion of posterior disk attachment on, 9, *12*, 21
  maximal, and condylar translation, 79, 91, *92*
    on plain radiography of TMJ, 79, 79–80
  muscles acting in, 15, 17
Orientation of head, by cephalostat, in plain
    radiography of TMJ, 77, *80*, *82*
  in tomography of TMJ, 86, *86*, 87
Osseous ankylosis, of temporomandibular joint, 66
  postoperative, 290–291, *291*
  spondylitis and, 310, *310*
Osseous components, of temporomandibular joint,
    3–7, *4*, 4(t). See also specific structures, e.g.,
    Mandibular condyle.

Osseous components (*Continued*)
  changes in, after diskectomy, 267, *269–271*, 270–
    271
    on MRI, 199, *201*, 209, *215*
    on plain radiography, 93, *93*, 94, *94*
  soft tissue cover of, 12
Osteoarthritis. See *Degenerative disease of TMJ.*
Osteochondroma, of mandibular condyle, *356*, 356–
    357
  vs. condylar hyperplasia, 355, 357
Osteochondrosis dissecans, and loose bodies in TMJ,
    345, 348–349, *348–349*

Panoramic views, on plain radiography of TMJ, 84, *85*
Partial disk displacement, 28, *32*, *33*. See also *Disk
    displacement.*
  arthrotomographic findings in, 155, *156*, 157
  MRI findings in, 191, *194*, *195*
  with reduction, 36–37. See also *Reduction.*
Patient positioning, for arthrography of TMJ, 105–
    106, *106*, 146
  for arthrotomography of TMJ, 114, *115*
  for computed tomography of TMJ, 224, *224*
  for plain radiography of TMJ, 74, *75*, 77, *80*, *82*
  for tomography of TMJ, 86, *86*, 88
Penetrating trauma, to temporomandibular joint, *364*,
    365
Perforation(s), involving disk or posterior disk
    attachment, 50, *50–52*, *51*
  arthrographic findings in, 132–133, *132–135*, 207,
    260, 353
  arthroscopic findings in, *372*, 380
  arthrosis (degenerative joint disease) and, 56, 59
  arthrotomographic findings in, *134*, 158–159, *160*,
    312
  disk displacement and, 50, *50*, *51*, 132–133, *132–
    135*, 135, 207
    clicking-associated, *246*
  disk displacement without reduction and, 132–
    133, *132–135*, 135, 207
  magnetic resonance imaging of, 205, *207*
    limitations of, 204–205, 208
  rheumatoid arthritis and, 311–312, *312*
Persistent joint space, after diskectomy, 265, *265*, 273
Petrotympanic fissure (squamotympanic fissure), 7
Pigmented villonodular synovitis, involving TMJ, 350–
    351
Plain radiography of TMJ, 73–85, 97, 398
  anteroposterior projection in, 80, *80–82*, 82–83
  bullet fragments on, *364*
  cephalostat used in, 77, *80*, *82*
  condylar fracture on, *330*, *364*
  condylar translation on, 79, 91, *92*
  lateral oblique transcranial projection in, 76, *76–80*,
    79
  lead markers used in, 74, *75*
  lead shield used in, *75*, 76
  mandibular ramus destruction on, metastatic cancer
    and, *358*, *359*
  open-mouth view on, 79, 79–80
  osseous changes on, 93, *93*, *94*
  panoramic views on, 84, *85*
  patient positioning for, 74, *75*, 77, *80*, *82*
  post-diskectomy findings on, *269*
  projections used in, 73–76, 74(t), *74–85*, 79–80, 82–
    84
    comparative value of, 76, *78*, 82–83, *84*

Plain radiography of TMJ *(Continued)*
   psoriatic arthropathy–associated changes on, *308*
   radiation dose in, 96
   subcondylar fracture on, *331*
   submentovertical projection in, *74*, 74–76, *75*
   technique of, 73–85
   total replacement implant on, *293*
   transcranial projection in, 76, *76–80*, 79
   transmaxillary projection in, 80, *80–82*, 82–83
   transpharyngeal projection in, *83*, 83–84
   vs. tomography, *78*
Planar radionuclide imaging, 237
   of face and neck, *241*
   of TMJ, 238, *239*, 240
Posterior disk attachment, 8, 21, 45, 48
   collagen fibers in, 43
   expansion of, on jaw opening, 9, *12*, 21
   fibrosis of, 48, *48*
   magnetic resonance imaging of, *170*, 186, *188*, 204,
     206
     remodeling and, 198–199, *199*
   perforation involving. See *Perforation(s), involving disk*
     or posterior disk attachment.
   remodeling of, MRI findings in, 198–199, *199*
   rupture of, 140
     arthrographic findings in, 140, *141*
   splitting of, in disk deformation, *47*
   thickening of, in disk deformation, 40, *40*, *41*, 43, *45*
     in disk displacement, 43, *44*
   vascularization of, 48, *49*
Posterior disk displacement, *31*, 38
   MRI findings in, 211, *216*
Postglenoid fossa, 7
Post-treatment imaging, 251–296, 400
   adhesions (scar tissue) on, 257, *260–263*, 261, *272*
   ankylosis on, 261, *263*, *264*, 290–291, *291*
   costochondral grafts on, 294, *294–296*, 296
   dermal grafts on, 290
   failed condylar fracture healing on, 292, *292*
   indications for, 251
   metallic artifacts on, 178, *178*, *291*, 291–292
   Proplast-Teflon TMJ implant on, *219*, 284, *284–289*,
     287, 289, 290, *293*. See also *Proplast-Teflon TMJ*
     implant.
   reparative TMJ changes on, in patients with arthritis
     or arthropathy, *308*
   results of splint therapy on, 194, *196*, 256. See also
     Protrusive splint therapy.
   silicone TMJ implant on, 233, *236*, *237*, 276, 278,
     279, *282*. See also *Silicone TMJ implant.*
   site of diskectomy on, 265, *265–275*, 267, 270–272,
     274–275, 276(t)
     implants and, 275–290. See also *Proplast-Teflon*
       TMJ implant; *Silicone TMJ implant.*
   surgically repositioned disk on, 161, 257, *258–264*,
     260(t), 261, 264–265
     adhesions (scar tissue) with, 257, *260–263*, 261
     fibrous ankylosis with, 261, *263*, *264*
   total joint replacement implant on, 292, *293*, 294
Prednisone pretreatment, in patient undergoing
   contrast studies, 104(t)
Premedication, for patient undergoing contrast studies,
   104(t)
Primary arthrosis, of TMJ, 54, 56. See also *Degenerative*
   disease of TMJ.
Progressive remodeling, 61. See also *Remodeling.*
Projections, in plain radiography of TMJ, 73–76, 74(t),
   74–85, 79–80, 82–84
   comparative value of, 76, *78*, 82–83, *84*

Proplast-Teflon TMJ implant, 283–284
   defects in, 283, *284*
   displacement of, *285*
   erosions associated with, 284, *285*, *286*
   fragmentation of, 287, *288*, *289*
   granulation tissue around, 284, 287, *287*, *288*, *289*
   imaging of, *219*, 284, *284–289*, 287, 289, 290, *293*
   results of treatment with, 283–284
   wearing of, 283, 284
Protrusive splint therapy, 251–252
   arthrographically assisted, 127, 129, *129*, 253, *253*
   MRI-assisted, 254, *254*
   results of, 254–255
     on MR imaging, 194, *196*, 256
   "therapeutic position" in, 252, *252*
Pseudogout (CPPD deposition disease), involving
   temporomandibular joint, 61–62, 349–350, *350*
Psoriatic arthropathy, involving TMJ, *306*, *308*, *314*,
   315, *322*
Pterygoid muscle(s), atrophy of, *63*
   lateral, 14(t), 15–17, *16*, *17*
     magnetic resonance imaging of, 186, *187*
   medial, 15
Pulse sequence, in magnetic resonance imaging, 171(t),
   174, *176*, 177(t), 183

Radiation dose, in plain radiography of TMJ, 96
   in tomography of TMJ, 96
Radiocontrast media, addition of epinephrine to, 111
   adverse reactions to, 104
     prophylaxis against, 104(t)
Radiography, contrast-aided, 101–162, 400. See also
   Arthrography of TMJ; *Arthrotomography of TMJ.*
   plain, 73–85, 97, 398. See also *Plain radiography of*
     TMJ.
Radionuclide imaging, of face and neck, *241*
   of TMJ, 237–240, 238(t), *239*, 398–399
Ramus of mandible, *354*
   costochondral graft at, 294, *294–296*
   destruction of, due to metastatic cancer, *358*, *359*
Recapture, of disk of TMJ, 124, *125*, 126, *126*, *253*
   arthrographically assisted, 127, *128*, 129, *129*
   MRI in assessment of, 194, *196*
   splinting and. See *Protrusive splint therapy.*
   staging of, 124, 126, *126*
Reciprocal clicking, 35, 123, 241
Reduction, disk displacement with, *34*, *35*, 35–36, *37*,
   123
     arthrographic findings in, 123
       vs. MRI findings, 191, *192*
     arthrotomographic findings in, *125*, 155, *155*
     clicking due to, 35, 122, 122(t), 123, *123*
     CT findings in, 231(t)
     definition of, 28(t)
     MRI findings in, 191, *192–194*, 212
     partial, 36–37
     TMJ sounds accompanying, 35, 122, 122(t), 123,
       123, 242, 243, *244*
   disk displacement without, *35*, 36, 129–130, *130*
     arthrographic findings in, *131*, 131–132
     arthrotomographic findings in, *136*, 158, *159*
     clicking due to, 122, 135, *136*
     CT findings in, *226*, 231(t)
     definition of, 28(t)
     MRI findings in, 194, *195*, *197*, 198, *198*, *199*,
       201, *202*, 207

Reduction *(Continued)*
    perforation accompanying, 132–133, *132–135*,
        135, *207*
    TMJ sounds accompanying, 122, 135, *136*, 242,
        243, *244*
    incomplete, disk displacement with, *37*, 37–38
Regressive remodeling, 61. See also *Remodeling.*
Remodeling, 56, *60*, 61
    changes in posterior disk attachment with, on MRI,
        198–199, *199*
    circumferential, 61
    definition of, 28(t), 56
    diskectomy and, 267, *269–271*, 270–271
    progressive, 61
    regressive, 61
    rheumatoid arthritis involving TMJ and, *309*
    tomographic findings in, 93, *93*, *270*
    vs. arthrosis (degenerative disease of TMJ), 56, *60*,
        61
Replacement, total, of temporomandibular joint, 292,
    293, 294
Repositioning therapy. See specific therapies, e.g.,
    Splinting; *Surgical repositioning.*
Rheumatoid arthritis, 303–304
    juvenile, 304
        TMJ involvement in, *309*, *311*, *312*, *313*, *315*, *316*,
            321
    pathologic abnormalities in, 303–304
    TMJ involvement in, *61*, 303–324
        anterior open bite associated with, *309*
        arthrotomographic findings in, 311–312, *312*, *313*
            vs. MRI findings, 314, *315–318*, 316–320, 320(t)
        condylar erosion accompanying, *305*, *307*, *316*,
            321, *323*
        CT findings in, 305, *306*, 307, *307*
            vs. MRI findings, 321
        disk position with, 312, 314
        MRI findings in, *311*, 312, *313*, 314, *317*, *319–321*
            vs. arthrotomographic findings, 314, *315–318*,
                316–320, 320(t)
            vs. CT findings, 321
            vs. tomographic findings, 321
        remodeling associated with, *309*
        tomographic findings in, 305, *305–309*, 307, *312*,
            316
            vs. MRI findings, 321
Rotational disk displacement, 28, *31*, 209, *209*
    "empty fossa" sign in, 209
    MRI findings in, 209, *211*
Rupture, of posterior disk attachment, 140
    arthrographic findings in, 140, *141*

Sagittal tomography of TMJ, 88, *89*. See also
    Tomography of TMJ.
Scintigraphy, of face and neck, *241*
    of TMJ, 237–240, 238(t), *239*, 398–399
Sclerotherapy, for TMJ hypermobility, 376, 384, *384*
    lysis-lavage-manipulation (LLM) with, 390, 390(t)
Secondary arthrosis, of TMJ, 54, 56. See also
    Degenerative disease of TMJ.
Sideways disk displacement, 28, 139–140, 209, *209*
    arthrographic findings in, 140, *141*, 209, *214*
    arthrotomographic findings in, *140*
    edge sign in, 140, *141*, 209, *214*
    "empty fossa" sign in, 209, *213*
    MRI findings in, 209, *210*, *213*, *214*

Signal averaging, and imaging time, in magnetic
    resonance imaging, 171(t), 174, *176*
Signal intensity determinants, in magnetic resonance
    imaging, 168(t)
Silicone TMJ implant, 275, 277
    cyst formation associated with, 278–279, *280*,
        283
    erosions associated with, 277–278, *277–279*
    fracture of, 278, *281*, *282*
    imaging of, 233, *236*, *237*, *276*, 278, 279, *282*
    results of treatment with, 278, 282(t)
    wearing of, 278, *281*
Simultaneous film exposure, in arthrotomography of
    TMJ, 151
    in tomography of TMJ, 87
Single-contrast arthrography of TMJ, 105–113. See
    also *Arthrography of TMJ.*
    complications of, 142
    equipment for, 105, *105*, 106
    errors in, 111, *112*, 116, *118*, 119, *119*
    joint puncture in, 106, *110*
        anesthetic injection for, 106, *109*
        identification and marking of site for, 106, *107*,
            108
    joint space injection in, 111, *112*, 113, *114*
        extravasation of radiopaque material following,
            111, *112*, 116, *118*
        needle positioning for, 106, 111, *111*, 113, *113*
            errors in, 111, *112*, 116, *118*, 119, *119*
    lower joint space injection in, 111, *112*
        needle positioning for, *111*
    patient positioning for, 105–106, *106*
    results of, 119–140
    technique of, 105–113, *105–114*
    upper joint space injection in, 113, *114*
        needle positioning for, 113, *113*
    vs. double-contrast arthrotomography of TMJ, *144*,
        145, 162
Single-contrast arthrotomography of TMJ. See
    Arthrotomography of TMJ.
Single-photon emission computed tomography
    (SPECT), of TMJ, 238, *239*, 240
Slice thicknesses, in magnetic resonance imaging,
    171(t), 172, 174, *175*, 220, *220*
    in tomography of TMJ, 87–88
Sodium tetradecyl sulfate, in sclerotherapy, 384
Soft tissue components, of temporomandibular joint,
    4(t), 7–13. See also *Disk, of temporomandibular
    joint.*
    imaging of. See *Arthrography of TMJ*; *Magnetic reso-
        nance imaging.*
Soft tissue cover, in temporomandibular joint, 12, 19
    appearance of, after diskectomy, 265, *265–267*,
        267, *269*
Sound analysis, of temporomandibular joint, 242, 242–
    247, *244–247*. See also *Temporomandibular joint,
    sounds made by.*
SPECT (single-photon emission computed
    tomography), of TMJ, 238, *239*, 240
Sphenomandibular ligament, 13(t)
Splinting, 251–252
    arthrographically assisted, 127, 129, *129*, 253,
        253
    MRI-assisted, 254, *254*
    results of, 254–255
        on MR imaging, 194, *196*, 256
    "therapeutic position" in, 252, *252*
Spondylitis, ankylosing, TMJ involvement in, 310, *310*,
    314

Squamotympanic fissure (petrotympanic fissure), 7

Staging, of disk recapture, 124, 126, *126*
  of internal TMJ derangements, 38, 39(t), 374, 375(t)

Steroid(s), intra-articular injection of, as adjunct to arthroscopic TMJ surgery, 383–384
  pretreatment with, in patient undergoing radiocontrast studies, 104(t)

Straight vs. oblique planes, in magnetic resonance imaging, *172, 173*

Stratum fibrosum, of temporomandibular joint capsule, 13

Stratum synoviale, of temporomandibular joint capsule, 13

Stylomandibular ligament, 13(t)

Subcondylar fractures, *331.* See also *Mandibular condyle, fractures of.*
  sequelae of, *333*

Submentovertical projection, in plain radiography of TMJ, *74,* 74–76, *75*

Suprahyoid muscles, 14, 15

Surgery, arthroscopic. See *Surgical arthroscopy of TMJ.*
  diskectomy. See *Diskectomy.*
  graft, 290, 294, *294–296,* 296
  imaging following, 255–296, 400
    adhesions (scar tissue) on, 257, *260–263,* 261, *272*
    bony ankylosis on, 290–291, *291*
    costochondral grafts on, 294, *294–296,* 296
    dermal grafts on, 290
    failed condylar fracture healing on, 292, *292*
    fibrous ankylosis on, 261, *263, 264*
    metallic artifacts on, 178, *178, 291,* 291–292
    Proplast-Teflon TMJ implant on, *219,* 284, *284–289,* 287, 289, 290, *293.* See also *Proplast-Teflon TMJ implant.*
    repositioned disk on, 161, 257, *258–264,* 260(t), 261, 264–265
    silicone TMJ implant on, 233, *236, 237,* 276, 278, 279, *282.* See also *Silicone TMJ implant.*
    site of diskectomy on, 265, *265–275,* 267, 270–272, 274–275, 276(t)
      implants and, 275–290. See also *Proplast-Teflon TMJ implant; Silicone TMJ implant.*
    total joint replacement implant on, 292, *293,* 294
  implantation. See *Implant(s).*
  repositioning. See *Surgical repositioning.*
  total joint replacement, 292, *293,* 294

Surgical arthroscopy of TMJ, 372–373, 382–383, 390–391
  care following, 384–385
  complications of, 385–388, 387(t)–389(t)
  indications for, 373(t), 373–374, 376
  lysis-lavage-manipulation (LLM) in, 389, 389(t)
    sclerotherapy with, 390, 390(t)
  results of, 388–390, 389(t), 390(t)
  steroid injection as adjunct to, 383–384

Surgical repositioning, of disk of TMJ, 255, 257
  adhesion (scar tissue) formation after, 257, *260–263,* 261
  fibrous ankylosis as complication of, 261, *263, 264*
  imaging after, 161, 257, *258–264,* 260(t), 261, 264–265

Synovial chondromatosis, and loose bodies in TMJ, 343, 345, *346–348*

Synovial fluid, in temporomandibular joint, 13

Synovitis, in rheumatoid arthritis. See *Rheumatoid arthritis.*
  on arthroscopy of TMJ, 377–378, *378*

Synovitis *(Continued)*
  villonodular, involving TMJ, 350–351

Temporal bone, articular tubercle of, 6
  erosion of, after diskectomy with Proplast-Teflon implant, 284, *285, 286*
  incoordination of, with mandibular condyle, 38–39
    and clicking, 135, 137, *137*
  soft tissue cover of, 19
    thickening of, 12
  protuberance rising from, 3-D computed tomography of, 233, *237*
  squamous part of, 6, 7

Temporal component, of temporomandibular joint, 6–7
  soft tissue cover of, 12

Temporalis muscle, 14(t), 14–15

Temporomandibular joint, 3–21
  anatomy of, 3–21
    functional, 21
    gross, 3–18
    microscopic, 18–21, *19*
    normal, 3–21
      on arthrography, 119, 121, *144, 188, 354*
      on arthrotomography, *120, 144,* 151–152, *152–154*
      on computed tomography, *225, 226, 227*
      on MRI, *185,* 185–186, *187, 188, 189*
  ankylosing spondylitis involving, 310, *310, 314*
  ankylosis of, 66, *138,* 360, *360*
    postoperative, 261, *263, 264,* 290–291, *291*
    spondylitis and, 310, *310*
  anomalies of, congenital/developmental, 64–65, *65*
  arthritis involving, 61, *61,* 303–324. See also *Rheumatoid arthritis, TMJ involvement in.*
    degenerative. See *Degenerative disease of TMJ.*
    diagnosis of, 142
      imaging in, 323–324, 324(t), 400–401
  arthrocentesis of, for vacuum phenomenon, 377
  arthrography of, 101–162, 400. See also *Arthrography of TMJ.*
  arthropathy involving, psoriatic, *306, 308, 314, 315, 322*
  arthroscopy of, 371–391. See also *Arthroscopy of TMJ.*
  arthrosis of. See *Degenerative disease of TMJ.*
  arthrotomography of. See *Arthrotomography of TMJ.*
  articular surfaces of, 12
  aseptic necrosis in, 62, 64
  blood supply to, 18
  bullet wound of, *364,* 365
  cancer metastatic to, 357, *358, 359*
  capsule of. See *Capsule of temporomandibular joint.*
  chondrocalcinosis (CPPD deposition disease, pseudogout) involving, 61–62, 349–350, *350*
  chondromalacia involving, 377
  chronic arthritis involving, 303–324. See also *Rheumatoid arthritis, TMJ involvement in.*
  clicking by. See *Temporomandibular joint, sounds made by.*
  compartments of. See *Compartments of temporomandibular joint.*
  computed tomography of, 223–233. See also *Computed tomography of TMJ.*
  congenital anomalies of, 64–65, *65*
  contrast studies of, 101–162, 400. See also *Arthrography of TMJ; Arthrotomography of TMJ.*
  crepitation from, 241, *247*

Temporomandibular joint (*Continued*)
　deformations of, 65
　degenerative disease of. See *Degenerative disease of TMJ.*
　derangements of, internal. See *Internal TMJ derangements.*
　developmental anomalies of, 64–65, *65*
　diagnostic imaging of, 398–401, *399*. See also specific modalities, e.g., *Arthrography of TMJ.*
　disk of. See *Disk, of temporomandibular joint.*
　disorders of, 25–67. See also specific conditions such as *Disk displacement.*
　　terminology applied to, 25
　disruption of, 65
　double-contrast studies of, 143–162. See also *Double-contrast* entries.
　dysplasia of, 65
　effusion in, 181, *181, 182,* 204, *204, 205*
　　and demonstration of perforation, 205, *207*
　　in psoriatic arthropathy, *322*
　　in rheumatoid arthritis, *320, 321*
　gout involving, 61
　grafts in, 290, 294, *294–296,* 296
　hypermobility of, sclerotherapy for, 376, 384, *384*
　　lysis-lavage-manipulation (LLM) with, 390, 390(t)
　hypocyclodial tomography of. See *Tomography of TMJ.*
　hypoplasia of, congenital, 65, *65*
　imaging of, 6. See also specific modalities, e.g., *Magnetic resonance imaging.*
　　diagnostic, 398–401, *399*. See also specific diagnostic aids, e.g., *Arthrography of TMJ.*
　　post-treatment, 251–296, 400. See also *Post-treatment imaging.*
　implant(s) in, 275–290, 292. See also *Implant(s), in TMJ.*
　infection of, 362, *363,* 365
　　arthroscopy and, 387
　inflammatory arthritis involving, 61, *61*
　　diagnosis of, 142
　　rheumatoid, *61,* 303–324. See also *Rheumatoid arthritis, TMJ involvement in.*
　innervation of, 18
　interarticular disk of. See *Disk, of temporomandibular joint.*
　internal derangements of. See *Internal TMJ derangements.*
　juvenile rheumatoid arthritis involving, *309, 311, 312, 313, 315, 316, 321.* See also *Rheumatoid arthritis.*
　lateral impingement of, 379–380
　ligaments related to, 13, 13(t)
　loose bodies in, 139, *139,* 343–349, *344*
　　osteochondrosis dissecans and, 345, 348–349, *348–349*
　　synovial chondromatosis and, 343, 345, *346–348*
　magnetic resonance imaging of, 179–220, 399–400. See also *Magnetic resonance imaging.*
　malformations of, 65
　mandibular condylar component of. See *Mandibular condyle.*
　metastases to, 357, *358, 359*
　muscles acting on, 13–18, 14(t), *14–17*
　osseous components of, 3–7, *4,* 4(t). See also specific structures, e.g., *Mandibular condyle.*
　　changes in, after diskectomy, 267, *269–271,* 270–271
　　　on MRI, 199, *201,* 209, *215*
　　　on plain radiography, 93, *93,* 94, *94*

Temporomandibular joint (*Continued*)
　soft tissue cover of, 12
　osteoarthritis involving. See *Degenerative disease of TMJ.*
　osteochondroma of, *356,* 356–357
　　vs. condylar hyperplasia, 355, 357
　pathology of, 25–67. See also specific conditions such as *Disk displacement.*
　　terminology applied to, 25
　persistent space in, after diskectomy, 265, *265, 273*
　plain radiography of, 73–85, 97, 398. See also *Plain radiography of TMJ.*
　post-treatment imaging of, 251–296, 400. See also *Post-treatment imaging.*
　psoriatic arthropathy involving, *306, 308, 314, 315, 322*
　radiography of, contrast-aided, 101–162, 400. See also *Arthrography of TMJ; Arthrotomography of TMJ.*
　　plain, 73–85, 97, 398. See also *Plain radiography of TMJ.*
　radionuclide imaging (scintigraphy) of, 237–240, 238(t), *239,* 398–399
　remodeling of. See *Remodeling.*
　rheumatoid arthritis involving, *61,* 303–324. See also *Rheumatoid arthritis, TMJ involvement in.*
　single-contrast arthrography of, 105–113, *105–114.* See also *Arthrography of TMJ.*
　　complications of, 142
　　results of, 119–140
　　vs. double-contrast arthrotomography of TMJ, *144, 145,* 162
　single-contrast arthrotomography of. See *Arthrotomography of TMJ.*
　single-photon emission computed tomography of, 238, *239,* 240
　soft tissue components of, 4(t), 7–13. See also *Disk, of temporomandibular joint.*
　　imaging of. See *Arthrography of TMJ; Magnetic resonance imaging.*
　soft tissue cover in, 12, 19
　　appearance of, after diskectomy, 265, *265–267, 267, 269*
　sounds made by, 122, 241–242
　　analysis of, *242,* 242–247, *244–247*
　　conditions associated with, 122, 122(t), 241, 241(t)
　　condyle-tubercle incoordination and, 135, 137, *137*
　　degenerative disease (arthrosis) and, *242, 247*
　　disk displacement with reduction and, 35, 122, 122(t), 123, *123,* 242, 243, *244*
　　disk displacement without reduction and, 122, 135, *136,* 242, 243, *244*
　　medial disk displacement with perforation and, *246*
　　myofascial pain-dysfunction syndrome and, 62
　　opening vs. closing, *242*
　　wave patterns of, 243, *245*
　spondylitis involving, ankylosing, 310, *310, 314*
　surgery of, imaging following, 255–296, 400. See also *Surgery, imaging following.*
　synovial fluid in, 13
　synovitis involving, arthroscopic findings in, 377–378, *378*
　　rheumatoid arthritis and. See *Rheumatoid arthritis.*
　　villonodular, 350–351
　temporal component of, 6–7
　　soft tissue cover of, 12
　three-dimensional CT studies of, 232–233, *234–237, 295, 334, 337*

Temporomandibular joint *(Continued)*
  tomography of. See *Arthrotomography of TMJ; Computed tomography of TMJ; Tomography of TMJ.*
  total replacement of, 292, *293*, 294
  trauma to, 327–342. See also *Mandibular condyle, fractures of.*
    imaging of, 138–139, 340, 342
    penetrating, *364*, 365
  tumors metastatic to, 357, *358*, *359*
Temporomandibular joint ligament, 13, 13(t)
"Therapeutic position," in splinting, 252, *252*
Three-dimensional computed tomography, 232–233
  condylar fracture sequelae on, *334*, *337*
  costochondral graft (at mandibular ramus) on, *295*
  craniofacial asymmetry on, 233, *234*
  mandibular trauma sequelae on, 233, *235*
  silicone TMJ implant on, 233, *236*, *237*
  temporal bone protuberance on, 233, *237*
TMJ. See *Temporomandibular joint.*
Tomography of TMJ, 86–89, 97, 398
  ankylosing spondylitis–associated changes on, *314*
  bony ankylosis on, postoperative, *291*
  cephalostat used in, 86, *86*, *87*
  computed. See *Computed tomography of TMJ.*
  condylar erosion on, after diskectomy with silicone implant, *277*, *278*
  condylar fracture and trauma sequelae on, *330*, *337*, *339*, *340*, *341*
  condylar position on, *90*, 90–91
    after diskectomy, 269
  contrast-aided. See *Arthrotomography of TMJ.*
  degenerative disease on, *353*
  frontal, 89, *90*
  lateral, 88–89
  limitations of, 96, *96*
  loose bodies on, *344*
  mandibular ramus on, *354*
  multifilm cassettes for, 87, *88*
  patient positioning for, 86, *86*, 88
  persistent joint space on, after diskectomy, *265*
  post-diskectomy findings on, *265*, *266*, *269*, *270*
    silicone implant and, *277*–*280*
  psoriatic arthropathy–associated changes on, *306*, *308*
  radiation dose in, 96
  remodeling on, 93, *93*
    after diskectomy, *270*
  rheumatoid arthritis–associated changes on, 305, *305*–*309*, 307, *312*, *316*
  sagittal, 88, *89*
  simultaneous film exposure in, 87
  slice thicknesses in, 87–88
  total replacement implant on, 292

Tomography of TMJ *(Continued)*
  vs. plain radiography, 78
Total replacement, of temporomandibular joint, 292, *293*, 294
Transcranial projection, in plain radiography of TMJ, 76, *76*–*80*, 79
Translation, condylar, at maximal mouth opening, 79, 91, *92*
Transmaxillary projection, in plain radiography of TMJ, 80, *80*–*82*, 82–83
Transpharyngeal projection, in plain radiography of TMJ, *83*, 83–84
Trauma, mandibular, 3-D computed tomography following, 233, *235*
  temporomandibular joint, 327–342. See also *Mandibular condyle, fractures of.*
    imaging of, 138–139, 340, 342
    penetrating, *364*, 365
  TMJ arthroscopy and, 386–387
Tubercle, articular, of temporal bone. See *Temporal bone, articular tubercle of.*
Tumors, condylar, 357
  metastatic to TMJ, 357, *358*, *359*

Upper temporomandibular joint compartment, 9, 11
  arthroscopic approach to, 381, *381*, 382
  arthroscopic visualization of, 382, *382*, *383*
  catheter insertion in, 147, *148*
  contrast injection into, 113, *114*, 149. See also *Arthrography of TMJ.*
    needle positioning for, 113, *113*
  vacuum phenomenon in, 377

Vagal response, during TMJ arthrography, 105, 142
Vascular injury, due to arthroscopy of TMJ, 386
Vascularization, of posterior disk attachment, 48, *49*
Vertical condylar angle, 5, 6
Villonodular synovitis, involving TMJ, 350–351

Wearing, of Proplast-Teflon TMJ implant, 283, 284
  of silicone TMJ implant, 278, *281*
Wilkes classification, of internal TMJ derangements, 38, 39(t), 375(t)

Zygomatic process of maxilla, interference with, by coronoid process of mandible, 66, *66*, 232, *233*